The Foot and Ankle in Rheumatology

The Foot and Ankle in Rheumatology

Edited By

Philip Helliwell
Professor of Clinical Rheumatology
Leeds Institute of Rheumatic and Musculoskeletal Medicine
University of Leeds
Leeds, UK

Mike Backhouse
York Trials Unit
Department of Health Sciences
University of York
York, UK

Heidi Siddle
Associate Professor and Honorary
Consultant Podiatrist
Leeds Institute of Rheumatic and Musculoskeletal Medicine
University of Leeds
Leeds, UK

OXFORD
UNIVERSITY PRESS

OXFORD
UNIVERSITY PRESS

Great Clarendon Street, Oxford, OX2 6DP,
United Kingdom

Oxford University Press is a department of the University of Oxford.
It furthers the University's objective of excellence in research, scholarship,
and education by publishing worldwide. Oxford is a registered trade mark of
Oxford University Press in the UK and in certain other countries

First Edition Published in 2019

Impression: 1

Published in the United States of America by Oxford University Press
198 Madison Avenue, New York, NY 10016, United States of America

British Library Cataloguing in Publication Data

Data available

Library of Congress Control Number: 2018962646

ISBN 978–0–19–873445–1

Printed in Great Britain by
Ashford Colour Press Ltd, Gosport, Hampshire

Foreword

I was pleased and honoured when approached to write a foreword to this excellent textbook on the foot and ankle in rheumatology. My initial thoughts were, 'why me and not an experienced orthopaedic surgeon or podiatrist?' The editors explained that it was the patient experience that they felt was needed, to remind the health professionals who will use this book, and of the impact that rheumatological foot disease can have on the lives of their patients. I hope that summarizing some of my experiences will be useful.

I was first diagnosed with severe seronegative polyarthritis at a young age (30). I am therefore one of a generation of patients with refractory disease, who were inadequately treated, even after visible bone erosions were apparent on X-ray. This was well before the advent of biologics, and the result has been considerable disability and having to undergo a huge amount of orthopaedic surgery. Four of my nineteen (to date) operations have been on my feet and ankles. My feet and ankles (as well as my neck and eyes) have caused me the most pain and distress in 37 years living with inflammatory polyarthritis.

Those who live with this awful disease are only too aware just how little attention is generally paid to feet and ankles, particularly as they are excluded from the DAS28 score, yet something like 90% of people with rheumatoid arthritis suffer foot/ankle problems at some point. Hopefully, as inflammatory arthritis is now much better understood and treated than when I was diagnosed, the percentage of people suffering severe foot/ankle disease should reduce over coming years.

I have huge respect and admiration for the clinicians who have treated my feet, none more so than my foot surgeon, who has operated on my feet, ankles, and assorted toes on four occasions. Each time I have had these surgeries, I have been 12 weeks non-weightbearing and off my biologic treatment, which of itself caused me problems, as pain in all my other joints got steadily worse the longer I was without treatment; this made recovery more challenging. Because of my fused wrists and replaced elbows, I cannot hop around on crutches, and this makes even the simplest everyday tasks really difficult.

In regard to the kind of routine foot care that is necessary for everyone with a musculoskeletal/ rheumatological condition, I am very fortunate to live close to one of the longest running providers of training in foot health in the UK and for many years have been able to access regular foot care from trainees working under supervision. This includes cutting toenails (which I can't do myself), attention to corns, and development of hard skin, which can cause real problems if ignored. This regular care has been beneficial. I have also had access, as needed, to the podiatry department at my hospital as part of the ongoing care from my rheumatology team; however, although I know how beneficial customized insoles can be for many with musculoskeletal conditions, I have found these to be less successful for me and my feet! Sadly, not all people with musculoskeletal conditions are able to access such regular podiatry care and this is a problem in the UK.

Owing to my foot and ankle problems I have had to change my wardrobe completely and could only wear trousers or long skirts as, for a long time, I was not able to wear shoes that would go with a knee-length dress or skirt. In recent years, however, because of the successful treatment I've had, I have, for the first time, been able to wear more trendy and attractive footwear (no heels of course!) and I can now also wear summer sandals and knee length boots, which most women take for granted, so I can now wear a dress! This means a lot.

Today I am able to walk further and stand for longer, although I continue to experience pain, use a wheelchair for distance, and on occasions get tenosynovitis, which can come on quite suddenly and acutely and be very disabling. However, the treatments I have received have made such a difference, including a lot less pain (unless I over-do it), and for this I will be forever grateful.

There is a lot more I could write, but I will finish by saying that foot/ankle pain interferes with almost every aspect of life, and such difficulties should not be ignored or underestimated. I hope that readers will use this book to improve the care of people with foot and ankle disease and appreciate the impact that such problems have on their lives.

Ailsa Bosworth MBE
Chief Executive, National Rheumatoid Arthritis Society
Maidenhead, 2017

Preface

The foot is an important anatomical structure and is a frequent site of pathology in rheumatic diseases. For health professionals who do not specialize in the foot and ankle, our experience suggests that it is unlikely to form part of a clinical examination unless patients specifically complain about their feet, which they often do. The widespread use of the 28-joint count is certainly complicit in encouraging this neglect. However, even if patients complain, generalists and specialists alike find the foot problematic. Why should this be so? We think there are several reasons underlying this aversion. The feet are often smelly and inaccessible. On a cold winter's day patients do not like to have to expose their feet by removing successive layers of protective clothing. If there is age and infirmity this becomes more of a challenge, and the garments still have to be put back on afterward. There is often a time pressure—if the consultation is taken up by this process, then little time is left to perform the other assessments and to formulate a plan. There is also an issue of training. For medical professionals in particular there is very little or no formal training on the examination and treatment of the foot and ankle.

From our experience in postgraduate education we know that rheumatologists and podiatrists feel in need of more knowledge and skills with respect to the foot in rheumatic disease. When all these factors are combined, they conspire to make complaints about the feet a bit of a black hole for health professionals not involved specifically in their care. This book should serve to cast away some of this darkness and uncertainty for that group, and as a companion text to any practical tuition that the reader can obtain. For foot specialists, who may have only had limited training in musculoskeletal diseases, the book will serve as an update on current thinking and will broaden the coverage of rheumatic disease impact.

It is our intention to make this book as evidence-based as possible. Inevitably, there will be areas where the evidence base is weak—in these instances we will be clear when we write from personal experience and practice. One point is clear: the evidence on which we base our evaluation and decisions is accumulating year on year. Since we published our book on the foot in rheumatoid arthritis (1) there have been many advances in this field and in most other diseases that can manifest in the foot. These updates will be highlighted in the following chapters.

The book opens with a chapter on current concepts in rheumatology, detailing the global epidemiology and impact of rheumatic disease. There follow two chapters giving the essentials on anatomy and normal function. We then discuss specific disease groups and how they can affect the foot. Each chapter is arranged to give essential details about the disease in general and then specific detail on how the foot is affected along with disease-specific treatment considerations. Specific chapters on assessment are followed by a generic management chapter, surgical considerations and, finally, a concluding chapter on organizing and evaluating care. The chapters are sufficiently referenced to enable the reader to seek appropriate further knowledge if required.

We hope this book will provide a substantial basis for any health professional who wishes to learn more about the foot in health and disease, and how to manage the problems that can occur.

Philip Helliwell
Mike Backhouse
Heidi Siddle
Leeds 2018

Reference

1. **Helliwell P, Woodburn J, Redmond A, Turner D, Davys HJ.** *The Foot and Ankle in Rheumatoid Arthritis: A Comprehensive Guide*. London: Churchill Livingstone: Elsevier; 2007.

Contents

Contributors

Begonya Alcacer-Pitarch
Post-doctoral Research Fellow, Leeds Institute of Rheumatic and Musculoskeletal Medicine, University of Leeds, Leeds, UK.

Principal Podiatrist, Leeds Teaching Hospitals NHS Trust.

Mike Backhouse
York Trials Unit, Department of Health Sciences, University of York, York, UK

Catherine Bowen
Professor in Podiatry, Faculty of Health Sciences, University of Southampton, Southampton, UK

Maya Buch
Professor of Rheumatology and Honorary Consultant Rheumatologist, Leeds Institute of Rheumatic & Musculoskeletal Medicine, University of Leeds, Leeds, UK

Graham Chapman
Head of Biomechanics Research Group, Leeds Institute of Rheumatic and Musculoskeletal Medicine, University of Leeds, Leeds, UK

Lindsey Cherry
National Institute for Health Research (NIHR) Clinical Lecturer in Podiatric Rheumatology, Faculty of Health Sciences, University of Southampton, Southampton, UK

Jordan Fletcher
Research Fellow, St Mark's Hospital, London

Lucy Gates
Postdoctoral Researcher in Epidemiology, Nuffield Department of Orthopaedics, Rheumatology and Musculoskeletal Sciences, University of Oxford, Oxford, UK

Andrew Grainger
Consultant Musculoskeletal Radiologist, Leeds Teaching Hospitals Trust and NIHR, Leeds Biomedical Research Centre, Leeds, UK

Nick Harris
Consultant Orthopaedic and Trauma Surgeon, Nuffield Health Leeds Hospital, Leeds, UK

Maggie Helliwell
Clinical Non-Executive Director,
Airedale NHS Foundation Trust,
West Yorkshire, UK

Philip Helliwell
Professor of Clinical Rheumatology, Leeds Institute of Rheumatic and Musculoskeletal Medicine, University of Leeds, Leeds, UK

Gordon Hendry
Senior Research Fellow, School of Health and Life Sciences, Glasgow Caledonian University, Glasgow, UK

Joseph Iaquinto
Research Health Science Specialist, VA Center for Limb Loss and MoBility, Seattle, USA

Rebecca Kearney
Associate Clinical Professor, Warwick Medical School, University of Warwick, Warwick, UK

Anne-Maree Keenan
Professor in Applied Research, School of Healthcare, University of Leeds, and Assistant Director and Training Lead, of the National Institute for Health Research (NIHR) Leeds Biomedical Research Centre, Leeds, UK

Karl B. Landorf
Associate Professor in the Discipline of Podiatry, La Trobe University, Melbourne, Australia

William Ledoux
Research Health Scientist, VA Puget Sound, Center for Limb Loss and MoBility (CLiMB), Seattle, WA, USA

Jane McAdam
Director of Prosthetics & Orthotics and Podiatry, University of Salford, Manchester, UK

Shannon Munteanu
Associate Professor in the Discipline of Podiatry, La Trobe University, Melbourne, Australia

James Pickering
Division of Anatomy, Leeds Institute of Medical Education, University of Leeds, Leeds, UK

Dave Roberts
Division of Anatomy, Leeds Institute of Medical Education, University of Leeds, Leeds, UK

Edward Roddy
Reader in Rheumatology and Honorary Consultant Rheumatologist, Keele University, Staffordshire, UK

Keith Rome
Professor of Podiatry, School of Clinical Sciences, Auckland University of Technology, Auckland, New Zealand

Emma Rowbotham
Consultant in Musculoskeletal Radiology, The Leeds Teaching Hospitals NHS Trust and NIHR, Leeds Biomedical Research Centre, Leeds, UK

Heidi Siddle
Associate Professor and Honorary Consultant Podiatrist, Leeds Institute of Rheumatic and Musculoskeletal Medicine, University of Leeds, Leeds, UK

Deborah Turner
Professor in Podiatry, School of Science and Health, Western Sydney University, Sydney, Australia

Edward Vital
Associate Professor and Honorary Consultant Rheumatologist, Leeds Institute of Rheumatic and Musculoskeletal Medicine, University of Leeds, Leeds, UK

Richard Wakefield
Senior Lecturer and Honorary Consultant Rheumatologist, Leeds Institute of Rheumatic and Musculoskeletal Medicine, University of Leeds, Leeds, UK

Chapter 1

Current concepts in rheumatology

Philip Helliwell

Epidemiology of rheumatic disease

Musculoskeletal disorders represent a significant proportion of the conditions contributing to the global burden of disease (1). Mostly, this is the so-called degenerative disorders: osteoarthritis and mechanical low back and neck pain. Together they cause significant morbidity. In the UK, low back and neck pain are the leading causes of disability-adjusted life years, with other musculoskeletal disorders coming in sixteenth (2). Globally, musculoskeletal disorders have an equivalent impact to depressive and behavioural disorders (3). However, there remain significant epidemiological challenges. Firstly, classification criteria for rheumatic diseases are evolving as new knowledge is accrued. Secondly, the ways in which criteria are applied across communities where a host of problems may be at work—language, geography, access, and politics are just some of the barriers. The World Health Organization (WHO) has, for some years, been supporting epidemiological studies in areas of the world where only rudimentary data are available. The Community-Oriented Program for Control of Rheumatic Diseases (COPCORD) initiative has provided valuable data on rheumatic disease prevalence in many previously uncharted communities (http://copcord.org/).

Osteoarthritis and other mechanical soft-tissue disorders are by far the most common cause of foot pain in the UK. Their management varies from resigned acceptance and self-modification of footwear to skilled intervention by health professionals. However, it is the less common inflammatory conditions that receive most attention in secondary care and that are the main focus of much of this book. In parallel, the majority of patients presenting to primary care physicians with musculoskeletal pain have osteoarthritis or soft-tissue disorders while the majority of patients seen in secondary care clinics have inflammatory musculoskeletal disorders (IMDs). Why should this be so when the burden of disease and disability is overwhelmingly with osteoarthritis and soft-tissue disorders? Essentially, IMDs are more likely to be destructive locally, to be polyarticular, and to have systemic features, thus requiring more complex medical management. Furthermore, diseases causing synovial inflammation, such as rheumatoid arthritis, commonly affect the foot, with over 90% of cases having foot involvement (4).

The concept of early treatment and the window of opportunity

Generally, and including the foot and ankle, it is believed there is a 'window of opportunity' in early inflammatory disease where aggressive early treatment might abort the processes that are causing inflammation, thus preventing joint damage and the chronic cycle of inflammatory change that might occur (5). The classic paradigm here is with rheumatoid arthritis where early and targeted treatment leads to better outcomes, but the same is likely true for other inflammatory

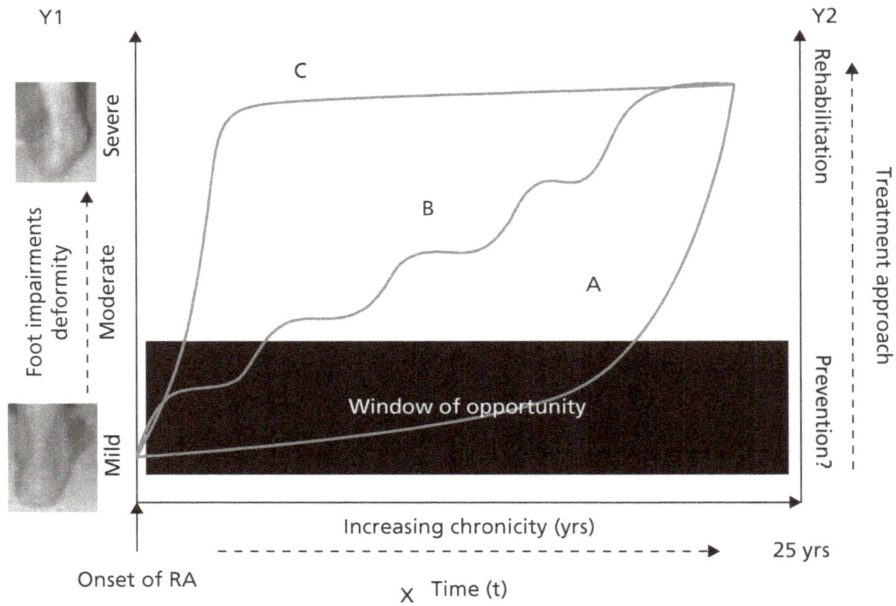

Figure 1.1 'Window of opportunity' in early inflammatory disease. The course of deformity (Y1) is plotted against time (X) from disease onset alongside treatment strategy (Y2). Patients who develop severe deformity within 5 years from disease onset (pathway C) have only a short time period in which to initiate preventative management. Others may develop progressive deformity (pathway B) following repeated inflammatory attacks (hence the 'saw-tooth' appearance). Finally, a smaller group (pathway A) resist cumulative damage and deformity until the later stages of disease and then rapid development of deformity occurs following some acute incident (perhaps rupture of tibialis posterior tendon). RA, Rheumatoid arthritis.

Reproduced from Helliwell P, Woodburn J, Redmond A, Turner D, Davys H. The Foot and Ankle in Rheumatoid Arthritis: A Comprehensive Guide. London: Churchill Livingstone: Elsevier; 2007.

diseases such as psoriatic arthritis (6). This trend to earlier treatment is reflected by the widespread adoption of early arthritis clinics, where the aim is to see and treat people before the disease becomes too established.

This concept has been nicely illustrated in the foot by Helliwell et al (Figure 1.1). The foot and ankle may well be a special case in terms of early intervention, as continued loading of inflamed structures may lead to early damage and deformity. This was illustrated by one of the first randomized controlled trials of functional foot orthoses in rheumatoid arthritis in a population who did not have particularly early disease but who had established, and partly reversible, deformity (7). As ever, the concept of joint protection in the foot is difficult to apply but should be acknowledged at an early stage.

There may be several reasons why delays occur before effective treatment can be given. The patient may not consult for a variety of reasons, including low expectations, poor availability of appropriate care, and a hope that things may settle with time. Once people consult, there may be disincentives to refer early, both financial and educational, and initial treatment may be symptomatic only. People consult a wide spectrum of health professionals and sorting out those who need early referral and treatment from those who don't is a challenge. A few simple 'rules' have been

Box 1.1 Clinical recommendations for early referral of rheumatoid arthritis

Rapid referral to a rheumatologist is advised in the event of clinical suspicion of rheumatoid arthritis, which may be supported by the presence of any of the following:

- Three or more swollen joints.
- Morning stiffness of more than 30 minutes.
- A positive metacarpal or metatarsal squeeze test.

Information sourced from Emery P, Breedveld FC, Dougados M, Kalden JR, Schiff MH, Smolen JS. Early referral recommendation for newly diagnosed rheumatoid arthritis: evidence based development of a clinical guide. *Annals of the Rheumatic Diseases*. 2002;**61**(4):290.

suggested (Box 1.1) (8). Whatever set of guidance is used, a low threshold of referral is necessary for treatment to be started early enough—within 3–6 months of symptom onset.

Delays at the secondary care institution could be minimized by appropriate triage and availability of clinic appointments. The development of new classification criteria, designed to permit earlier identification and treatment, may well help earlier identification and treatment in this disease (Table 1.1) (9).

If a true biologic marker was available diagnosis would be much more straightforward for all concerned. A biologic marker usually has pathological relevance, and for some time it was thought that rheumatoid factor fulfilled this role in rheumatoid arthritis. However, it later became clear that rheumatoid factor is present in only about 75% of cases of rheumatoid arthritis. Further biologic markers have been sought. Antibodies to keratin, in particular anti-citrullinated protein antibodies (ACPAs), have been found to be more specific (95%) for rheumatoid arthritis than rheumatoid factor. However, this occurs at the cost of lower sensitivity (67%) (10). This test may, however, be of more use in situations where it is desired to have a very low rate of false positives. Are new ways of imaging helpful? For example, magnetic resonance imaging (MRI) is a very sensitive technique for detecting inflammation. Joints not inflamed clinically may, nevertheless, show extensive inflammation on MRI. The same is true for ultrasound (US), especially power Doppler US. Both these techniques are discussed in Chapter 12. The point to be made here is that using these new techniques may change the way we diagnose and treat inflammatory diseases such as rheumatoid arthritis. MRI is costly but US is cheaper, is becoming widely available, and may permit much earlier diagnosis.

Treatment approaches: pharmacological therapies

The treatment of IMDs has seen many significant changes over the past 15 years, with the concept of tight control and the introduction of biologic drugs. The biologic drugs, the logical end-product of the science of inflammation, have transformed the treatment of inflammatory disease, and may even yet be found to be of use in other musculoskeletal disorders. With the advent of biologic drugs has come an escalation of costs, making the rheumatology department one of the most expensive in the hospital setting. However, traditional approaches must not be forgotten. Small molecules such as hydroxychloroquine, methotrexate, and corticosteroids remain the cornerstone of treatment and are cheap and readily available across all societies. Biologic drugs, given systemically, may be 'rationed' (https://www.nice.org.uk/guidance/ta375, accessed 25 January 2016) but are generally widely available in the UK, if needed. It is also worth remembering that IMDs are

Table 1.1 The 2010 classification criteria for rheumatoid arthritis. These criteria apply to people who have at least one joint with synovitis and no other plausible explanation for the condition (e.g., someone with psoriatic arthritis)

Add scores of categories A to D. Interpretation: a score of ≥6 indicates that this person can be classified as having rheumatoid arthritis	
A. Joint involvement	
Criterion	*Score*
1 large joint (hip, knee, ankle, shoulder, elbow)	0
2–10 large joints	1
1–3 small joints (excludes distal interphalangeal joints, first carpometacarpal joint, and first metatarsophalangeal joint)	2
4–10 small joints	3
>10 joints (includes at least one small joint)	5
B. Serology	
Criterion	*Score*
Negative rheumatoid factor (RF) and negative anti-citrullinated protein antibody (ACPA)	0
Low positive RF or low positive ACPA	2
High positive RF or high positive ACPA	3
C. Acute phase reactants	
Criterion	*Score*
Normal C-reactive protein (CRP) and normal erythrocyte sedimentation rate (ESR)	0
Abnormal CRP and abnormal ESR	1
D. Duration of symptoms	
Criterion	*Score*
<6 weeks	0
≥6 weeks	1

Reproduced from Aletaha D, Neogi T, Silman AJ et al. 2010 Rheumatoid arthritis classification criteria: an American College of Rheumatology/European League Against Rheumatism collaborative initiative. *Annals of the Rheumatic Diseases*. 2010;**69**(9):1580–8 with permission from Wiley.

still potentially chronic disabling disorders, without a cure, and that treatment of patients with these conditions should involve much more than just pharmacotherapy, although that does provide the starting point. The multidisciplinary team, consisting of physicians, nurses, physiotherapists, occupational therapists, podiatrists, pharmacists, and psychologists, is still important to the patient in the delivery of their care.

Tumour necrosis factor (TNF) inhibitors have proven to be the benchmark of biologic therapies across the disease spectrum, particularly in rheumatoid arthritis and the spondyloarthropathies. Clearly TNF is a key cytokine in the process of inflammation and abrogation of this molecule will result in significant, and often life-changing, improvements for patients. The initial fears of adverse events—and in particular neoplasm and infection—have been less prominent than expected but, of course, remain a threat and can be catastrophic for some patients. TNF inhibitors probably work better for spondyloarthropathy than rheumatoid arthritis, for which they were initially designed, but there is a significant proportion of patients in whom the drug does not work and in whom the drug does work but subsequently becomes ineffective. In the latter group it may help to switch to another TNF inhibitor, but there is little benefit in so doing with the former group. Those who never respond to TNF inhibitors may be driven by other cytokines—interleukin (IL)-17, for example—and an alternative approach to disease management is required in this group.

Other cytokine inhibitors that are now available or becoming available are inhibitors of IL-6, the IL-17 inhibitors, the IL-12/23 (and IL-23 alone) inhibitors, and there are a host of others in development. The cytokines (IL-17 and IL-23) are clearly more important in spondyloarthropathy and will in time completely change our treatment options for these disorders. IL-17 inhibition may work for TNF-resistant rheumatoid arthritis, but early results are not promising. For rheumatoid arthritis IL-6 seems to be important and this is now an important alternative treatment for patients with rheumatoid arthritis who have never responded to TNF inhibitors or for whom several have failed.

There are other biologic drugs targeted not at cytokines but at cell lines or cell–cell interaction. Of these, rituximab, targeting a surface molecule on B cells (which produce antibodies and autoantibodies such as rheumatoid factor and ACPA), has proven to be very effective in rheumatoid arthritis and systemic lupus. Abatacept, targeting T cell surface molecules, is an alternative treatment of rheumatoid arthritis and has been used in psoriatic arthritis. Other ways of selectively blocking inflammatory pathways are under development or are about to be introduced and we can expect new, and biosimilar, drugs to appear regularly in the future. Indeed, new small molecules have been developed that target immune cellular pathways. Of these the Janus kinase (JAK) inhibitors and inhibitors of phosphodiesterase-4 look promising.

For all these powerful disease-modifying drugs it is worth remembering that the normal immune system also uses these pathways so that lowered immunity means that infection is a constant risk. If infection occurs, it can spread locally extremely fast and become a systemic infection with all the gravity of that situation. As clinicians we should keep a low threshold of detection and management of infection, particularly in the foot, in people on any antirheumatic drug, but particularly biologic drugs. The patient should be advised to stop the drug and seek immediate treatment for the infection—usually a combination of local and systemic therapy (Box 1.2) (11).

Box 1.2 Guidelines for podiatrists treating patients on biologic therapies

- Patients who are being managed with biologic therapies should have immediate access to a specialist podiatrist if they present with foot ulceration or other infections affecting the foot.
- Podiatrists should contact the patient's consultant/rheumatology nurse *immediately* if the patient is being managed with biologic therapy and develops an ulcer and/or infection.
- Optimum ulcer management for any patient can only be achieved by a holistic and integrated multidisciplinary approach.
- Consultant advice should be taken on ingrown nails if the patient is being managed with a biologic therapy and where there are signs of clinical infection and/or the need for nail surgery.

Adapted from Williams A. et al. Guidelines for the management of foot health problems associated with rheumatoid arthritis. *Musculoskelet Care*. 2011;**9**:86–92 with permission from Wiley.

Treatment approaches: non-pharmacological therapies

As noted above, although biologic therapies may have a dramatic impact, there is much more to the delivery of care. In recent years the importance of the multidisciplinary team in disease management has been highlighted in the UK by the National Institute of Health and Care Excellence (NICE) and by the Arthritis and Musculoskeletal Alliance (ARMA) (https://www.nice.org.uk/guidance/cg79 and http://arma.uk.net/wp-content/uploads/pdfs/ia06.pdf). There is evidence that this model has not been widely adopted from the point of view of podiatry care (http://arma.uk.net/wp-content/uploads/pdfs/musculoskeletalfoothealthproblems.pdf). To what extent is the multidisciplinary approach to care evidence-based? There is burgeoning evidence for individual contributions: nursing, podiatry, occupational therapy, physiotherapy (7, 12, 13)—and for education provided across the multidisciplinary team (14).

Care may effectively be delivered in the context of a combined multidisciplinary clinic (15, 16). Such a method of delivering care has been described for the foot across a spectrum of disease, providing anecdotal evidence of improved outcomes and cost savings (15). This approach is not always practical, though: an alternative might be a weekly multidisciplinary meeting to discuss problems and approaches to management of shared patients. Even this approach may provide a challenge in some situations. What is clear is that lines of communication should be established between members of the team so that patient management can be shared—one approach in Bradford, UK is to have a single electronic record shared between the primary and secondary care teams, and to which all relevant parties can contribute.

Economic impact and treatment cost-effectiveness

In most healthcare systems there are finite resources. In the National Health Service typical cost savings of up to 20% have to be made year on year. At the same time, wages are rising, technology and the drugs we use are becoming more expensive. Arguments have been made that the cost/benefit analysis should be wider than just at the individual and local level. In societal terms, the introduction of effective, but expensive, treatments, such as TNF inhibitors, will not only alleviate individual suffering but prevent work loss and increase productivity, to the benefit of the wider community. Nevertheless, in the UK, there is 'rationing' of a subtle kind, and this rationing may vary from location to location (the so-called post code lottery). The UK entrusts the guidance on the use of biologics and other new drugs and technologies to NICE. The process by which such judgements are made is a thorough and fair appraisal of the cost/benefit equation. NICE have an unstated threshold of about £30,000 per quality-adjusted life year (QALY). The means by which this is calculated and the projections made in the modelling may have some uncertainties but, equally, the quality of the data provided for the assessments may not always be appropriate. More collaboration between trialists and bodies such as NICE might overcome some of these difficulties, as might new approaches to economic modelling.

The changing role of the multidisciplinary team

With the emergence of new data, foot health management has moved into an evidence-based specialty, and this has in turn led to more prominence in the infrastructure and pathways for treating rheumatic diseases (http://arma.uk.net/wp-content/uploads/pdfs/musculoskeletalfoothealthproblems.pdf). At the same time, the treatment paradigm has become aligned with that of rheumatology in general: early detection and treatment prevents subsequent deformity and disability.

This has meant that the podiatrist is now much more proactive and treats to prevent rather than to react. Of course, there are still situations where 'reaction' is important and treatment of established inflammatory and degenerative diseases will still be a large part of podiatry care.

This early intervention role is mirrored by the approaches taken. There is now much more assessment of the foot as a complex biomechanical structure and less emphasis, especially in early disease, on the skin and nails. Gait analysis, from qualitative assessment to full quantitative studies performed in the laboratory, is an essential part of the role, as well as an appreciation of the contribution of the different soft-tissue structures to the normal function of the foot. Many health professionals are also now becoming skilled at US, so that more precise assessments of ligamentous stability and inflammatory activity can be made, as well as targeted injections.

The podiatrist is also now, as a member of the multidisciplinary team, thinking beyond the foot to the disease as a whole, albeit inflammatory or non-inflammatory. In particular, podiatrists perform an important role in surveillance for potential infection for patients on biologics and for ulceration in rheumatoid arthritis and connective tissue disease. As the role develops it is likely that more and more podiatrists will partake in integrated care in outpatient settings with seamless communication and education links to primary care teams. This role will of course be extended into the wider multidisciplinary team providing care across different settings. Podiatrists will no longer gaze at feet, and never stray above the ankle, but will look beyond to the rest of the patient, as physicians must learn to look below the upper limb to the feet.

References

1. **Hoy D, Smith E, Cross M, et al.** Reflecting on the global burden of musculoskeletal conditions: lessons learnt from the Global Burden of Disease 2010 Study and the next steps forward. *Ann Rheum Dis.* 2015;**74**:4–7.
2. **Murray C, Vos T, Lozano R, et al.** Disability-adjusted life years (DALYs) for 291 diseases and injuries in 21 regions, 1990–2010: a systematic analysis for the Global Burden of Disease Study 2010. *Lancet.* 2012;**380**:2197–223.
3. **Vos T, Flaxman A, Naghavi M, et al.** Years lived with disability (YLDs) for 1160 sequelae of 289 diseases and injuries 1990–2010: a systematic analysis for the Global Burden of Disease Study 2010. *Lancet.* 2012;**380**:2163–96.
4. **Vainio K.** The rheumatoid foot. A clinical study with pathological and roentgenological comments. *Clin Orthop Relat Res.* 1991;**265**:4–8.
5. **Woodburn J, Hennessy K, Steultjens M, McInnes I, Turner D.** Looking through the 'window of opportunity': is there a new paradigm of podiatry care on the horizon in early rheumatoid arthritis? *J Foot Ankle Res.* 2010;**3**:8.
6. **Coates LC, Moverley AR, McParland L, et al.** Effect of tight control of inflammation in early psoriatic arthritis (TICOPA): a UK multicentre, open-label, randomised controlled trial. *Lancet.* 2015;**386**:2489–98.
7. **Woodburn J, Barker S, Helliwell PS.** A randomised controlled trial of foot orthoses in rheumatoid arthritis. *J Rheumatol.* 2002;**29**(7):1377–83.
8. **Emery P, Breedveld FC, Dougados M, Kalden JR, Schiff MH, Smolen JS.** Early referral recommendation for newly diagnosed rheumatoid arthritis: evidence based development of a clinical guide. *Ann Rheum Dis.* 2002;**61**(4):290–7.
9. **Aletaha D, Neogi T, Silman AJ, et al.** 2010 Rheumatoid arthritis classification criteria: an American College of Rheumatology/European League Against Rheumatism collaborative initiative. *Ann Rheum Dis.* 2010;**69**(9):1580–8.

10. **Nishimura K, Sugiyama D, Kogata Y, et al.** Meta-analysis: diagnostic accuracy of anti-cyclic citrullinated peptide antibody and rheumatoid factor for rheumatoid arthritis. *Ann Intern Med.* 2007;**146**(11):797–808.
11. **Williams A, Davies S, Graham A, et al.** Guidelines for the management of the foot health problems associated with rheumatoid arthritis. *Musculoskelet Care.* 2011;**9**:86–92.
12. **Bird H, Le Gallez P, Hill J.** *Combined Care of the Rheumatic Patient.* London: Springer-Verlag; 1985.
13. **Hammond A, Freeman K.** The long-term outcomes from a randomized controlled trial of an educational–behavioural joint protection programme for people with rheumatoid arthritis. *Clin Rehab.* 2004;**18**(5):520–8.
14. **Helliwell PS, O'Hara M, Holdsworth J, Hesselden A, King T, Evans P.** A 12-month randomized controlled trial of patient education on radiographic changes and quality of life in early rheumatoid arthritis. *Rheumatology.* 1999;**38**(4):303–8.
15. **Helliwell PS.** Lessons to be learned: review of a multidisciplinary foot clinic in rheumatology. *Rheumatology.* 2003;**42**(11):1426–7.
16. **Siddle HJ, Backhouse MR, Monkhouse R, Harris NJ, Helliwell PS.** Joint orthopaedic and rheumatology clinics: evidence to support the guidelines. *Musculoskelet Care.* 2011;**9**(3):180–3.

Chapter 2

Anatomy of the foot and ankle

Dave Roberts, James Pickering, and Jordan Fletcher

The human foot and ankle are uniquely adapted to support the entire weight of the body and provide a platform through which propulsive forces are transmitted to the ground beneath. Far from being passive elements, however, the foot and ankle together represent a dynamic, reactive, and force-generating structure containing a complex arrangement of bones held in inherently unstable configurations by an array of ligaments and muscle tendons. This anatomical complexity, together with the biomechanical demands placed on them, make the foot and ankle particularly susceptible to a variety of injuries and disease processes.

Bones of the foot

The skeleton of the foot is comprised of 26 non-sesamoid bones that can be conveniently considered in three groups: the bones of the rearfoot, those of the midfoot, and those of the forefoot (Figure 2.1).

The rearfoot includes just two bones, the talus above and the calcaneus below. The talus of the rearfoot articulates with the distal ends of the tibia and fibula of the leg at the ankle joint. It is important to appreciate that no other joints contribute to the ankle joint. In particular, it should be noted that the subtalar joint, which lies between the talus above and the calcaneus below, is *not* part of the ankle joint.

The skeleton of the midfoot is comprised of the navicular, the three cuneiform bones lying in a row immediately anterior to it, and the laterally positioned cuboid bone. The bones of the midfoot and rearfoot articulate at the talocalcaneonavicular and calcaneocuboid joints. A line drawn through these joints delineates the boundary between the two regions; this boundary is called the transverse tarsal line.

The forefoot includes the five metatarsals and their associated phalanges. The metatarsals of the forefoot articulate with the bones of the midfoot at the tarsometatarsal joints. A line drawn through these joints, the tarsometatarsal line, defines the boundary between the midfoot and the forefoot.

The ankle joint

The ankle joint proper is a strong and stable synovial joint formed between the talus of the rearfoot and the distal ends of the tibia and fibula (Figure 2.1). The joint, which is also known as the talocrural joint, resembles a mortice and tenon in arrangement, with the mortice formed mainly by the ends of the fibula and tibia, and the tenon by the wedge-shaped body of the talus. The joint is easily located, as the medial and lateral malleoli of the tibia and fibula provide prominent bony landmarks at the distal end of the leg. It is a hinge joint, limited almost entirely to flexion

(a)

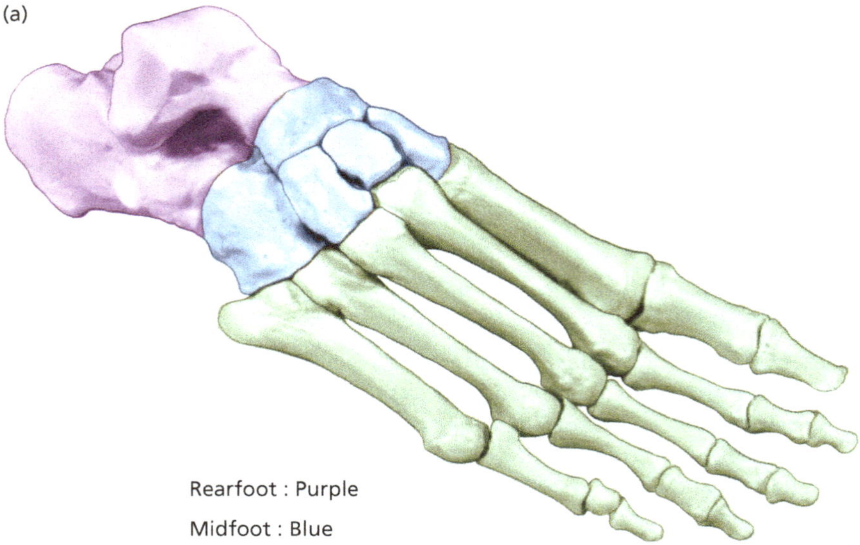

(b)

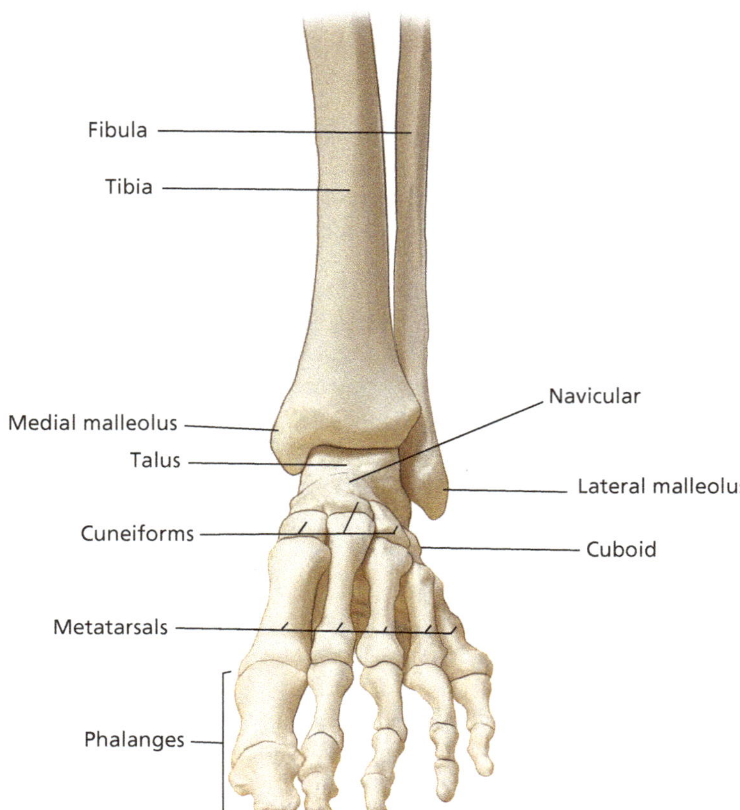

Figure 2.1 Bones of the foot and ankle. (a) Oblique view. (b) Anterior view. (c) Posterior view. (d) Lateral view. (e) Medial view.

(c)

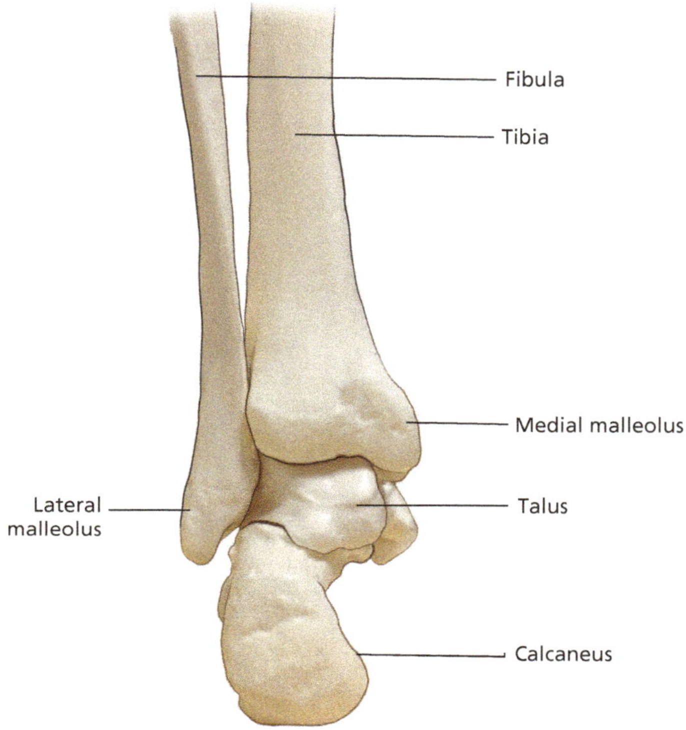

(d)

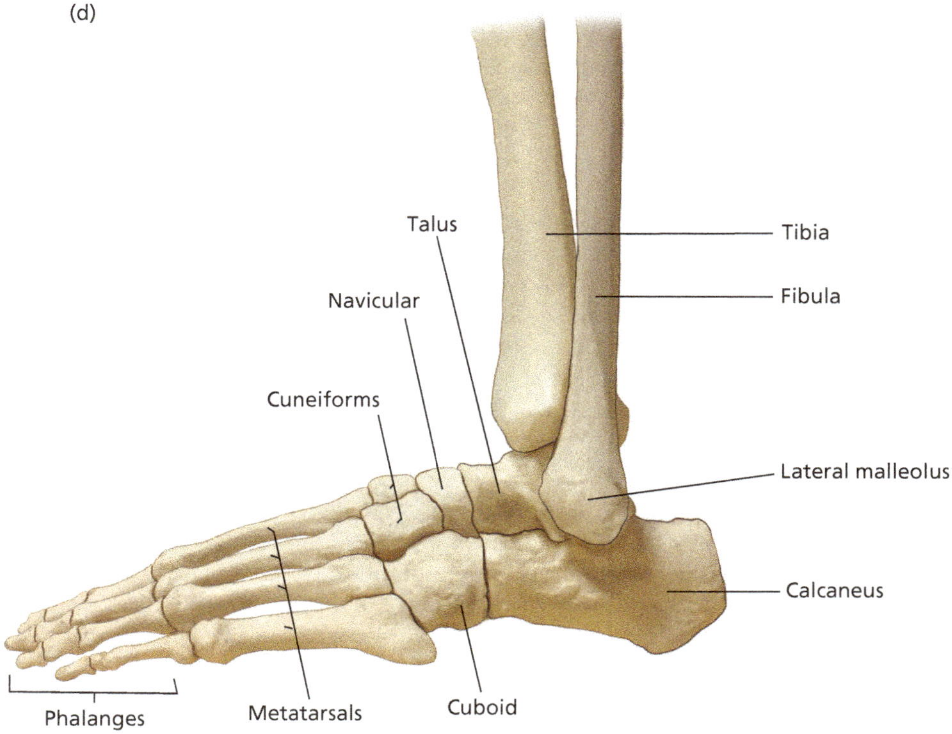

Figure 2.1 Continued

(e)

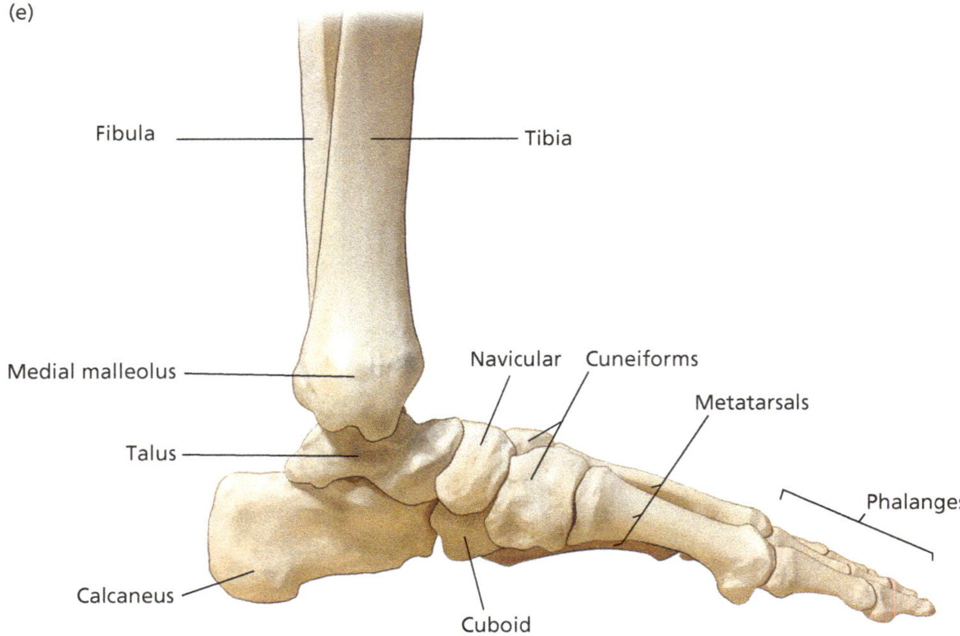

Figure 2.1 Continued

(dorsiflexion) and extension (plantar flexion) around a near-horizontal axis that passes through the tip of the lateral malleolus and somewhat inferior to the medial malleolus.

The ankle joint is topographically and functionally associated with the inferior tibiofibular joint. This fibrous joint is found between the distal end of the fibula and the fibular notch on the lateral side of the tibia. It is supported by a number of ligaments, principally the interosseous ligament, which is continuous with the interosseous membrane of the leg, and the transverse tibiofibular ligament. The latter contributes directly to the mortice of the ankle joint, along with the two bones that it joins.

The fibrous nature of the inferior tibiofibular joint imparts the joint with a degree of flexibility that contributes directly to ankle joint stability. During dorsiflexion, the wider, anterior part of the articular surface of the talus is forced between the distal ends of the tibia and fibula, tending to separate them. The limited expansion allowed by the tibiofibular joint ensures a snug, stabilizing fit that helps to hold the talus in the mortice of the ankle joint during dorsiflexion. During plantar flexion, the joint becomes less stable as the narrower posterior articular surface of the talus occupies the joint. As a result, the majority of ankle injuries occur when the joint is plantar flexed.

Capsule and ligaments

The capsule completely encloses the ankle joint with its fibrous layer attaching superiorly to the articular margins of the tibia and fibula and inferiorly around those of the talus. The capsule is thin anteriorly and posteriorly, facilitating smooth, unobstructed movement of the joint. Medially and laterally, it blends with the strong collateral ligaments of the joint. The latter include the deltoid ligament on the medial aspect and three separate collateral ligaments on the lateral side of the joint (Figure 2.2). These ligaments both stabilize the joint and help to define the limits of its movement.

The deltoid (medial collateral) ligament of the ankle joint is large and strong. It attaches to the inferior tip of the medial malleolus and spreads distally to attach to the talus, calcaneus, and navicular. Although it is a single discrete structure, the ligament has four named parts, defined by their distal attachments:

- Anterior tibiotalar band
- Posterior tibiotalar band
- Tibiocalcaneal band
- Tibionavicular band.

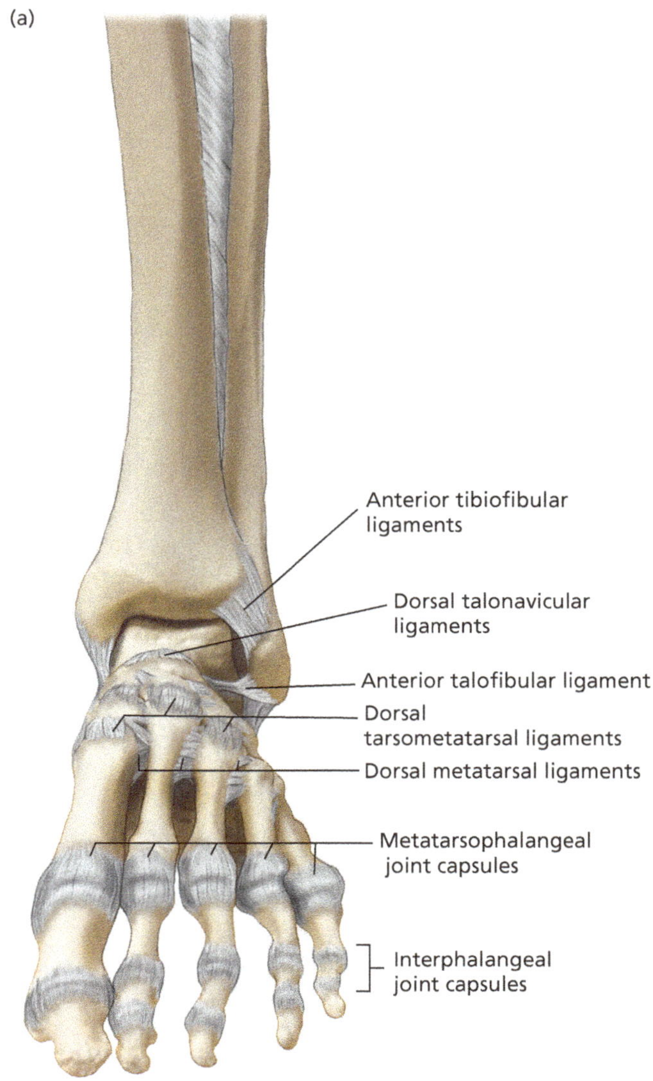

Figure 2.2 Major ligaments of the foot and ankle. (a) Anterior view. (b) Posterior view. (c) Lateral view. (d) Medial view.

(b)

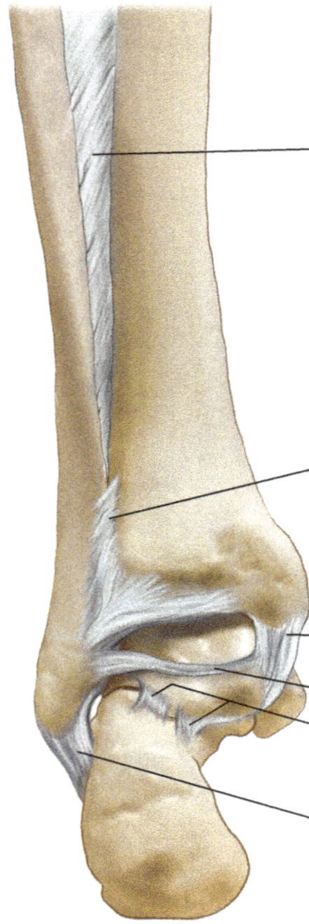

Figure 2.2 Continued

The lateral side of the ankle joint is stabilized by the anterior talofibular, the posterior talofibular, and the calcaneofibular ligaments (Figure 2.2). These three discrete lateral collateral ligaments correspond to three of the four bands of the deltoid ligament lying on the medial aspect of the joint. The joint is less stable on its lateral side, so most sprains are associated with inversion, rather than eversion, of the foot.

Dorsiflexion of the joint is controlled, in part, by the posterior components of the collateral ligaments (posterior talofibular ligament and posterior tibiotalar band of the deltoid ligament). Plantar flexion is controlled by the anterior components (anterior talofibular ligament and anterior tibiotalar band). It should be appreciated, however, that other factors, both within and external to the joint, play a role in limiting the range of these movements.

The restriction of normal ankle joint movement almost entirely to dorsiflexion and plantar flexion is largely a consequence of the mortice and tenon-like arrangement of the bones involved. However, the tibiocalcaneal and tibionavicular bands of the deltoid ligaments assist by limiting abduction of the talus, whilst the calcaneofibular ligament limits its adduction.

(c)

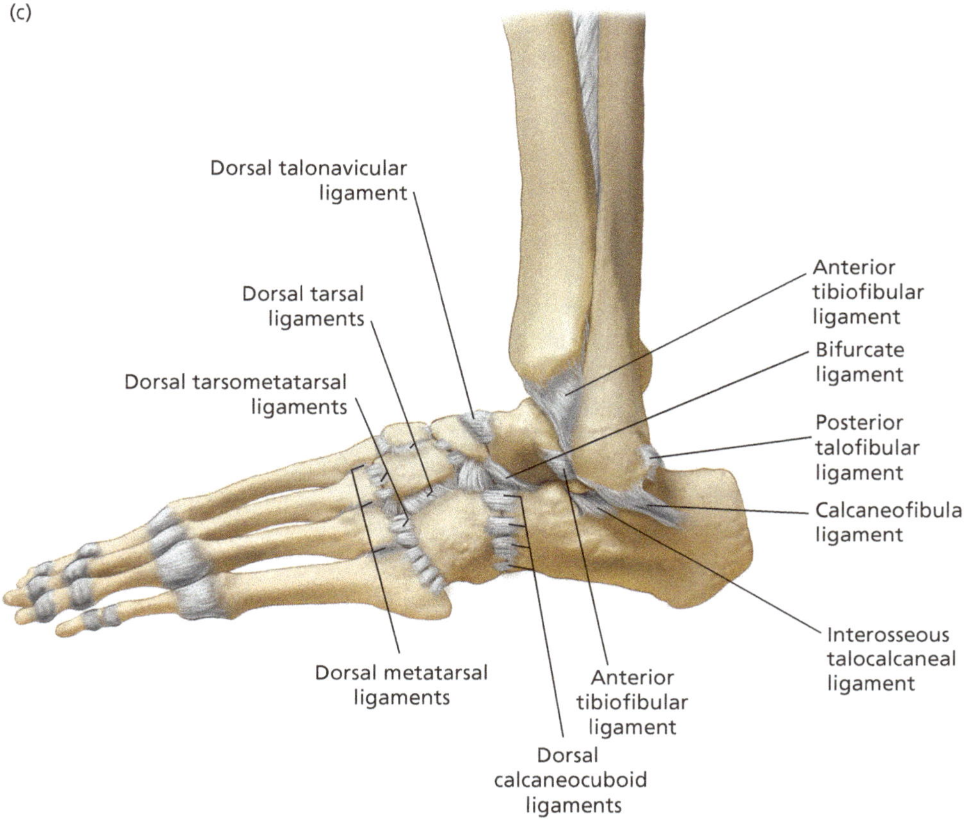

(d)

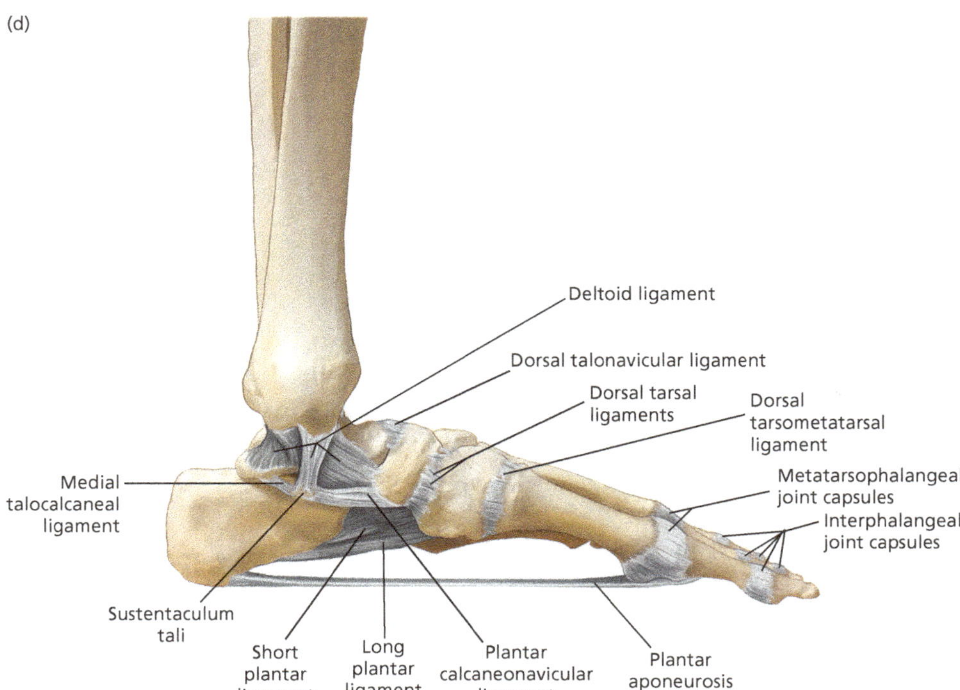

Figure 2.2 Continued

Articular cartilage

Most of the articular surfaces of the foot and ankle are covered with hyaline cartilage. This creates a near-frictionless surface to facilitate articulation, weightbearing, and shock absorption during movement. It is avascular, aneural, and alymphatic. It receives its nourishment from the fluid produced by the synovial membrane that lines the fibrous joint capsule.

Hyaline cartilage is comprised of a dense extracellular matrix containing sparsely distributed chondrocytes. The latter are specialized, highly metabolic cells responsible for producing and maintaining the matrix that ultimately entraps them. They are the only differentiated cell type present in hyaline cartilage.

The extracellular matrix is mainly composed of water, collagen, and proteoglycans. The predominant fibre type is type II collagen, the triple helical structure of which provides the cartilage with its ability to resist shearing and tensile forces. The main proteoglycan is aggrecan, a large macromolecule with interacts with hyaluronan to form extensive proteoglycan complexes. These large aggrecan complexes, which occupy the spaces between the collagen fibrils, are osmotically active. As such, they are responsible for imparting the hyaline cartilage with its impressive ability to resist compressive loads.

Tendons, retinacula, and synovial sheaths

The ankle joint is crossed by several tendons as they pass to their insertions on the bones of the foot (Figure 2.3). These tendons can be considered in four broad groups, depending on their position relative to the joint:

- Anterior
  - Extensor hallucis longus
  - Tibialis anterior
  - Extensor digitorum longus
  - Peroneus tertius (where present)
- Posteromedial
  - Tibialis posterior
  - Flexor digitorum longus
  - Flexor hallucis longus
- Posterolateral
  - Peroneus longus
  - Peroneus brevis
- Posterior
  - The calcaneal tendon (the fused tendon of gastrocnemius, soleus and, usually, plantaris).

With the exception of the calcaneal tendon, all of these tendons are held in place by thickenings of the deep fascia known as retinacula.

Tendons passing anterior to the ankle joint would have a tendency to 'bowstring' during dorsiflexion unless bound down by the extensor retinacula. The superior extensor retinaculum is located just above the joint, running transversely between the tibia and fibula. All of the anterior tendons pass immediately deep to this layer, although the tibialis anterior tendon may pass through a canal in the retinaculum rather than deep to it. At this level, only the tibialis anterior tendon is surrounded by a synovial sheath, a fluid-filled, double-layered covering of synovial membrane that reduces friction between the sliding tendon and the structures around it.

(a)

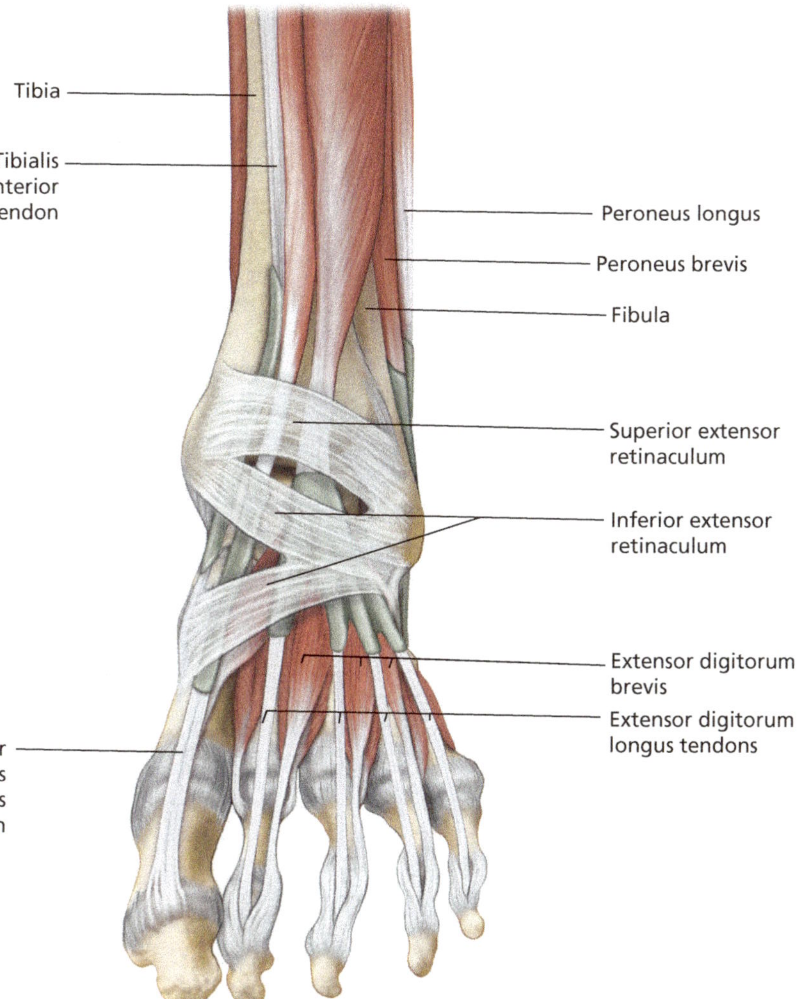

Figure 2.3 Tendons and retinacula associated with the ankle joint. (a) Anterior view. (b) Medial view. (c) Lateral view.

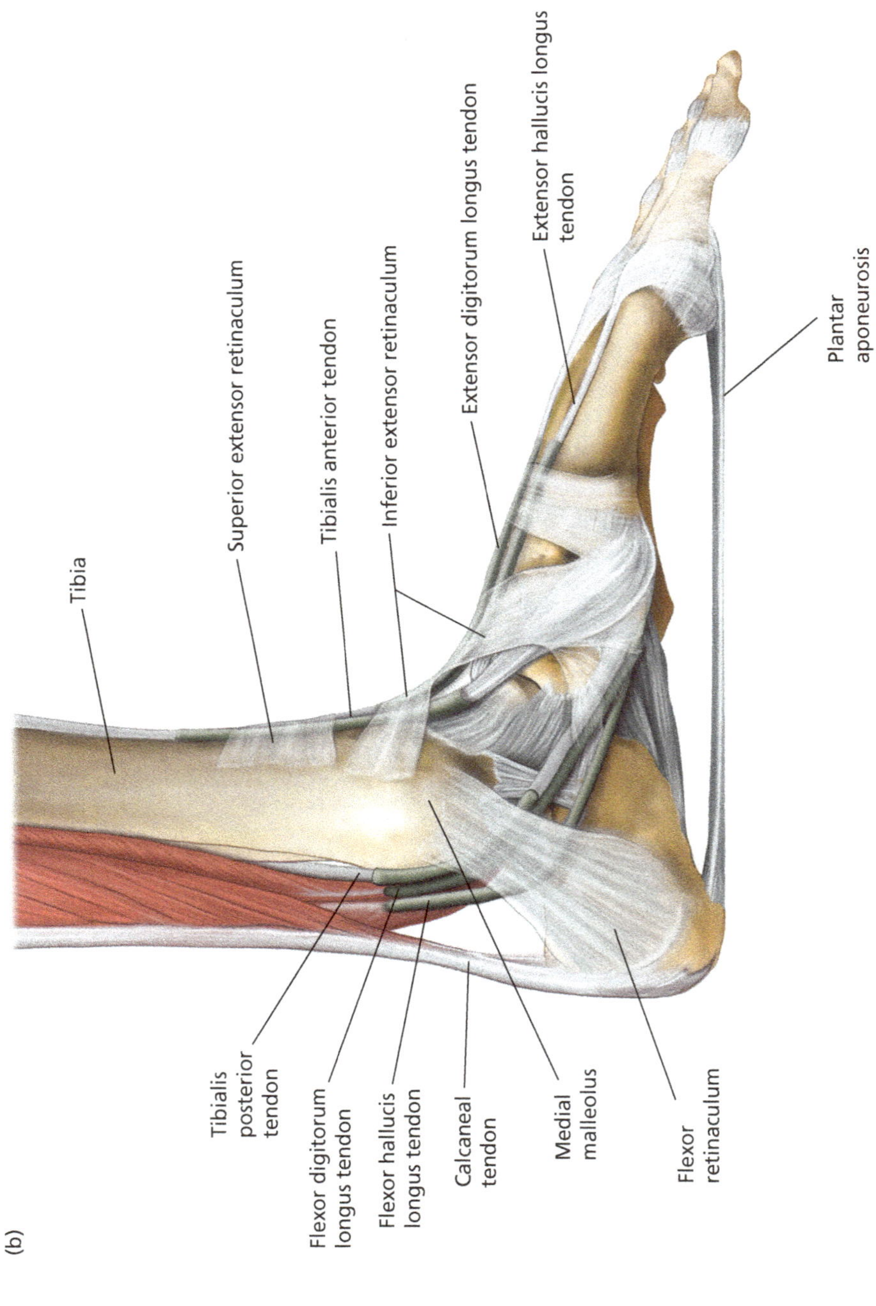

Figure 2.3 Continued

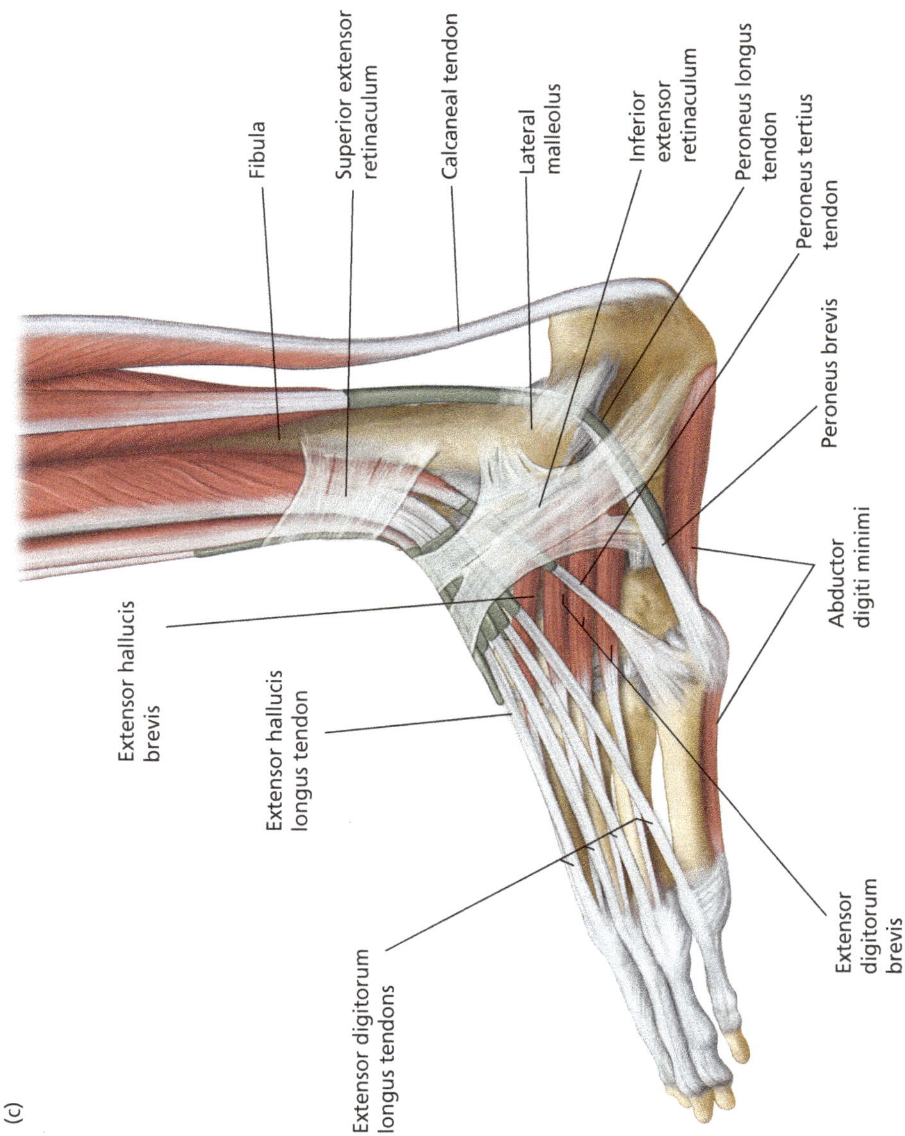

Figure 2.3 Continued

The inferior extensor retinaculum is a Y-shaped band running lateral-to-medial across the proximal aspect of the dorsum of the foot. The tibialis anterior and extensor hallucis longus tendons pass through separate tunnels in the retinaculum, surrounded by their own individual synovial sheaths. The four tendons of the extensor digitorum longus and that of the peroneus tertius pass though a common tunnel in the retinaculum, enveloped in a single, shared, synovial sheath.

The tendons lying posteromedial to the ankle joint all pass deep to the flexor retinaculum. This is attached to the medial malleolus of the tibia superiorly and the calcaneus inferiorly. Fibrous septa pass from the deep aspect of the retinaculum to the ankle joint capsule and tibia, producing four tunnels, one for each of the three tendons and another for the neurovascular bundle of the tibial nerve. Each tendon has its own synovial sheath at this point.

The tendons of peroneus longus and brevis are retained by the peroneal retinacula. The superior peroneal retinaculum passes from the lateral malleolus to the calcaneus, immediately superficial to the two tendons, which, at this point, share a common synovial sheath. The inferior retinaculum provides separate tunnels for the tendons as they pass lateral to the calcaneus, now enclosed in separate synovial coverings.

The gastrocnemius and soleus muscles, the chief plantar flexors of the foot, attach as a single fused tendon to the posterior surface of the calcaneus. This calcaneal tendon passes posterior to the ankle joint without any retinacular binding or synovial covering. It is the thickest tendon in the body, reflecting the substantial forces that gastrocnemius and soleus can generate during propulsion. Despite its very substantial nature, it has elastic properties that permit it to absorb strain and thereby generate recoil forces with the potential to assist plantar flexion.

The rearfoot

The subtalar joint and sinus tarsi

The undersurface of the talus presents three articular surfaces for articulation with corresponding surfaces on the dorsal aspect of the calcaneus. On both bones, the anterior and middle articular surfaces are closely related, whilst the posterior surface is separated from them by a deep groove, or sulcus. Together, the sulcus tali above and the sulcus calcanei below form the sinus tarsi, a channel that runs from posteromedial to anterolateral through the skeleton of the rearfoot.

The three sites of articulation between the talus and the calcaneus form what is clinically and functionally considered to be a single joint, the subtalar joint. Although the three articulations are enclosed by two distinct capsules, they have a common axis of motion and cannot move independently of one another.

The anterior and middle articulations of the subtalar joint share a joint capsule that attaches posteriorly to the roof and floor of the sinus tarsi. The anterior aspect of the discrete capsule around the posterior articulation makes similar attachments. As a result, the two capsules lie adjacent to each other in the sinus tarsi, where they are thickened to form the strong intraosseous talocalcaneal ligament of the subtalar joint. This ligament plays a central role in stabilizing the joint.

At the lateral end of the sinus tarsi is the cervical ligament. This strong fibrous band, which attaches to the talus above and the calcaneus below, plays a particular role in limiting inversion of the foot.

The capsule of the posterior articulation of the joint is not only thickened anteriorly, but also laterally, medially, and posteriorly. These thickenings form the lateral, medial, and posterior talocalcaneal ligaments, respectively (Figure 2.2).

In addition to the stability conferred by the intrinsic ligaments of its capsules, the subtalar joint is supported by the medial and lateral collateral ligaments of the ankle and by the long tendons of muscles crossing it on their way from the leg to the foot. As a result, the subtalar joint is very robust and rarely dislocated.

The calcaneal enthesis

The insertion of the calcaneal tendon into the calcaneus is the archetypal example both of a fibrocartilaginous enthesis and of the closely related concept of the enthesis organ.

An enthesis is the site of insertion of a tendon, ligament, or joint capsule into bone. There are two types of such insertion, fibrous and fibrocartilaginous. Fibrous entheses are typified by the insertion of muscle tendons into the diaphyses of long bones, and characterized by a purely fibrous connection between the bone and the structure attaching to it. In contrast, fibrocartilaginous entheses, which are found at sites including the epiphyses and apophyses of long bones, have a more complex and more organized structure, with layers of fibrocartilage present at the heart of the insertion. Fibrocartilaginous entheses are generally considered to be the more important, in part because they are more numerous but, in particular, because they are far more frequently involved in disease or injury.

A fibrocartilaginous enthesis such as the insertion of the calcaneal tendon, is made up of four zones of tissue:

1. Dense fibrous tissue indistinguishable from tendon
2. Un-ossified fibrocartilage
3. Ossified fibrocartilage
4. Bone.

As the first and fourth zones are indistinguishable from the structures that the enthesis joins, it is impossible to define exactly where the interface begins and ends. However, what is clear is that the junction between un-ossified (soft) and ossified (hard) tissue occurs in the fibrocartilaginous core of the enthesis. This junction is clearly visible microscopically as a straight basophilic line. In contrast to the very straight demarcation of un-ossified and ossified fibrocartilage, the boundary between the fibrocartilage and the underlying bone is more irregular, possibly adding mechanical stability to the union. Interestingly, there is little or no cortical bone at the point of insertion; it has been suggested that direct interaction with the trabecular bone may serve to anchor the enthesis, with the bony trabeculae acting analogously to the roots of a tree.

As the ankle is flexed and extended through its full range of motion, the calcaneal enthesis undergoes significant changes in insertion angle. This is typical of fibrocartilaginous entheses, which, at least in part, appear to have evolved to cope with such changes. The un-ossified fibrocartilaginous zone of the insertion appears to dampen down stress caused by the bending of collagen fibres in the enthesis; this layer tends to be thicker in sites that have a greater range of insertion angles.

During maximal dorsiflexion, the most inferior part of the calcaneal tendon tends to impinge on the posterior surface of the calcaneus. As a result, layers of fibrocartilage develop on the deep surface of the tendon adjacent to the bone (the sesamoid fibrocartilage) and on the involved surface of the bone itself (the periosteal fibrocartilage). These layers move closer together as the ankle is dorsiflexed, and apart as it is plantar flexed. Between them is a bursa, which facilitates movement between the tendon and the bone (the retrocalcaneal bursa) and the tip of a fat pat (the Kager fat pad), which moves into and out of the bursa as the ankle moves, thereby maintaining the pressure of the lubricating synovial fluid inside the bursa.

The calcaneal enthesis, together with its associated sesamoid and periosteal fibrocartilage layers, bursa, and fat pad, have been described as the prototypical example of a functional collection of tissues dubbed the 'enthesis organ'. Such 'organs' are found throughout the body, including at other sites in the foot.

Functional entheses of the rearfoot

The long tendons that run posteromedial and posterolateral to the ankle joint undergo a significant change in direction as they course through the rearfoot. On the medial surface of the calcaneus, for example, the sustentaculum tali guides the tendon of flexor hallucis longus through an angle of around 90° at rest. The other tendons are similarly guided by a combination of retinacula and bony projections.

Where tendons are deflected by bone, there is a tendency for each of the two interacting surfaces to develop a protective covering of fibrocartilage. In general, the tendons will also be enclosed in fluid-filled synovial sheaths at these points of directional change. Bone and tendon separated by two protective layers of fibrocartilage and an intervening synovial compartment represent a structure that is clearly reminiscent of the enthesis organs described earlier. In contrast to the enthesis organ, there is no union of one structure with another at such sites, which have been named 'functional entheses'.

Bursae

The retrocalcaneal bursa of the calcaneal enthesis organ is the only bursa consistently found in association with the rearfoot and ankle joint. Adventitious bursae can develop in the soft tissues covering the posterior surface of the calcaneal tendon, the inferior surface of the calcaneus, and the malleoli. These bursae arise in response to external forces to provide additional protection to the underlying structures.

The midfoot

The midfoot is comprised of the navicular, cuboid, and three cuneiforms (Figure 2.1). The navicular and cuboid are located directly anterior to the talus and calcaneus, and form the talocalcaneonavicular and calcaneocuboid joints with them, respectively.

The talocalcaneonavicular joint is a synovial ball-and-socket joint involving the head of the talus and the posterior surface of the navicular. It also includes the anterior and middle articulations between the talus and calcaneus described above as part of the subtalar joint. The joint is reinforced by three ligaments: the dorsal talonavicular, the plantar calcaneonavicular, and the bifurcate ligament (Figure 2.2).

It should be noted that, although the capsule of the talocalcaneonavicular joint encloses all three of its articulations in a single joint cavity, for clinical purposes the joint is often considered as separate talonavicular and talocalcaneal joints.

The plantar calcaneonavicular, or spring, ligament (Figure 2.2) has particular functional importance as it helps to maintain the overall shape of the foot. It is particularly strong and extends from the anterior aspect of the sustentaculum tali of the calcaneus to the inferior and medial aspects of the navicular. The superior surface of the ligament runs adjacent to the head of the talus, where it contributes a fibrocartilaginous facet to one of the articular surfaces of the talocalcaneonavicular joint. It is important in transferring force from the talus into the more distal elements of the foot.

The calcaneocuboid joint is also a synovial joint with a single fibrous joint capsule reinforced by three ligaments. The bifurcate ligament, which is shared with the talocalcaneonavicular joint, originates from the upper region of the calcaneus and splits to form attachments with the upper surfaces of both the cuboid and the navicular. The short plantar (plantar calcaneocuboid) ligament is a strong band passing from the anterior tubercle on the undersurface of the calcaneus to the plantar surface of the cuboid (Figure 2.2). It is separated from the more superficial long plantar ligament by adipose tissue. The long plantar ligament extends from the plantar surface of the calcaneus to the bases of the third, fourth, and fifth metatarsals and the plantar aspect of the cuboid bone. As it approaches the metatarsals, it passes superficial to the peroneus longus tendon. As well as reinforcing the calcaneocuboid joint, the short and long plantar ligaments both play a functionally critical role in maintaining the overall form of the foot.

The talocalcaneonavicular and calcaneocuboid joints together form the junction between the rearfoot and midfoot as delineated by the transverse tarsal line. Together with the subtalar joint, these so-called transverse talar joints are the main sites facilitating inversion and eversion of the foot. Inversion (a combination of adduction and supination, usually accompanied by plantar flexion of the ankle) is mainly brought about by the tibialis anterior and posterior muscles of the leg. Eversion (a combination of abduction and pronation, usually accompanied by dorsiflexion of the ankle) is produced by the peroneal muscles.

The three cuneiforms of the midfoot are located anterior to the navicular and medial to the cuboid bone (Figure 2.1). Identified as medial, intermediate, and lateral, they articulate via synovial joints and are held together mainly by the strong interosseous and plantar intercuneiform ligaments. Distally, each articulates with the base of one or more metatarsals.

The cuboid articulates with the lateral cuneiform at the cuneocuboid joint, which is supported by dorsal, interosseous, and plantar ligaments. It also articulates with the two lateral metatarsals.

The forefoot

The forefoot is comprised of five metatarsals and fourteen phalanges (Figure 2.1). The first three metatarsals articulate with the cuneiform bones, whilst the two most lateral metatarsals articulate with the cuboid bone. These five tarsometatarsal joints define the junction between the midfoot and the forefoot.

Each tarsometatarsal joint is reinforced by plantar and dorsal tarsometatarsal ligaments (Figure 2.2). Additional, interosseous, ligaments connect the medial cuneiform to the second metatarsal, and the lateral cuneiform to the fourth metatarsal. Lying close by, between the bases of the second to the fifth metatarsals, are the intermetatarsal joints. These small synovial joints are supported by yet more plantar, dorsal, and interosseous ligaments. The interosseous intermetatarsal ligaments, which pass between the bases of adjacent metatarsals, help to maintain the overall shape of the foot.

The extensive array of ligaments and a mortice-like interlocking arrangement at the base of the second metatarsal limits movement at the tarsometatarsal joints. As a group, they contribute to inversion and eversion of the foot.

The convex head of each metatarsal articulates with the concave base of the respective proximal phalanx. These metatarsophalangeal joints are condyloid synovial joints with individual joint capsules supported by collateral and plantar ligaments. Dorsally, the extensor tendons reinforce the joints (Figure 2.3). The deep transverse metatarsal ligament joins all the metatarsophalangeal joints mediolaterally (Figure 2.4). These joints permit plantar flexion and dorsiflexion, as well as limited abduction, adduction, and circumduction.

The great toe has only two phalanges; all the others have three (Figure 2.1). Each individual phalanx is comprised of a base, a shaft, and a head. An interphalangeal hinge joint is located between the head of each phalanx and the base of the next in the series. Each joint is enclosed by an individual joint capsule supported by collateral ligaments, a thick plantar ligament and, where present, a dorsal extensor tendon expansion. The only movements permitted are plantar flexion and dorsiflexion.

Bursae

The main bursae of the forefoot lie immediately superior to the deep transverse metatarsal ligament, in the distal aspect of each intermetatarsal space (Figure 2.4). In the second, third, and fourth spaces, these synovial intermetatarsal bursae are bounded on each side by the interosseous tendons and the collateral ligament complexes of the respective metatarsophalangeal joints. The relations of the first intermetatarsal bursa are similar, except that its medial aspect is bounded by collateral ligaments and the tendon of the adductor hallucis muscle.

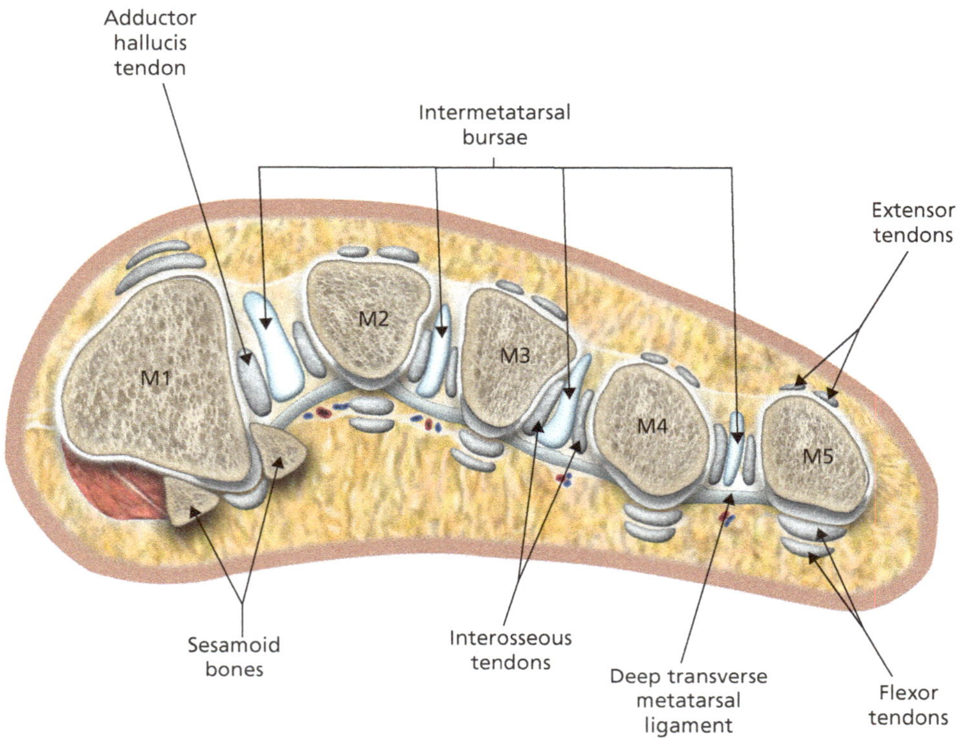

Figure 2.4 Bursae of the forefoot. Simplified diagram of a section through the foot at the level of the metatarsal heads (M1–M5). The intermetatarsal bursae lie immediately superior to the deep transverse metatarsal ligament, sandwiched between the tendons of short intrinsic muscles of the foot.

In the first and fourth space, the bursae do not extend beyond the distal border of the deep transverse metatarsal ligament. Consequently, they remain separated from the respective neurovascular bundle, which runs inferior to this ligament (Figure 2.4).

In the second and third intermetatarsal spaces, the bursae extend beyond the distal extent of the deep transverse metatarsal ligament to lie between the bases of the associated proximal phalanges; at this point, they lie close to the neurovascular bundle of the respective space.

As in the rearfoot, non-synovial adventitious bursae can develop in the forefoot in response to external forces. These are particularly likely to be found in association with the plantar surfaces adjacent to the metatarsal heads and in the soft tissue overlying the medial aspect of the first metatarsal head.

Arches of the foot

To fulfil its purpose as an active, force-transmitting interface between the body and the ever-changing substrate it is travelling over, the foot has to be both stable and adaptable at the same time. To this end, its many interconnected bones are arranged into a series of flexible arches that are created and maintained by the actions of ligaments and muscles. The bones at each end of an arch are known as its pillars.

The medial longitudinal arch

The medial longitudinal arch runs along the medial border of the foot and includes the calcaneus, talus, and navicular, the three cuneiforms, and the first three metatarsals. Its pillars are the posterior aspect of the calcaneus and the heads of its metatarsals.

The form of the medial longitudinal arch is almost entirely dependent on the actions of ligaments and muscles. Of particular importance is the plantar aponeurosis, a dense, superficial collagenous sheet of tissue attaching to the inferior surface of the calcaneus posteriorly and the ligamentous structures around the metatarsophalangeal joints and proximal phalanges anteriorly (Figures 2.2 and 2.3). This acts as a tie-beam between the two pillars of the arch.

The plantar calcaneonavicular (spring) ligament (Figure 2.2) also plays a critical role in maintaining the medial arch as it helps to support the talus and ties the calcaneus and navicular together. If it fails, the talus adopts an abnormally low position, compromising the arch-like configuration on the medial aspect of the foot.

Muscles with a particular role in maintaining the medial arch are the flexor hallucis longus, tibialis posterior, and tibialis anterior (Figure 2.3). Others with lesser roles include flexor digitorum longus, abductor hallucis, and part of flexor digitorum brevis.

The lateral longitudinal arch

The lateral longitudinal arch includes the calcaneus, the cuboid, and the lateral two metatarsals. Its pillars are the calcaneus and the heads of its two metatarsals.

The shape of the lateral longitudinal arch is, like that of the medial arch, dependent on ligaments and muscles. The most important ligaments in this regard are the plantar aponeurosis along with the long and short plantar ligaments (Figure 2.2). The peroneus longus muscle has a particularly important role, assisted by flexor digitorum longus, flexor accessorius, part of flexor digitorum brevis, and abductor digiti minimi (Figure 2.3).

The lateral longitudinal arch is considerably shallower and more rigid than its medial equivalent, providing a firm base for contact with the ground.

The transverse arch

The transverse arch runs across the foot. It involves the cuboid, cuneiforms, and the bases of all five metatarsals. Its pillars are the first cuneiform and the base of the first metatarsal medially, and the cuboid and base of the fifth metatarsal laterally.

The transverse arch is stabilized by the ligaments connecting the plantar aspect of its bones together, principally the interosseous intermetatarsal ligaments and the intercuneiform ligaments. The peroneus longus, the tendon of which crosses lateral to medial across the base of the foot, is the main muscle involved in maintaining this arch.

Surface anatomy of the foot and ankle joint

The surface of the foot and ankle is characterized by the underlying bony structures, ligaments, and tendons. Some of these can be palpated through the skin, especially when the relevant muscles are tensed against resistance.

The ankle joint is easily located thanks to the two prominent malleoli that form its lateral and medial margins (Figure 2.1). The sustentaculum tali (Figure 2.2) can be palpated around 2 cm below the tip of the medial malleolus. The navicular tuberosity is easily felt as a prominence 2–3 cm anterior to the sustentaculum tali, with the calcaneonavicular, or spring, ligament palpable between these two bony landmarks, particularly when the foot is everted. The tendon of tibialis anterior is particularly obvious, running anterior to the medial malleolus and superior to the navicular tuberosity (Figure 2.3).

The calcaneal tendon is easily palpated in the midline of the limb posterior to the ankle joint as it approaches its insertion on the posterior surface of the calcaneus (Figure 2.3).

On the lateral aspect of the foot, the calcaneus can be felt forming its joint with the cuboid bone, particularly when the foot is inverted. Eversion permits the peroneal tendons (Figure 2.3) to be felt running toward the base of the fifth metatarsal, which forms a very obvious bony prominence on the lateral aspect of the foot. The thin skin on the dorsum of the foot makes the paths of the extensor digitorum longus and extensor hallucis longus tendons clearly visible; the pulse of the dorsalis pedis artery is easily felt by light palpation between them.

Chapter 3

Normal function and movement

William Ledoux and Joseph Iaquinto

The foot and ankle are critical components of the human locomotive system, as with each step the weight of the entire body must be borne and distributed over the ground. In a well-functioning foot (i.e., a 'normal, healthy' foot), the complex system of bones, cartilage, plantar fat, ligaments, tendons, and muscles works together to adapt to the ground and accept body weight before propelling forward for the next step. It is recognized that there is variability in the morphology of feet, and that 'normal' feet are part of a continuum of arch heights. In general, feet that have too low an arch are considered flat feet (i.e., pes planus) and often include an everted hindfoot and abducted forefoot, while feet with too high an arch are described as high-arched (i.e., pes cavus) and often have an inverted hindfoot and adducted forefoot. These definitions do not consider symptomatic versus non-symptomatic feet (e.g., there are many flat feet that are not painful) nor the position of other, non-arch-related foot joints (e.g., the first metatarsal phalangeal joint in a foot with hallux valgus). For the purposes of this chapter, a normal, healthy foot will be considered to be pain-free, with a neutral hindfoot (neither everted nor inverted) and forefoot (neither abducted nor adducted) and neutrally aligned joints. A normal functioning foot allows for pain-free ambulation at varying speeds and across variable terrains. Should pathology arise, then walking can become painful, inefficient, and difficult.

In this chapter, we will begin with a basic overview of the principles of human movement, anatomy, and function, before discussing the foot structure–function relationship. We will then briefly review the principles and techniques of gait analysis, followed by a review of walking and the gait cycle and the response of ankle cartilage during gait. Next, a description of normal movement and foot function, reviewing tissue- and joint-specific function, as well as complex systematic foot function, will be given. Finally, a review of some specialized techniques for studying foot function, including computational modelling, biplane fluoroscopy, and cadaveric gait simulation, will be provided.

Principles of human movement

Introduction

Human beings are systems of parts that experience complex forces and motions. To understand such complexity, an introduction to the fundamentals of classical mechanics is required. A subset of physics, classical mechanics is traditionally separated into three branches:

- *Static equilibrium:* the study of objects at rest and the forces involved.
- *Kinematics:* the study of objects in motion, without regard to the forces involved.
- *Dynamics:* the study of objects in motion, with regard to the forces involved.

These branches provide several ways to study structures and systems within the human body.

Static equilibrium, kinematics, and dynamics

Classical mechanics is also called Newtonian mechanics, as Newton's laws describe how objects interact with one another. Objects are defined as containing matter; the amount of matter in the object is defined as mass; this quantifies how an object will resist motion. Force is an interaction that will alter the motion of an object. One commonly experienced force is gravity, which results from the mutual attraction between two objects of mass.

- Newton's first law states that objects at rest will remain at rest unless external forces act upon them, and that objects in motion will remain in motion, in a straight line and at a constant speed, unless external forces act on them.
- Newton's second law states that the sum of forces acting on an object will accelerate that object by an amount proportional to the mass (i.e., $\vec{F} = m \cdot \vec{a}$).
- Newton's third law states that, when an object exerts a force onto a second object, the second object exerts a force onto it equal in magnitude and opposite in direction.

With this framework it is possible to quantify object motion and the standard unit system for this is the International System (SI). *Time* is given the unit of second (s) and *length* the unit of meter (m). *Mass* is given the unit of kilogram (kg) and force is given the unit of newton (N), and, where 1 N accelerates 1 kilogram of mass at 1 meter per second per second, then 1 N = 1 kg m s^{-2}.

Static equilibrium

An object is considered to be in a static state when the net sum of forces acting on that object is zero and thus imparts no change to the object (Figure 3.1).

We encounter countless examples of static equilibrium daily. When typing, the force of each keystroke against the keyboard is perfectly opposed by a force exerted on the bottom of the keyboard by the desk. A well-maintained locked door will not budge when pulled on because the hinges, lock, frame, and door knob all act to counteract the pull of the door. The air pressure within a car's tires presses equally against all interior tire surfaces and with a total force equal to the weight of the car. These are all examples of a static state; in all cases there are forces acting in opposition to one other to maintain a net force of zero.

Kinematics

In the field of kinematics, the primary measures of interest are position and its subsequent derivatives. Velocity is the instantaneous change (strictly, the derivative) of position and acceleration is the instantaneous change (derivative) of velocity (or the second derivative of position). Like position and velocity, acceleration may also not be constant. The derivative of acceleration yields instantaneous jerk. Higher derivatives are also defined (with such whimsical names as snap, crackle,

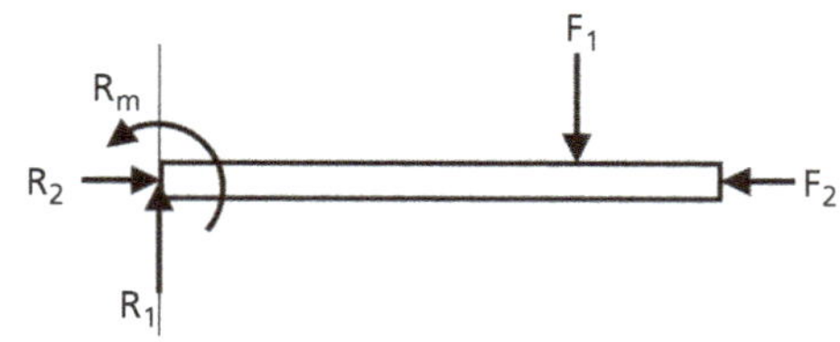

Figure 3.1 Free body diagram of a beam in static equilibrium, fixed on its left side, experiencing external loads in the downward direction F_1 and into the unfixed side F_2. These forces are being perfectly opposed by reactions on the fixed side. R_1 is opposing F_1 and R_2 is opposing F_2. Additionally, a bending moment (R_m) exists to counteract a rotation of the beam due to F_1.

and pop), but in the domain of human kinematics, terms beyond the second derivative (acceleration) rarely appear, although jerk appears fairly commonly in concussion research.

Dynamics

The field of dynamics allows us to describe systems of moving objects which interact and transfer energy in ways that alter their motion. Consider this example of dynamic motion. A pool cue striking the cue ball is a system where there is a net external force (imparted by the pool cue) acting on an object (the ball). In this case, the cue ball rapidly accelerates, changing its velocity and therefore position on the table. When it encounters another object, such as the 8-ball, it may impart some or all of its energy (minus frictional losses due to the air and the table felt) into the 8-ball. Like kinematics, position, velocity, and acceleration are important, but with the addition of mass and force (i.e., Newton's second law).

Anatomical motion

The anatomically neutral position provides a common reference point to describe poses and motions. Traditionally, the anatomical position consists of the face and palms facing forward, hands at the sides and legs together with the toes pointing down (Figure 3.2, left). We can superimpose three orthogonal planes onto this position, each of which bisect the body. The transverse plane divides the body into superior (top) and inferior (bottom) halves, the sagittal plane divides the body into left and right halves, and the coronal plane divides the body into anterior (front) and posterior (back) halves (Figure 3.2, left). When we consider developing local anatomical planes for the foot and ankle, the ankle joint is typically repositioned into the neutral position, with the ankle joint at 90° (as opposed to with the toes pointing down; Figure 3.2, right) such that the bottom surface of the foot is parallel to the transverse plane, while the long axis of the calf is directed superiorly towards the knee. With the foot in a neutral position, there are several common motions available (Figure 3.3).

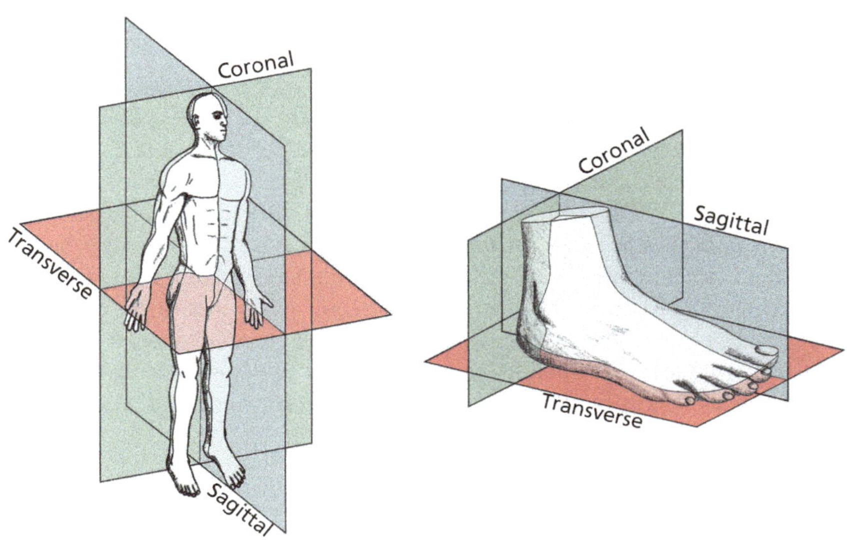

Figure 3.2 Anatomical position, with primary anatomical planes: sagittal, coronal, and transverse (left). Common anatomical planes of the foot, with the ankle at 90° (right).

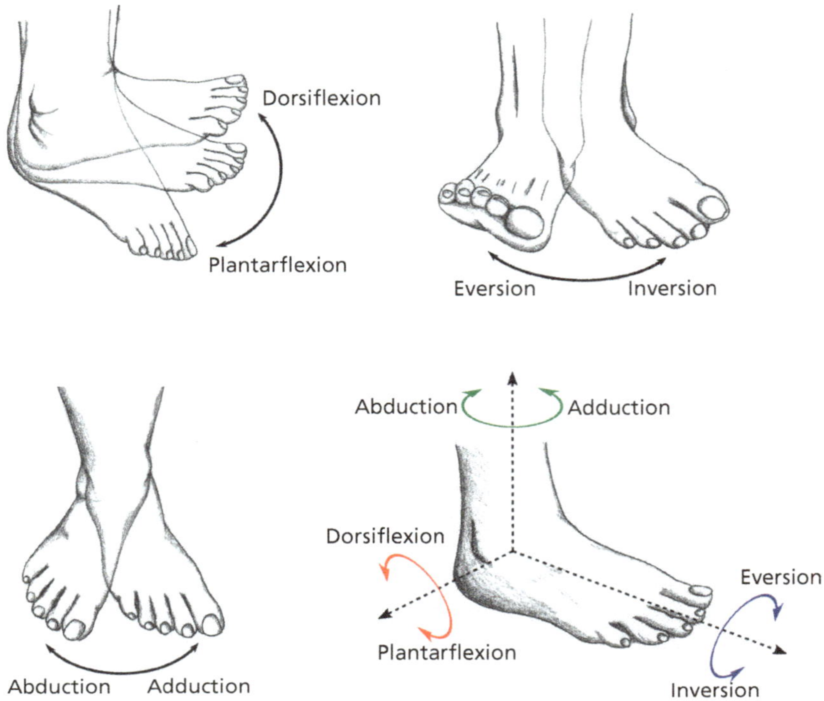

Figure 3.3 Common motions of the foot and ankle. Sagittal plane motion (dorsiflexion and plantarflexion, upper left); coronal plane motion (eversion and inversion, upper right); transverse plane motion (abduction and adduction, lower left); and these common movements with respect to the three anatomical axes (lower right).

Anatomical function

Motion of the human body is derived from the interaction of the bony framework of the musculoskeletal system, articulating through joint cartilage, constrained by ligaments and sometimes tendons, and moved by muscles to impart or prevent motion via the application of force. Briefly, as more detail is provided elsewhere (see Chapter 2), the bones are relatively rigid structures capped with cartilage at their articulations. Both the bone and cartilage at these sites are shaped to promote and guide specific movements, e.g., the hinge-like nature of the ankle joint. Ligaments further constrain joints by preventing them from moving beyond their ideal envelope of motion. Muscles exert force during contractions. They can only pull, not push, but can do this while lengthening (eccentric contraction), remaining at the same length (isometric contraction), or shortening (concentric contraction). Tendons determine how muscle acts on bones relative to joints, both by where they insert into bones and how they wrap around bony features.

Structure–function relationship

Analyzing the motion present at a joint (function) requires knowledge of the geometry of the bones and articulations, the locations of muscle insertions, and the effect of nearby soft tissue (structure). Consider the following simple free body diagram, and its relation to a toe of the foot (Figure 3.4). In this model, the toe is modelled as a series of mass segments connected by hinge

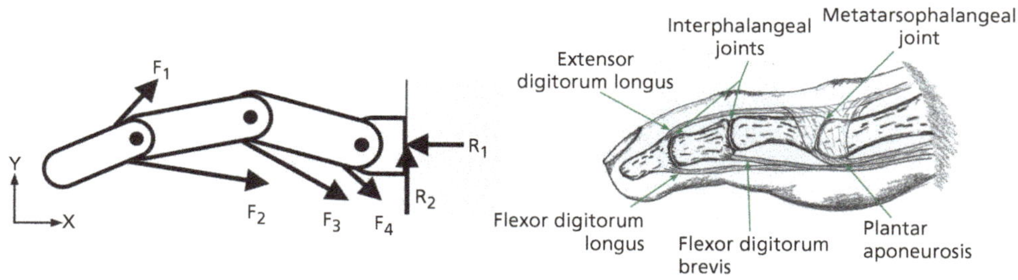

Figure 3.4 Representative free body diagram of a lesser toe with multiple linkages and external forces consisting of a combination of global X and Y components (left). Anatomical diagram of a lesser toe, showing the bony anatomy and several tendon insertions (right). Note the similarity between applied forces and tendon insertions. (No ligaments are shown in either diagram.)

joints with force applied at each segment. While a toe can potentially be described using such a simple model, the complete foot and ankle is much more complicated and would require a more sophisticated model to understand its function. Nevertheless, the concepts are the same—namely, that structure (e.g., tendon insertions [anatomy] and bone shape [morphology]) dictates function. For example, the structure of the subtalar joint encompasses the shapes and relative positions of the cartilage-covered articulating facets between the calcaneus and talus, while ligaments attach to and support these two bones, and tendons insert on or wrap around these bones; together, these aspects cause the subtalar joint to invert and evert. This level of complexity, and more, is present throughout human anatomy. All of these structural characteristics must be incorporated into the model if foot function (i.e., joint motion) is to be properly understood.

Principles of gait analysis

Introduction

Gait analysis is the quantification of the kinematics and kinetics of the lower extremity. One common purpose for gait analysis studies is to understand how pathological motion differs from normal motion, and to develop and evaluate various conservative and surgical treatment options. Perhaps the greatest challenge in gait analysis is attempting to understand bone motion and joint loads while being unable to directly measure either of these non-invasively. Instead, we track limb motion with skin-mounted markers, measure forces beneath the foot, and conduct an inverse dynamic analysis to estimate joint forces and moments.

Techniques for motion analysis

A detailed summary of the various motion analysis techniques is presented elsewhere in this book (see Chapter 11), so only a cursory, generalized review will be given here. The most widely used systems for motion capture employ optical, retro-reflective, marker-based techniques (Figure 3.5). The markers are then taped to the subject's skin both individually or in clusters to reduce extraneous marker motion. The markers are used to define body segments, such as the thigh, and create joint coordinate systems; anthropometric measurements are also commonly made to estimate inertial properties. To improve anatomical descriptions, static calibration trials are often collected with additional markers or apparatuses that are removed prior to dynamic trials. The subject then moves through a calibrated space while a set of synchronized cameras capture marker reflections in the visible, or commonly, infrared, spectrum. Often 10 or more

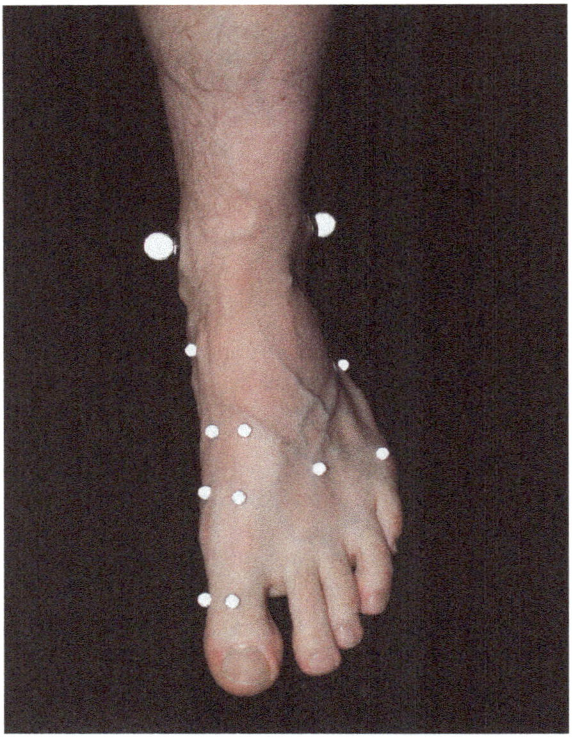

Figure 3.5 A left foot with kinematic markers placed on several bones. Given the small size and close proximity of the bones of the foot, it is not possible to attach three markers to each bone to create a coordinate system. (Note that markers on the foot are smaller to avoid blending together owing to their closeness during motion capture.)

cameras are used depending on the size of the space. Once data are collected, post-processing allows for marker identification in 3D space and filtering, rigid body tracking, transformations from global coordinate systems to anatomical coordinate systems, and, finally, joint kinematic and kinetic curves. A closely related technique involves using active LED-based markers in place of retro-reflective markers for easier marker identification.

The main limitation of motion capture systems is soft-tissue artifact (STA), defined as motion seen at the marker that is caused by the intervening soft tissues between the marker and the bone. STA has been quantified and addressed in a variety of ways, such as repeatability studies (1–3), estimating skin motion over anatomical landmarks (4, 5), and direct measurement of bone pin markers versus skin markers (6, 7). More advanced imaging modalities have also been used to analyse STA directly by measuring marker movements between static positions with magnetic resonance imaging (MRI) (8) and fluoroscopy (9), as well as determining the alignment of skin markers with respect to bony anatomy (10). A second limitation is that, owing to the small size and close proximity of the bones of the foot, it is often impossible to mount three markers on each bone to create a coordinate system for that bone. Hence, assumptions must be made and multiple bones are often grouped together as 'rigid' bodies.

In addition to traditional marker-based techniques, other methods do exist. Markerless motion capture allows for data collection without attaching anything to the body and without being constrained to a laboratory environment. This technique has demonstrated promising results (11), but it is less accurate than marker-based systems. Electromagnetic-based systems are both accurate and precise, and do not require a line of site as do optical marker systems. However, these systems typically have small ranges, are tethered, are affected by metal, and have large sensors that can also suffer from STA (12). Inertial measurement units (IMUs) can also be used for motion capture. IMUs have been shown to deviate from optical systems in the sagittal plane on the order of only 3° at the knee and 1° at the ankle (13). Finally, biplane fluoroscopy techniques have been used to obtain accurate and precise kinematic data for various joints of the lower extremity, including the knee (14–16) and the foot and ankle (17–19). More details of the use of this technique for the foot and ankle are provided below (see section on 'Specialized techniques for quantifying foot function').

Techniques for force and pressure analysis

Force plates are either strain gauge-based or piezoelectric-based platforms used to quantify the reaction forces between the foot and the ground. Typically, these devices have multiple sensors arrayed at various locations within the plate, and sensor readings are combined to calculate the vertical ground reaction force, the anterior/posterior, and medial/lateral shear forces (Figure 3.6). The free moment or the moment of the foot generated about an axis normal to the top surface of the force plate can also be measured using force plates. Strain gauge force plates are better suited for longer measurement protocols, while piezoelectric force plates are ideal for high-frequency applications.

In addition to measuring ground reaction forces, clinicians and researchers often wish to quantify the distribution of loads across the foot. Our discussion of load distributions will be limited to plantar pressure, as shear sensors are not commercially available and remain research-based. Pressure sensors either take the form of a platform (stepped on by the barefoot/shod subject) or an insole (worn within the shoe). Typically these sensors are capacitive- or resistive-based; the former are thicker and more stable over time, while the latter are thinner and require more frequent calibration. Parameters of interest include peak plantar pressure and the pressure–time integral (a measure of dosage) at specific locations beneath the foot. The center of pressure (CoP) and, in particular, the path that CoP takes relative to the plantar surface of the foot, is also a desirable output (Figure 3.7).

Other technologies and techniques

It is beyond the scope of the chapter to describe the following technologies in any great detail, but it is worth noting that, in addition to motion analysis and force/pressure analysis, there are also methodologies for quantifying muscle activity (using electromyography [EMG]), metabolic oxygen consumption, limb accelerations, total steps, as well as temporal (e.g., cadence) and spatial (e.g., step width) characteristics of gait. Treadmills and stair-climbers can be used to study multiple steps, and remote monitor systems can be used outside the laboratory environment. Additionally, X-ray systems, like biplane fluoroscopy, can be used to quantify foot bone motion to a high degree of accuracy (see section on 'Specialized techniques for quantifying foot function'). Further, while most gait analyses occur over three or four steps during straight, over ground walking, there are techniques for studying turning, ergonomic activities (e.g., scanning groceries), and/or sports-related activities (e.g., pitching a baseball).

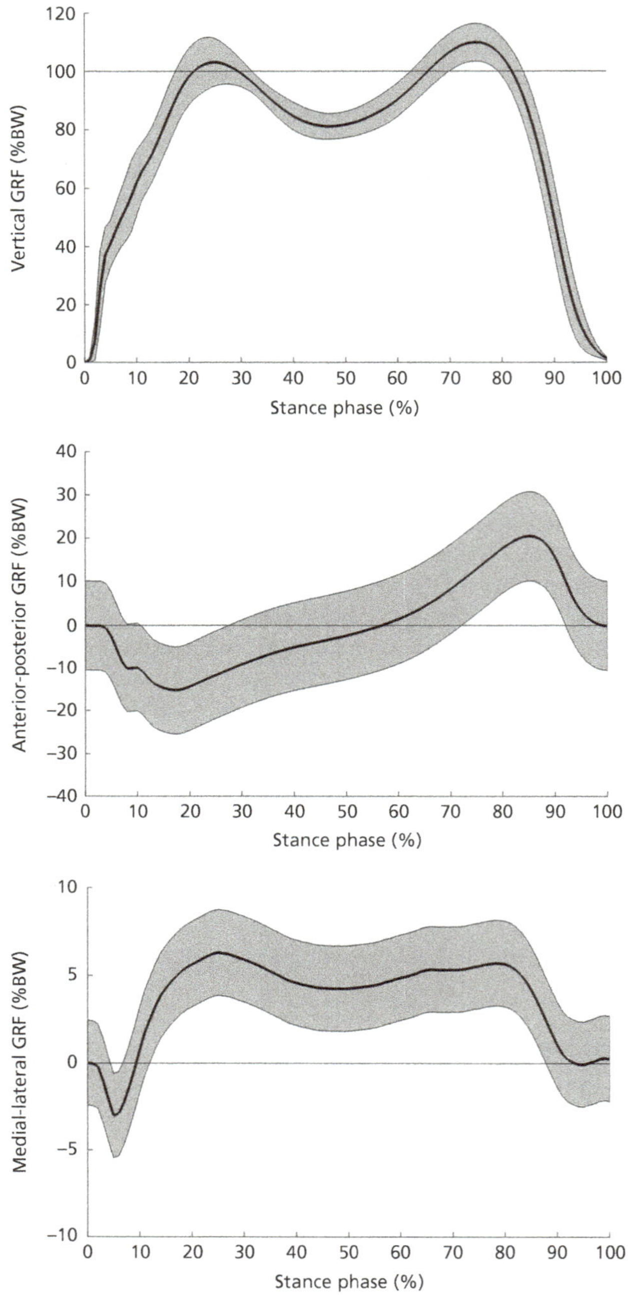

Figure 3.6 Vertical, anterior/posterior, and medial/lateral characteristic ground reaction force (GRF) curves for neutrally aligned feet (*n*=10). Curves are presented normalized by body weight (%BW). The abscissa is in units of stance phase, i.e., the duration over which the foot is in contact with the ground.

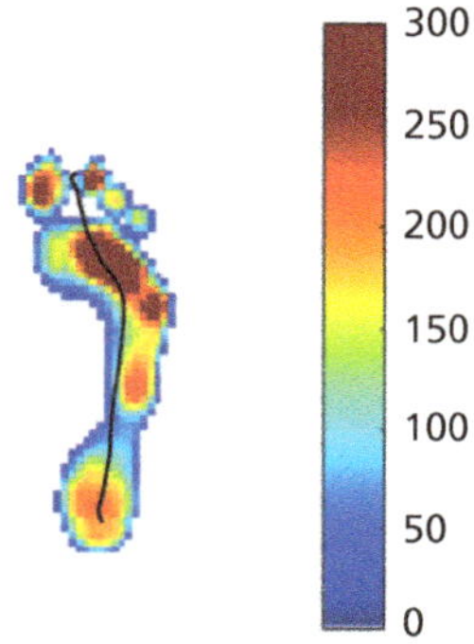

Figure 3.7 Peak plantar pressure distribution (kPa) and center of pressure (in black) progression for a neutrally aligned foot. Pressure (colored bar on right) is given in units of kilopascals (kPa).

Walking and the normal gait cycle

Introduction

The gait cycle is a dynamic interplay of events with purposes such as stability, propulsion, efficiency, and rhythm. During gait, the foot must engage the ground in a controlled fashion, accepting body weight, propelling the body forward, and, finally, recovering for the next step. The phases of the normal, double-support gait cycle are re-occurring, or periodic. At each phase, features such as timing, motion, muscular activation, ground reaction force, and center of pressure are similar from step to step.

Terminology and overview of the gait cycle

Multiple phases exist within a single gait cycle. The common terminology for these phases are (in chronological order): initial contact, loading response, mid-stance, terminal stance, pre-swing, initial swing, mid-swing, and terminal swing (20).

There are some distinct events within the gait cycle that relate to the foot's contact with the ground:

- *Heel-strike* occurs in the initial contact phase when the heel first contacts the ground.
- *Foot-flat* occurs during the loading response when the forefoot contacts the ground.
- *Heel-off* occurs in the terminal stance phase when the heel leaves the ground.
- *Toe-off* occurs during pre-swing when the toes leave the ground.

The gait cycle itself can be separated into two higher-level phases:

- *Stance* is the period between heel-strike and toe-off (the foot is in contact with the ground).
- *Swing* is the period between toe-off and that foot's next heel-strike (the foot is not in contact with the ground).

These various points in the gait cycle can be readily distinguished in a graph of the vertical ground reaction force (GRF), i.e., the force exerted onto the foot from the floor, over time (Figure 3.8). The GRF curve exhibits two local peaks within the stance period; this bimodal 'double hump' shape is a characteristic of normal walking. There is also often a distinct spike very early in stance—this is known as the heel-strike transient, but it is not present in either of our example plots (Figures 3.6 and 3.8).

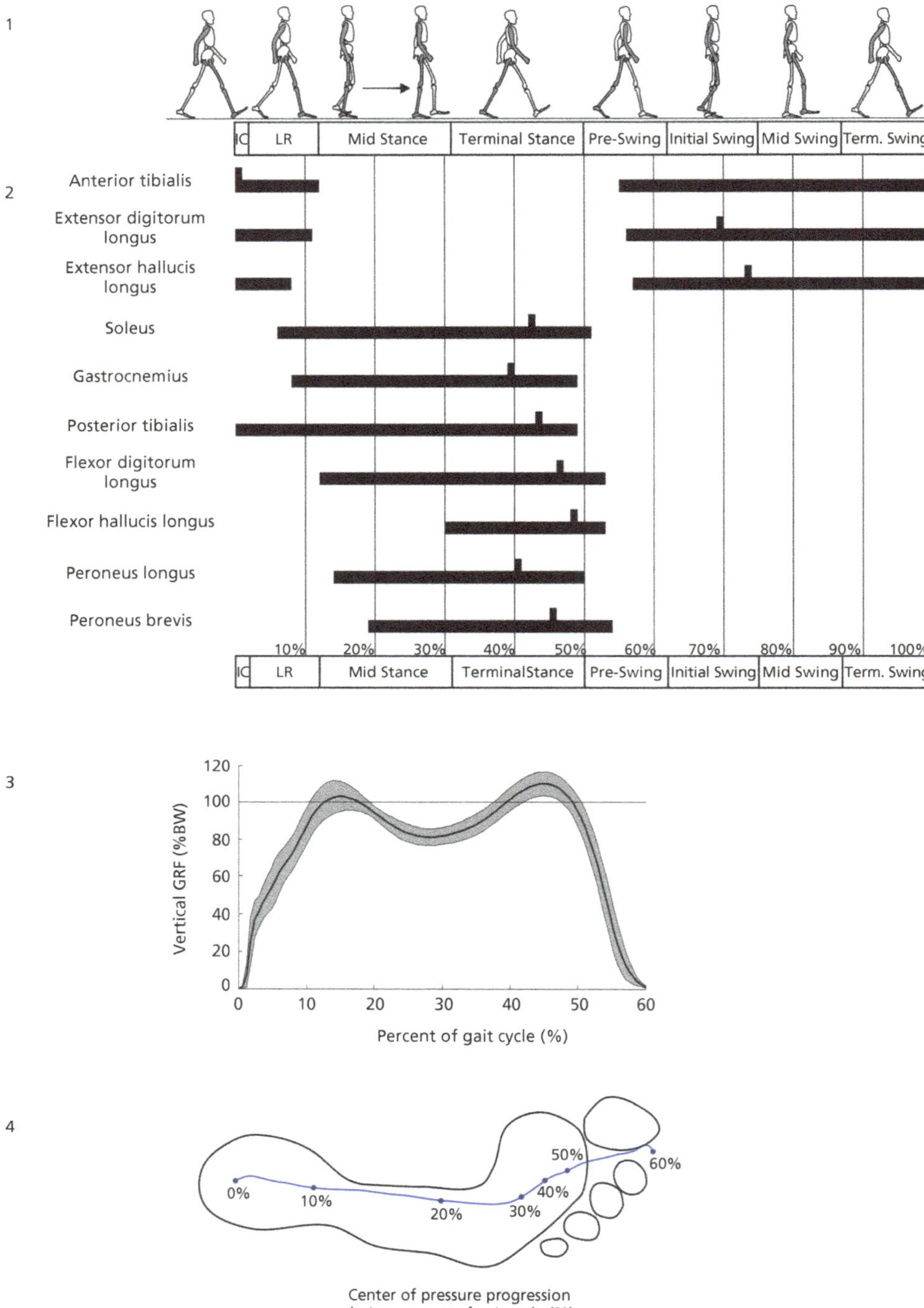

Figure 3.8 A vertical comparison of several concurrent aspects of gait, aligned by phase and 10% increment. Starting from top: (1) diagram of body position during each major phase of gait—nearest leg is the limb of interest; (2) major muscle on/off activation time during gait, notch in activation bar denotes peak muscle activity; (3) vertical ground reaction force (GRF) plot during the stance phase; (4) plantar footprint, with center of pressure trajectory. BW, Body weight; IC, initial contact; LR, loading response.

During the gait cycle there is a complex interplay of motion, muscular activity, and ground contact. Each phase has distinct features with variable complexity. The phases of gait, and the corresponding GRFs, muscle activations, and center of pressure (CoP) progression under the foot are shown in Figure 3.8.

The gait cycle, in depth

Initial contact

Duration: the first approximately 2% of the gait cycle (20).
Pose: the limb is straight and forward of the midline of the body, positioned to touch the ground with the heel. Body and opposite limb (still planted on the ground) trail behind.
Activity: the ankle dorsiflexors (tibialis anterior, extensor digitorum longus, and extensor hallucis longus) are firing and the plantarflexors (soleus, gastrocnemius, flexor digitorum longus, and flexor hallucis longus) are quiet (20, 21).
Ground contact: during this time, the heel makes forceful contact with the ground, generating a heel-strike transient in the GRF (~10% stance phase) (20, 22). The CoP under the foot is located at the heel (23).

Loading response

Duration: from approximately 2–12% of the gait cycle (20).
Pose: the heel is in contact with the ground and the ankle rotates to engage the forefoot with the ground (foot-flat). The body trails behind the foot and the opposing limb begins its swing phase.
Activity: the ankle dorsiflexors continue to fire to control the rotation of the ankle into foot-flat and prevent 'foot slap' (20, 21). Towards the end of the loading response, the plantarflexors activate.
Ground contact: the load on the limb increases during weight acceptance, peaking above body weight near the end of the loading response. With the foot flat and the plantarflexors firing, the CoP moves slightly anteriorly and laterally within the heel region (23).

Mid-stance

Duration: occurring during approximately 12–31% of the gait cycle (20).
Pose: the foot is flat and the tibia is rotating over the ankle joint. The body's center of mass passes from the heel forward into the forefoot. The opposing limb swings past.
Activity: the plantarflexors are firing but have not yet peaked (20, 21).
Ground contact: following weight acceptance, as the body's center of mass moves forward the load against the ground drops to slightly less than body weight. The CoP moves from the heel anteriorly and arcs slightly laterally through the midfoot before approaching the mid-sagittal plane as it nears the forefoot (23).

Terminal stance

Duration: occurring during approximately 31–50% of the gait cycle (20).
Pose: the heel rises from the ground. The body's center of mass has passed over the foot and the opposing limb is outstretched and preparing for initial contact.
Activity: the plantarflexors all reach peak activation during this phase; first the soleus and gastrocnemius and then the extensor digitorum longus/hallucis longus (20, 21).
Ground contact: the foot is now driving the body forward and upward, and thus the load applied to the ground rises again above body weight, creating the second peak characteristic of gait's bimodal shape. The CoP is located under the forefoot near the second metatarsal head (23).

Pre-swing

Duration: the final contact phase takes place during 50–62% of the gait cycle (20).
Pose: the forefoot and toes rise off the ground in this phase (toe-off), fully lifting the foot clear. Most of the body's mass is now in front of the limb and the opposing foot is in its loading response phase.
Activity: with the removal of the foot from the ground, the plantarflexors cease their activity, and concurrently the dorsiflexors re-engage to prevent the toes from dragging against the ground during swing (20, 21).
Ground contact: Limb load against the ground falls to zero as the CoP completes at the great toe (23).

Swing

Swing itself can be divided into three subphases (initial, mid, terminal) but, as the limb is unloaded in these phases, they are of less interest to this discussion and will be considered together for simplicity.
Duration: swing encompasses the final 38% of the gait cycle (20).
Pose: the lifted limb flexes slightly at the knee to clear the ground, with toes dorsiflexed. The limb is then flexed at the hip to pull it forward and past the planted opposing limb. The limb then straightens in preparation for initial contact.
Activity: the dorsiflexors are active continually during this period, with peaks both at the beginning to clear the ground and at the end of swing. Other notable activities include knee and hip flexion for advancement of the limb and for stability (20).
Ground contact: none.

Ankle cartilage and the gait cycle

The aim of this chapter is to inform the reader about the behavior of the foot and ankle, and the role of the cartilage in normal and pathological function. This requires an understanding of the biomechanics of the ankle during gait. As mentioned in the introduction part of the section on 'Principles of gait analysis', gait analysis has the inherent difficulty of being unable to measure bone motion and joint loads directly. This problem is compounded at the ankle, as the depth of the talus causes difficulty with placing skin-based markers near it. Despite an inability to measure ankle cartilage behaviour using non-invasive methods, there are research efforts being made to measure and model the function of the ankle joint. Consider the following two studies, both of which specifically focus on ankle joint cartilage during gait. These studies represent novel methods of inferring the environment to which ankle cartilage is exposed by using cutting edge techniques in simulation, image segmentation, and image registration.

Study 1: articular contact stress–computational simulation

Finite element (FE) analysis has been used to evaluate patient-specific intra-articular contact (24). This study modelled patient-specific ankle joint geometry using computed tomography (CT) scans, with surfaces extruded to represent cartilage. Each model underwent a series of static loading conditions, which represented 13 successive tibiotalar poses and axial load scenarios present during gait. The major findings were that controls exhibited a more uniform distribution of cartilage load, with peak stresses between 9 and 14 MPa. Patients with incongruous tibial plafond fractures were found to have more varied focal stress distributions, with stress magnitudes peaking at 18 MPa. The authors acknowledged a number of limitations to this work; however, their use of patient-specific models and gait phase simulations yielded a methodology to evaluate relative differences in anatomy during a simulated dynamic activity (Figure 3.9).

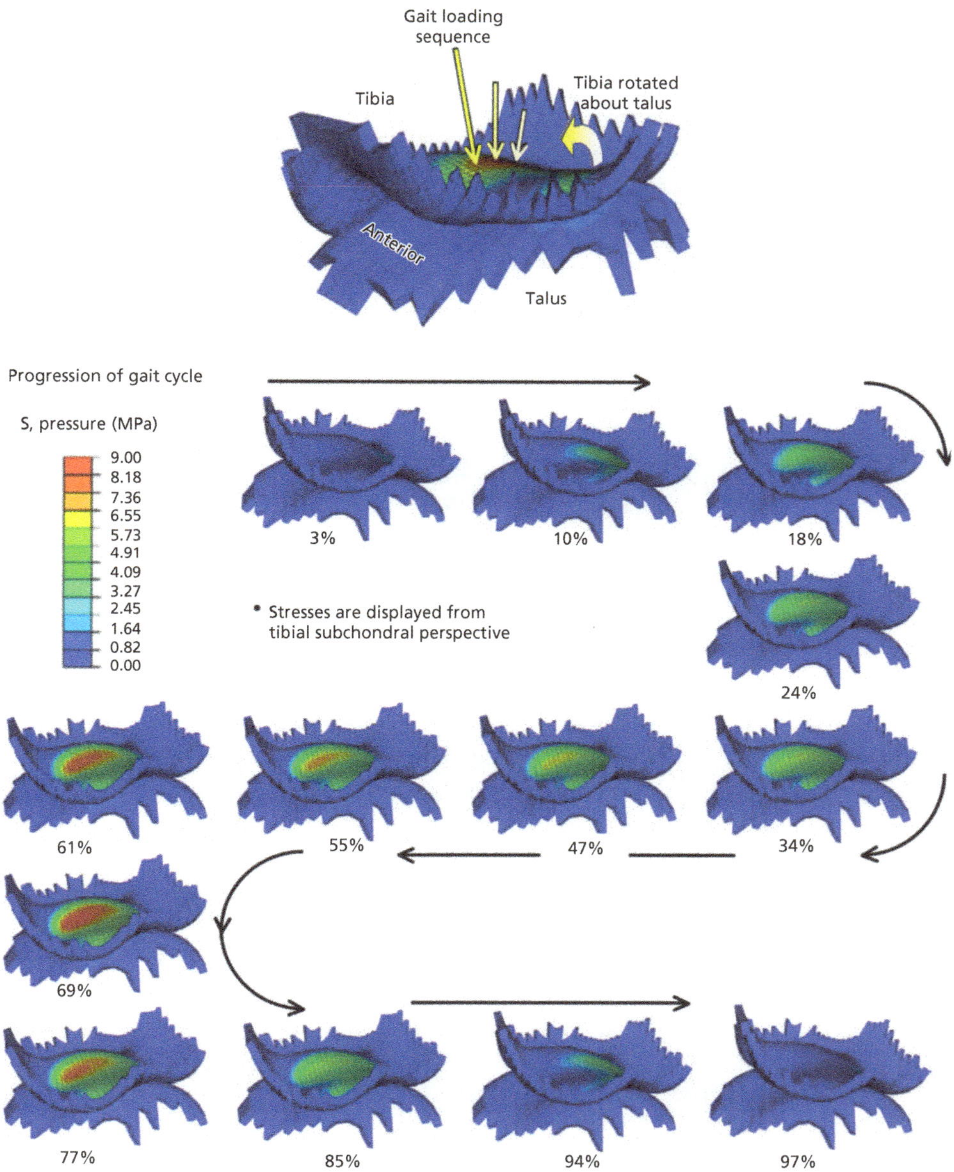

Figure 3.9 Tibial articular contact stresses during a simulated stance phase of gait. Simulation of the stance phase involved solving the sequence of 13 successive loading increments displayed (axial loads ranged from 10 to 2800 N, applied tibial flexions ranged from 5° plantarflexion to 9° dorsiflexion). Each increment/solution is labelled based on its percentage of the stance phase progression. *Note:* since the talus is free to rotate, except about the flexion–extension axis, ankle rotation is not about a fixed axis.

Adapted from 'Intra-articular Contact Stress Distributions at the Ankle throughout Stance Phase – Patient-Specific Finite Element Analysis as a Metric of Degeneration Propensity' by D.D. Anderson, 2006, *Biomech Model Mechanobiol*, **5**(2–3): pp. 82–89. Copyright 2006 by Springer International Publishing AG, with permission from Springer Verlag.

Study 2: articular contact area–dynamic in vivo imaging

Ankle cartilage contact has also been measured from in vivo poses of gait phases using an X-ray method (25). Subjects assumed static poses representing heel-strike, mid-stance, and toe-off while being imaged in a dual X-ray system. Cartilage contact was determined by evaluating the overlap between modelled subject cartilage (obtained with MR) during the phasic poses. This method allowed the researchers to map the areas of contact on both the tibial and talar articular surfaces of the ankle (Figure 3.10). The cartilage coverage area was averaged for nine ankles. Cartilage area was 964.9 ± 156.1 mm^2 on the distal tibia and 1304.8 ± 208.4 mm^2 on the proximal talus. The cartilage contact between both sides of the talocrural joint averaged 272.7 ± 61.1 mm^2 at heel-strike, 416.8 ± 51.7 mm^2 at mid-stance, and 335.7 ± 64.5 mm^2 at toe-off. While this study also had limitations, the methods described are a novel and promising approach to measuring in vivo cartilage contact (26). This group is currently working toward methods to measure deformity and strain in the cartilage.

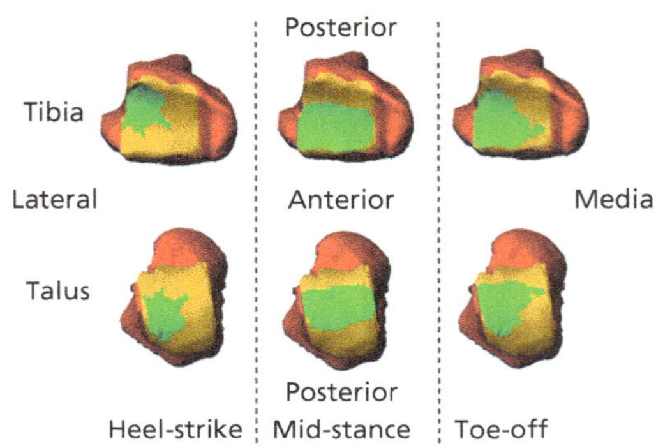

Figure 3.10 In vivo cartilage contact patterns of a left foot during the simulated stance phase of walking for a typical talocrural joint. Red denotes non-articulating bone surfaces, yellow denotes the talocrural articular surfaces, and green denotes the portion of the talocrural articular surfaces that are in contact during each phase of gait.

Adapted from 'Determination of in-vivo articular cartilage contact areas of human talocrural joint under weightbearing conditions' by L. Wan, 2006, *OsteoArthritis and Cartilage* **14**: pp. 1294–1301. Copyright 2006 by the Osteoarthritis Research Society International. Adapted with permission from Elsevier.

Normal movement and function of the foot

Introduction

Foot function can be considered at the tissue, joint, or systematic level.

Tissue-specific function

Bones

The 28 bones in the foot form the rigid structure that supports the other tissues. As evidenced by the internal structure of the foot bones (i.e., the trabecular pattern), compressive forces are borne from the tibia, through the talus, and into both the calcaneus and the forefoot. The morphology of the foot bones also dictates the basic function of the joints of the foot, as discussed below.

Muscles

We will limit the discussion here to the 20 intrinsic muscles of the foot, which are organized into a dorsal layer and four plantar layers. As with skeletal muscle elsewhere in the body, these muscles apply tensile forces only. The primary functions of the intrinsic muscles are to stabilize the arch of the foot during loading and to control the motion of the toes.

Tendons

There are 11 extrinsic muscle tendons in each foot from 12 extrinsic muscles—the Achilles' tendon is the combined insertion of the soleus and gastrocnemius. The Achilles' tendon applies the propulsive force during each step required for locomotion. Other major tendon functions include the tibialis anterior, which applies a force early in stance to prevent foot slap, the tibialis posterior, which is the primary dynamic stabilizer of the medial arch of the foot and maintains heel position during plantarflexion, while the flexor hallucis longus wraps around the talus providing posterior support to a bone without tendinous insertions.

Ligaments

The over 100 ligaments in the foot have a wide range of functions. The lateral collateral ankle ligaments help prevent the ankle and subtalar joints from moving beyond their normal range of motion and are often injured during inversion sprains. Interosseous ligaments, such as the interosseous talocalcaneal ligament, tightly connect adjacent surfaces of bones. One specialized ligament, called the spring or plantar calcaneonavicular ligament, has two components, the superomedial and the inferior, that support the head of the talus on the medial and plantar aspects. The long plantar ligament and the plantar aponeurosis, which is technically a ligament, are also both key structures in maintaining arch height.

Cartilage

The joints of the foot are synovial (cartilaginous); thus every osseous contact surface is covered in hyaline cartilage. The cartilage serves to reduce friction at the joints and to distribute loads across surfaces.

Other tissue

Another important tissue in the foot is plantar fat, which absorbs shock and distributes load with each step. Several retinacula serve to hold the extrinsic tendons against the foot and prevent the tendons from bowing out. Tendon sheaths allow various tendons to glide with little friction. Finally, skin is thick on parts of the plantar surface and serves to cover, support, and protect all other tissues in the foot.

Joint functions

Talocrural

As there are over 55 joints in the foot, only some of the major ones will be discussed here. The talocrural, or ankle, joint is the articulation between the tibia, fibula, and talus. The primary axis of rotation is in the sagittal plane (i.e., dorsiflexion and plantarflexion), but the axis is, on average, inverted 18° in the coronal plane and externally rotated 16° in the transverse plane (Figure 3.11) (27). The primary function of the ankle joint is to allow the body to rotate over the fixed foot during locomotion. A secondary function is to maintain sagittal plane position during quiet stance. Since the talus is wider anteriorly than it is posteriorly, this joint is more stable in dorsiflexion as the talus becomes firmly wedged into the tibial plafond.

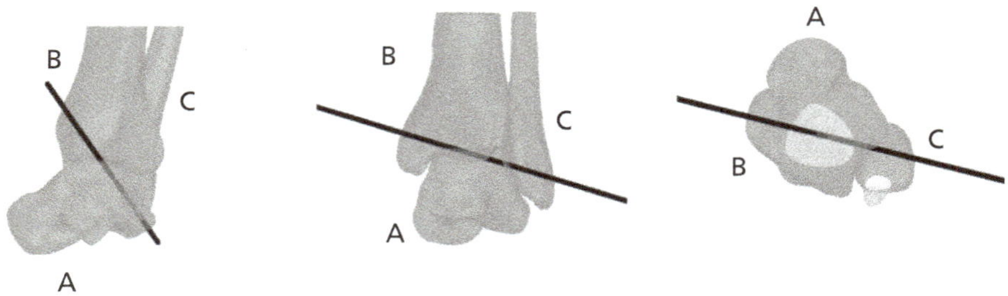

Figure 3.11 The axis of rotation of the talocrural joint of a right foot in the sagittal plane, medial view (left), coronal plane, posterior view (middle), and transverse plane, superior view (right). A, talus; B, tibia; C, fibula.

Talocalcaneal

The talocalcaneal, or subtalar, joint is the articulation between the talus and the calcaneus. The axis of rotation is, on average, dorsiflexed 43° in the sagittal plane and externally rotated 21° in the transverse plane (Figure 3.12) (27). The posterior, middle, and anterior facets guide the relative motion of these bones.

Talonavicular

The talonavicular joint, which shares a common joint capsule with the middle and anterior facets of the subtalar joint, has a similar axis of rotation as the talocalcaneal joint; that is, dorsiflexed 35° on average in the sagittal plane and externally rotated 10° in the transverse plane (Figure 3.13) (27). Together, these two joints function such that the mostly sagittal plane motion of the ankle joint becomes a triplanar motion within the foot itself. This motion ranges from plantarflexion, inversion, and internal rotation to dorsiflexion, eversion, and external rotation.

Other joints

The calcaneocuboid joint is saddle-shaped. Together with the talonavicular joint, it is often called the midtarsal or Chopart's joint. Progressing anteriorly, the joints between the cuneiforms and cuboid proximally and the metatarsals distally (i.e., between the midfoot and forefoot) are collectively known as the tarsometatarsal or Lisfranc's joint. The midtarsal and tarsometatarsal joints give the foot great flexibility and allow the foot to adapt to uneven terrain. Finally, the first metatarsophalangeal joint, or great toe joint, is the articulation between the first metatarsal and hallux. This joint can have up to 90° of range of motion in healthy subjects, but is also one of the most frequent joints to develop osteoarthritis (28).

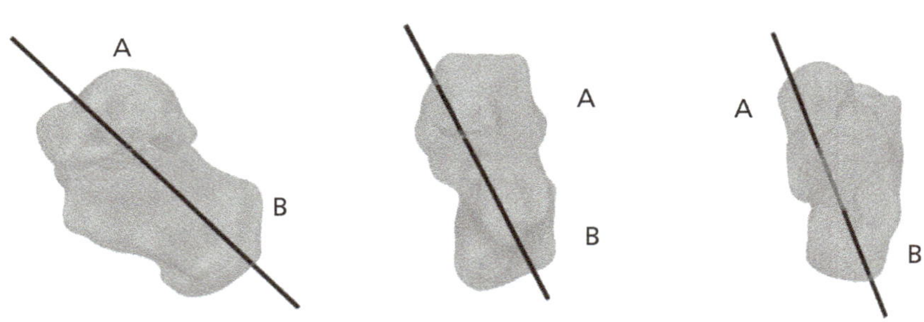

Figure 3.12 The axis of rotation of the talocalcaneal joint of a right foot in the sagittal plane, medial view (left), coronal plane, posterior view (middle), and transverse plane, superior view (right). A, talus; B, tibia.

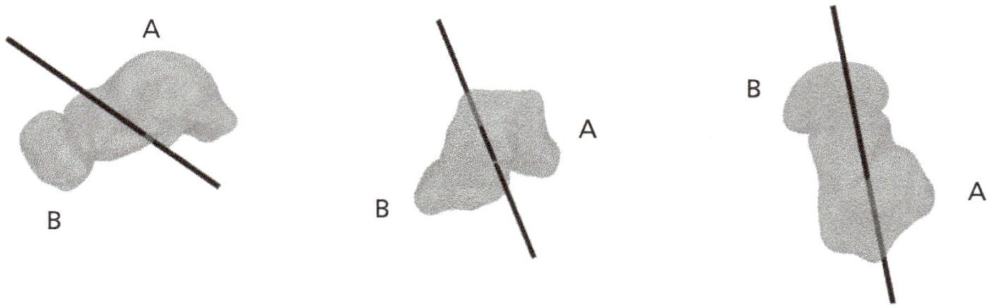

Figure 3.13 The axis of rotation of the talonavicular joint of a right foot in the sagittal plane, medial view (left), coronal plane, posterior view (middle), and transverse plane, superior view (right) planes. A, talus; B, navicular.

More complex functions

Foot type

Foot morphology exists along a continuum, but can, for the most part, be categorized as high-arched (pes cavus), neutrally aligned, or flat (pes planus). As noted above, cavus feet tend to have an adducted forefoot, a high arch, and an inverted hindfoot, while planus feet tend to have an abducted forefoot, a low arch, and an everted hindfoot. Pes planus is the most common foot condition, affecting patients of all ages in the USA (29, 30). Pes cavus is often seen in patients with neurological disorders, and may be congenital.

During each step, the loading path or CoP has a characteristic shape relative to the plantar surface of the foot (Figure 3.14) and differs by foot type. For heel-strikers (as opposed to midfoot or forefoot strikers), the CoP typically progresses monotonically from posterior to anterior. For neutral feet, after heel-strike the CoP moves laterally, before shifting medially later in stance. Compared to neutrally aligned feet, the CoP of cavus subjects is, in general, more lateral, while the CoP of planus subjects is more medial, often not inverting at all.

Windlass mechanism

The windlass mechanism relates to the effect of passive toe extension on arch height and foot length (31). When the first metatarsophalangeal joint is extended, the plantar aponeurosis, which has fibers that extend to the hallux, is tightened. This is turn applies an anteriorly directed force to the calcaneus via the plantar aponeurosis insertion. The applied force leads to a decrease in foot length and an increase in arch height (32). This mechanism can be observed

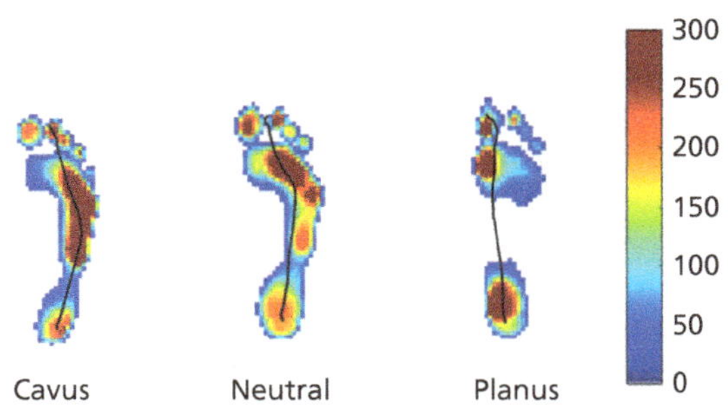

Figure 3.14 Peak plantar pressure distribution (kPa) and center of pressure (in black) progression for a cavus (left), neutrally aligned (middle), and planus (right) foot. Pressure (colored bar on right) is given in units of kilopascals (kPa).

by extending one's great toe while resting the foot against the ground to see the arch of the foot become more pronounced. Functionally, this occurs during late stance during every step, when maximum great toe joint dorsiflexion occurs. This mechanism helps to preserve the foot arch during toe-off.

Midtarsal joint 'locking' mechanism

One of the unique functions of the foot and ankle is that they can both adapt to uneven terrain during weight acceptance and also serve as a rigid lever for propulsion during push-off. In other words, the foot changes from a flexible to stiff platform and then back again in less than a second with each step. This capability has been attributed to the function of the midtarsal joint, which consists of the calcaneocuboid and talonavicular joints. The proposed theory states that the primary axes of rotation of the two joints are well aligned when the hindfoot is everted, and become more skewed when the hindfoot is inverted (33), leading to the so-called midtarsal joint 'locking' and a more stiff foot at push-off. More recently, a cadaveric study provided indirect support of the theory by determining that the range of motion of the forefoot in the sagittal plane was significantly greater when the calcaneus was maximally everted than when the calcaneus was maximally inverted (34). However, this study did not determine the specific process by which the foot became stiffer. Finally, direct exploration of this mechanism was achieved using dynamic cadaveric gait simulation to determine quantitative joint axes of rotation (35). Contrary to the proposed theory, this study demonstrated that, while the midtarsal joint everted early in stance and inverted late in stance, there was still continuous motion at the joints, i.e., the midtarsal joint was not 'locked'. The study's authors speculated that muscular forces play a larger role in stiffening the foot than previously thought.

Specialized techniques for quantifying foot function

Because the foot has many small, intricately-shaped bones, it is impossible for traditional motion analysis techniques to track individual foot bone motion. Hence researchers often lump the foot bones into groups, thus modelling the foot as three or four segments (36). This limits the ability to study the effects of clinical treatments (e.g., ankle arthrodesis) on individual foot joints. Alternative approaches include the insertion of radio-opaque beads (37) or bone pins with retro-reflective markers (38); both of these are very accurate but also highly invasive. Owing to these limitations, these approaches will likely never progress beyond research-based techniques into standard clinical care.

Biplane fluoroscopy

One technique that has shown increasing promise is biplane fluoroscopy, whereby dual X-ray sources, in combination with a 3D representation of the subject's foot anatomy (derived from CT or MR imaging), are used to track foot bone motion. Dual C-arms have been used to study ankle motion (17, 18, 25, 39); however, the set-up of the two C-arms required non-ideal data collection as subjects were not able to walk unfettered through the field of view, as the C-arms constrained the available travel of the subjects. One group has conducted preliminary validation of a custom biplane system for the foot and ankle (40), but full gait data have yet to be reported (Figure 3.15). Others have developed specialized walkways to allow for oblique imaging of the hindfoot, but limitations on camera sampling frequency have limited the study from 9% to 86% of stance (41). More recently, the accuracy and feasibility of a biplane split belt treadmill system was explored and interesting results for the ankle and subtalar joint were collected (42). Using biplane fluoroscopy to study foot bone kinematics is an area of future foot and ankle research.

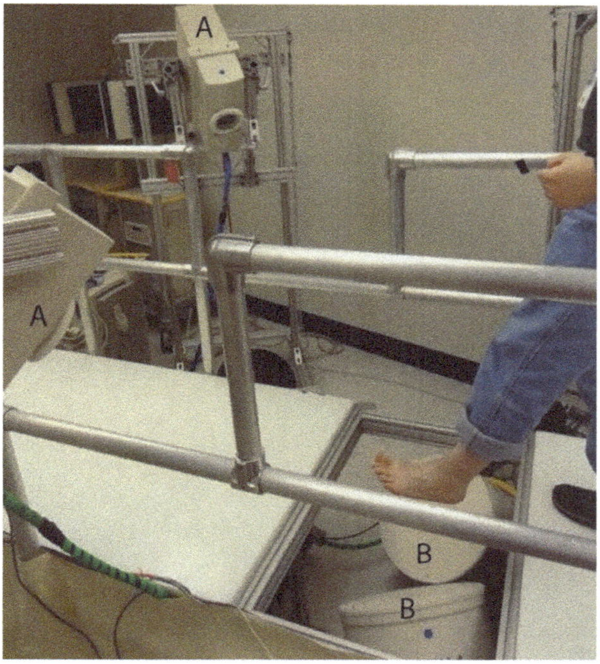

Figure 3.15 A custom biplane system based on two BV Pulsera C-arms disarticulated and mounted to adjustable posts. Stock cameras have been replaced with high-speed (1000 Hz) cameras and synchronized. The two X-ray sources are on the upper left (A and A), while the two image intensifiers are on the lower right (B and B). The carbon fiber flooring has been removed for illustrative purposes.

Cadaveric gait simulation

Lower limb dynamic cadaveric gait simulators are a useful alternative to investigate the biomechanics of the foot and ankle. The first such simulator was developed by Sharkey et al. (43) and has been used to address many clinical questions related to the lower extremity, including metatarsal strain (44), ankle kinematics after malleolar fracture (45), normal foot kinematics (46, 47), flexor hallucis function (48, 49), and multi-segment foot model evaluation (7). Several other research groups have developed cadaveric gait simulators of varying degrees of complexity (50–58). One system in particular, the robotic gait simulator (RGS), developed at the VA Puget Sound Health Care System and the University of Washington, utilizes a 6-degrees of freedom parallel robot to recreate the relative tibia-to-ground motion (Figure 3.16). The RGS has been used to study prosthetic feet (59), flat feet (60), surgical correction of flat feet (61), the effect of great toe fusion angle (62), the effect of a long second metatarsal (63), surgical treatment for a long second metatarsal (64), and foot bone kinematics (65).

Computational models

Computational models of the foot and ankle have shown promise for studying foot function. They are especially useful when studying parameters that cannot be readily measured, such as

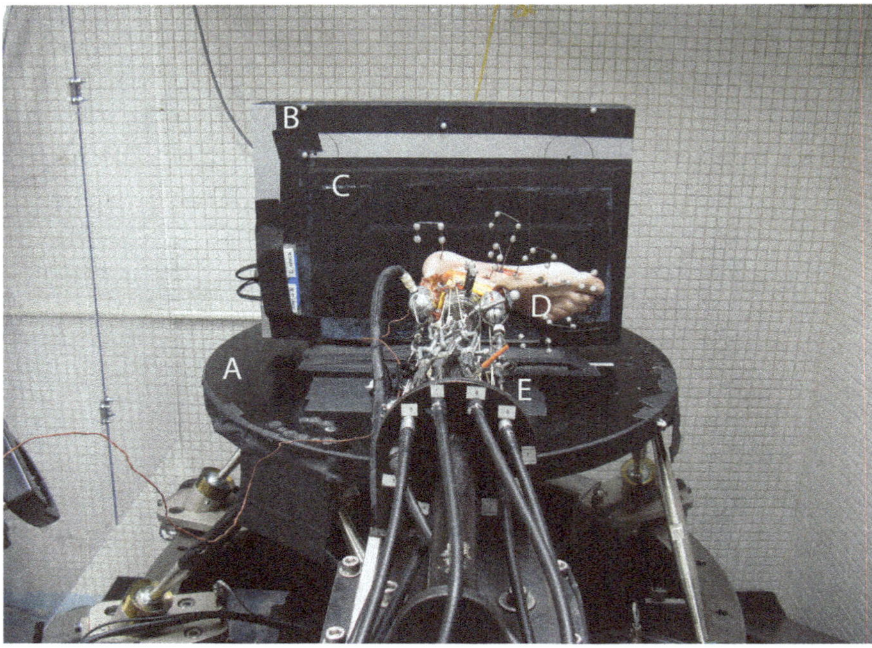

Figure 3.16 The robotic gait simulator, consisting of the hexapod robot (A) with a force plate (B) and pressure mat (C) mounted to the top plate. The force plate is the 'ground' that moves relative to a fixed tibia of the cadaver foot (D) while muscle forces are applied via tendon clamps (E) and actuators (not shown). Foot model kinematics are tracked with a motion capture system using retro-reflective markers.

muscle activation patterns or internal stresses. However, in general, these models are limited by either the lack of anatomical detail (e.g., limited degrees of freedom in the foot musculoskeletal models [66]) or, conversely, by the model's complexity (e.g., patient-specific, anatomically detailed FE models are difficult to validate [67]). One of the most comprehensive efforts on FE foot modelling is the work of Cheung et al., who have modelled the effects of plantar fascia release (68, 69), insole design (70, 71), stiff plantar soft tissue (72), Achilles' tendon loading (73), sock friction (74), and high heels (75). Cavanagh et al. have made extensive progress on their FE foot modelling efforts, including a second metatarsal model to explore the effect of insole and tissue thickness on plantar pressure (76), an inverse FE model to determine the material properties of the plantar soft tissue (77), a parametric analysis on insole conformity, thickness, and material (78), a first ray model to explore hallux limitus and hallux varus (79), a multi-layer inverse FE forefoot model (80), and a simplified patient-specific model for improved orthotic prescription (81). Recently, Ledoux et al. have generated patient-specific material properties from MRI scans (82, 83) that can be incorporated into patient-specific FE models and used to predict internal tissue stresses (Figure 3.17) (67).

Conclusion

This chapter has reviewed several concepts related to normal foot function and movement. First, by way of an introduction, basic mechanics were reviewed, as were the anatomical planes and motions. Next, gait analysis, including the techniques for motion analysis, and for force and pressure

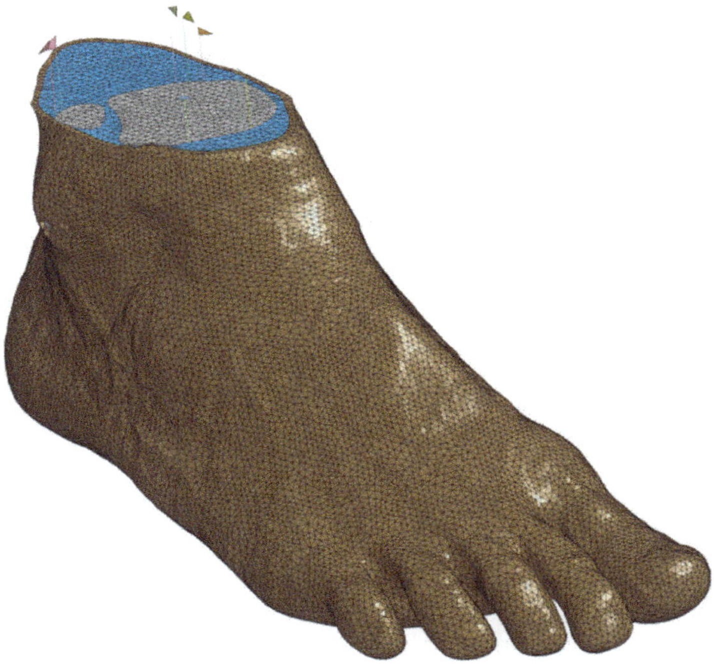

Figure 3.17 A finite element model of the foot and ankle, including bones, ligaments, tendons, muscle, plantar fat, and skin.

analyses, were reviewed. A detailed overview of the gait cycle was then presented, followed by a review of normal movement and foot function.

Acknowledgements

The authors would like to acknowledge the editorial contributions of Christina Stender and Matthew Kindig. Additionally, Matthew Kindig and Eric Thorhauer generated several of the figures.

References

1. **Wright CJ, Arnold BL, Coffey TG, Pidcoe PE.** Repeatability of the modified Oxford foot model during gait in healthy adults. *Gait Posture*. 2011;**33**:108–12.
2. **Peters A, Sangeux M, Morris ME, Baker R.** Determination of the optimal locations of surface-mounted markers on the tibial segment. *Gait Posture*. 2009;**29**:42–8.
3. **Caravaggi, P, Benedetti MG, Berti L, Leardini A.** Repeatability of a multi-segment foot protocol in adult subjects. *Gait Posture*. 2011;**33**:133–5.
4. **Cappello A, Stagni R, Fantozzi S, Leardini A.** Soft tissue artifact compensation in knee kinematics by double anatomical landmark calibration. performance of a novel method during selected motor tasks. *IEEE Trans Biomed Eng*. 2005;**52**:992–8.
5. **Tranberg R, Karlsson D.** The relative skin movement of the foot: a 2-D roentgen photogrammetry study. *Clin Biomech (Bristol, Avon)*. 1998;**13**:71–6.
6. **Nester C, Jones RK, Liu A, et al.** Foot kinematics during walking measured using bone and surface mounted markers. *J Biomech*. 2007;**40**:3412–23.

7. **Okita N, Meyers SA, Challis JH, Sharkey NA.** An objective evaluation of a segmented foot model. *Gait Posture.* 2009;**30**:27–34.
8. **Sangeux M, Marin F, Charleux F, Durselen L, Ho Ba Tho MC.** Quantification of the 3D relative movement of external marker sets vs. bones based on magnetic resonance imaging. *Clin Biomech (Bristol, Avon).* 2006;**21**:984–91.
9. **Shultz R, Kedgley AE, Jenkyn TR.** Quantifying skin motion artifact error of the hindfoot and forefoot marker clusters with the optical tracking of a multi-segment foot model using single-plane fluoroscopy. *Gait Posture.* 2011;**34**:44–8.
10. **Long JT, Wang M, Winters JM, Harris GF.** A multisegmental foot model with bone-based referencing: sensitivity to radiographic input parameters. *Conf Proc IEEE Eng Med Biol Soc.* 2008;**2008**:879–82.
11. **Mundermann L, Corazza S, Andriacchi TP.** The evolution of methods for the capture of human movement leading to markerless motion capture for biomechanical applications. *J Neuroeng Rehabil.* 2006;**3**:6.
12. **Audenaert EA, Vigneron L, Van Hoof T, et al.** In vitro validation and reliability study of electromagnetic skin sensors for evaluation of end range of motion positions of the hip. *Med Biol Eng Comput.* 2011;**49**:1405–12.
13. **Seel T, Raisch J, Schauer T.** IMU-based joint angle measurement for gait analysis. *Sensors (Basel).* 2014;**14**:6891–909.
14. **Bey MJ, Kline SK, Tashman S, Zauel R.** Accuracy of biplane x-ray imaging combined with model-based tracking for measuring in-vivo patellofemoral joint motion. *J Orthop Surg.* 2008;**3**:38.
15. **Giphart JE, Zirker CA, Myers CA, Pennington WW, LaPrade RF.** Accuracy of a contour-based biplane fluoroscopy technique for tracking knee joint kinematics of different speeds. *J Biomech.* 2012;**45**:2935–8.
16. **Anderst W, Zauel R, Bishop J, Demps E, Tashman S.** Validation of three-dimensional model-based tibio-femoral tracking during running. *Med Eng Phys.* 2009;**31**:10–16.
17. **de Asla RJ, Wan L, Rubash HE, Li G.** Six DOF in vivo kinematics of the ankle joint complex. Application of a combined dual-orthogonal fluoroscopic and magnetic resonance imaging technique. *J Orthop Res.* 2006;**24**:1019–27.
18. **Caputo AM, Lee JY, Spritzer CE, et al.** In vivo kinematics of the tibiotalar joint after lateral ankle instability. *Am J Sports Med.* 2009;**37**:2241–8.
19. **Peltz CD, Haladik JA, Hoffman SE, et al.** Effects of footwear on three-dimensional tibiotalar and subtalar joint motion during running. *J Biomech.* 2014;**47**:2647–53.
20. **Perry J.** *Gait analysis. Normal and Pathological Function*, 2nd edn. Thorofare, NJ: SLACK Incorporated, 2010.
21. **Liu MQ, Anderson FC, Schwartz MH, Delp SL.** Muscle contributions to support and progression over a range of walking speeds. *J Biomech.* 2008;**41**:3243–52.
22. **Verdini F, Marcucci M, Benedetti MG, Leo T.** Identification and characterisation of heel strike transient. *Gait Posture.* 2006;**24**:77–84.
23. **Chiu MC, Wu HC, Chang LY.** Gait speed and gender effects on center of pressure progression during normal walking. *Gait Posture.* 2013;**37**:43–8.
24. **Anderson DD, Goldsworthy JK, Shivanna K, et al.** Intra-articular contact stress distributions at the ankle throughout stance phase-patient-specific finite element analysis as a metric of degeneration propensity. *Biomech Model Mechanobiol.* 2006;**5**:82–9.
25. **Li G, Wan L, Kozanek M.** Determination of real-time in-vivo cartilage contact deformation in the ankle joint. *J Biomech.* 2008;**41**:128–36.
26. **Wan L, de Asla RJ, Rubash HE, Li G.** Determination of in-vivo articular cartilage contact areas of human talocrural joint under weightbearing conditions. *Osteoarthritis Cartilage.* 2006;**14**:1294–301.
27. **Fassbind MJ, Rohr ES, Hu Y, et al.** Evaluating foot kinematics using magnetic resonance imaging: from maximum plantar flexion, inversion, and internal rotation to maximum dorsiflexion, eversion, and external rotation. *J Biomech Eng.* 2011;**133**:104502.

28. **van Saase JL, Vandenbroucke JP, van Romunde LK, Valkenburg HA.** Osteoarthritis and obesity in the general population. A relationship calling for an explanation. *J Rheumatol.* 1988;**15**:1152–8.
29. **Gould N, Schneider W, Ashikaga T.** Epidemiological survey of foot problems in the continental United States: 1978–1979. *Foot Ankle.* 1980;**1**:8–10.
30. **Ledoux WR, Shofer JB, Ahroni JH, Smith DG, Sangeorzan BJ, Boyko EJ.** Biomechanical differences among pes cavus, neutrally aligned, and pes planus feet in subjects with diabetes. *Foot Ankle Int.* 2003;**24**:845–50.
31. **Hicks JH.** The mechanics of the foot II. The plantar aponeurosis and the arch. *J Anat.* 1954;**88**:25–31.
32. **Stolwijk NM, Koenraadt KL, Louwerens JW, Grim D, Duysens J, Keijsers NL.** Foot lengthening and shortening during gait: a parameter to investigate foot function? *Gait Posture.* 2014;**39**:773–7.
33. **Elftman H.** The transverse tarsal joint and its control. *Clin Orthop.* 1960;**16**:41–5.
34. **Blackwood CB, Yuen TJ, Sangeorzan BJ, Ledoux WR.** The midtarsal joint locking mechanism. *Foot Ankle Int.* 2005;**26**:1074–80.
35. **Okita N, Meyers SA, Challis JH, Sharkey NA.** Midtarsal joint locking. New perspectives on an old paradigm. *Journal of Orthopaedic Research. Official Publication of the Orthopaedic Research Society.* 2013;**32**(1):110–15.
36. **Leardini A, Benedetti MG, Berti L, Bettinelli D, Nativo R, Giannini S.** Rear-foot, mid-foot and fore-foot motion during the stance phase of gait. *Gait & Posture.* 2007;**25**:453–62.
37. **Lundberg A.** Kinematics of the ankle and foot. In vivo roentgen stereophotogrammetry. *Acta Orthop Scand Suppl.* 1989;**233**:1–24.
38. **Lundgren P, Nester C, Liu A, et al.** Invasive in vivo measurement of rear-, mid- and forefoot motion during walking. *Gait Posture.* 2008;**28**:93–100.
39. **Wan L, de Asla RJ, Rubash HE, Li G.** In vivo cartilage contact deformation of human ankle joints under full body weight. *J Orthop Res.* 2008;**26**:1081–9.
40. **Iaquinto JM, Tsai R, Haynor DR, Fassbind MJ, Sangeorzan BJ, Ledoux WR.** Marker-based validation of a biplane fluoroscopy system for quantifying foot kinematics. *Med Eng Phys.* 2014;**36**:391–6.
41. **Koo S, Lee KM, Cha YJ.** Plantar-flexion of the ankle joint complex in terminal stance is initiated by subtalar plantar-flexion. A bi-planar fluoroscopy study. *Gait Posture.* 2015;**42**:424–9.
42. **Wang B, Roach KE, Kapron AL, et al.** Accuracy and feasibility of high-speed dual fluoroscopy and model-based tracking to measure in vivo ankle arthrokinematics. *Gait Posture.* 2015;**41**:888–93.
43. **Sharkey NA, Hamel AJ.** A dynamic cadaver model of the stance phase of gait: performance characteristics and kinetic validation. *Clin Biomech (Bristol, Avon).* 1998;**13**:420–33.
44. **Donahue SW, Sharkey NA.** Strains in the metatarsals during the stance phase of gait. Implications for stress fractures. *J Bone Joint Surg Am.* 1999;**81A**:1236–44.
45. **Michelson JD, Hamel AJ, Buczek FL, Sharkey NA.** Kinematic behavior of the ankle following malleolar fracture repair in a high-fidelity cadaver model. *J Bone Joint Surg Am.* 2002;**84A**:2029–38.
46. **Hamel AJ, Sharkey NA, Buczek FL, Michelson J.** Relative motions of the tibia, talus, and calcaneus during the stance phase of gait. a cadaver study. *Gait Posture.* 2004;**20**:147–53.
47. **Okita N, Meyers SA, Challis JH, Sharkey NA.** Segmental motion of forefoot and hindfoot as a diagnostic tool. *J Biomech.* 2013;**46**:2578–85.
48. **Kirane YM, Michelson JD, Sharkey NA.** Evidence of isometric function of the flexor hallucis longus muscle in normal gait. *J Biomech.* 2008;**41**:1919–28.
49. **Kirane YM, Michelson JD, Sharkey NA.** Contribution of the flexor hallucis longus to loading of the first metatarsal and first metatarsophalangeal joint. *Foot Ankle Int.* 2008;**29**:367–77.
50. **Hurschler C, Emmerich J, Wulker N.** In vitro simulation of stance phase gait part I. Model verification. *Foot Ankle Int.* 2003;**24**:614–22.
51. **Wulker N, Hurschler C, Emmerich J.** In vitro simulation of stance phase gait part II. Simulated anterior tibial tendon dysfunction and potential compensation. *Foot Ankle Int.* 2003;**24**:623–9.

52. **Nester CJ, Liu AM, Ward E, et al.** In vitro study of foot kinematics using a dynamic walking cadaver model. *J Biomech.* 2007;**40**:1927–37.
53. **Kim KJ, Kitaoka HB, Luo ZP, et al.** In vitro simulation of the stance phase of gait. *J Musculoskel Res.* 2001;**5**:113–21.
54. **Noble LD Jr., Colbrunn RW, Lee DG, van den Bogert AJ, Davis BL.** Design and validation of a general purpose robotic testing system for musculoskeletal applications. *J Biomech Eng.* 2010:**132**:025001.
55. **Lee DG, Davis BL.** Assessment of the effects of diabetes on midfoot joint pressures using a robotic gait simulator. *Foot Ankle Int.* 2009;**30**:767–72.
56. **Erdemir A, Sirimamilla PA, Halloran JP, van den Bogert AJ.** An elaborate data set characterizing the mechanical response of the foot. *J Biomech Eng.* 2009;**131**:094502.
57. **Natsakis T, Peeters K, Burg F, Dereymaeker G, Vander Sloten J, Jonkers I.** Specimen-specific tibial kinematics model for in vitro gait simulations. *Proceedings of the Institution of Mechanical Engineers. Part H, Journal of Engineering in Medicine.* 2013;**227**:454–63.
58. **Natsakis T, Burg J, Dereymaeker G, Jonkers I, Vander Sloten J.** Inertial control as novel technique for in vitro gait simulations. *J Biomech.* 2015;**48**:392–5.
59. **Aubin PM, Cowley MS, Ledoux WR.** Gait simulation via a 6-DOF parallel robot with iterative learning control. *IEEE Trans Biomed Eng.* 2008;**55**:1237–40.
60. **Jackson LT, Aubin PM, Cowley MS, Sangeorzan BJ, Ledoux WR.** A robotic cadaveric flatfoot analysis of stance phase. *J Biomech Eng.* 2011;**133**:051005.
61. **Vaudreuil NJ, Ledoux WR, Roush GC, Whittaker EC, Sangeorzan BJ.** Comparison of transfer sites for flexor digitorum longus in a cadaveric adult acquired flatfoot model. *J Orthop Res.* 2014;**32**:102–9.
62. **Bayomy AF, Aubin PM, Sangeorzan BJ, Ledoux WR.** Arthrodesis of the first metatarsophalangeal joint. a robotic cadaver study of the dorsiflexion angle. *J Bone Joint Surg Am.* 2010;**92**:1754–64.
63. **Weber JR, Aubin PM, Ledoux WR, Sangeorzan BJ.** Second metatarsal length is positively correlated with increased pressure and medial deviation of the second toe in a robotic cadaveric simulation of gait. *Foot Ankle Int.* 2012;**33**:312–19.
64. **Trask DJ, Ledoux WR, Whittaker EC, Roush GC, Sangeorzan BJ.** Second metatarsal osteotomies for metatarsalgia: a robotic cadaveric study of the effect of osteotomy plane and metatarsal shortening on plantar pressure. *J Orthop Res.* 2014;**32**:385–93.
65. **Whittaker EC, Aubin PM, Ledoux WR.** Foot bone kinematics as measured in a cadaveric robotic gait simulator. *Gait Posture.* 2011;**33**:645–50.
66. **Delp SL, Loan JP, Hoy MG, Zajac FE, Topp EL, Rosen JM.** An interactive graphics-based model of the lower extremity to study orthopaedic surgical procedures. *IEEE Transactions on Biomedical Engineering.* 1990;**37**:757–67.
67. **Isvilanonda V.** *Finite Element Modeling of the Foot.* Washington: University of Washington, 2015.
68. **Cheung JT, Zhang M, An KN.** Effects of plantar fascia stiffness on the biomechanical responses of the ankle-foot complex. *Clin Biomech (Bristol, Avon).* 2004;**19**:839–46.
69. **Cheung JT, An KN, Zhang M.** Consequences of partial and total plantar fascia release: a finite element study. *Foot Ankle Int.* 2006;**27**:125–32.
70. **Cheung JT, Zhang M.** A 3-dimensional finite element model of the human foot and ankle for insole design. *Arch Phys Med Rehabil.* 2005;**86**:353–8.
71. **Cheung JT, Zhang M.** Parametric design of pressure-relieving foot orthosis using statistics-based finite element method. *Med Eng Phys.* 2008;**30**:269–77.
72. **Cheung JT, Zhang M, Leung AK, Fan YB.** Three-dimensional finite element analysis of the foot during standing—a material sensitivity study. *J Biomech.* 2005;**38**:1045–54.
73. **Cheung JT, Zhang M, An KN.** Effect of Achilles tendon loading on plantar fascia tension in the standing foot. *Clin Biomech (Bristol, Avon).* 2006;**21**:194–203.
74. **Dai XQ, Li Y, Zhang M, Cheung JT.** Effect of sock on biomechanical responses of foot during walking. *Clin Biomech (Bristol, Avon).* 2006;**21**:314–21.

75. **Yu J, Cheung JT, Fan Y, Zhang Y, Leung AK, Zhang M.** Development of a finite element model of female foot for high-heeled shoe design. *Clin Biomech (Bristol, Avon).* 2008;**23**(Suppl. 1):S31–38.
76. **Lemmon DR, Shiang TY, Hashmi A, Ulbrecht JS, Cavanagh PR.** The effect of insoles in therapeutic footwear. A finite-element approach. *J Biomech.* 1997;**30**:615–20.
77. **Erdemir A, Viveiros ML, Ulbrecht JS, Cavanagh PR.** An inverse finite-element model of heel-pad indentation. *J Biomech.* 2006;**39**:1279–86.
78. **Goske S, Erdemir A, Petre M, Budhabhatti S, Cavanagh PR.** Reduction of plantar heel pressures. Insole design using finite element analysis. *J Biomech.* 2006;**39**:2363–70.
79. **Budhabhatti SP, Erdemir A, Petre M, Sferra J, Donley B, Cavanagh PR.** Finite element modeling of the first ray of the foot: a tool for the design of interventions. *J Biomech Eng.* 2007;**129**:750–6.
80. **Petre M, Erdemir A, Panoskaltsis VP, Spirka TA, Cavanagh PR.** Optimization of nonlinear hyperelastic coefficients for foot tissues using a magnetic resonance imaging deformation experiment. *J Biomech Eng.* 2013;**135**:61001–12.
81. **Spirka TA, Erdemir A, Ewers Spaulding S, Yamane A, Telfer S, Cavanagh PR.** Simple finite element models for use in the design of therapeutic footwear. *J Biomech.* 2014;**47**:2948–55.
82. **Williams ED, Stebbins MJ, Cavanagh PR, et al.** The design and validation of a magnetic resonance imaging-compatible device for obtaining mechanical properties of plantar soft tissue via gated acquisition. *Proc Inst Mech Eng H.* 2015;**229**:732–42.
83. **Williams ED, Stebbins MJ, Cavanagh PR, et al.** A preliminary study of patient-specific mechanical properties of diabetic and healthy plantar soft tissue from gated magnetic resonance imaging. *Proc Inst Mech Eng H.* 2017;**231**(7):625–33.

Chapter 4

Osteoarthritis

Anne-Maree Keenan and Shannon Munteanu

An overview of osteoarthritis

Defining osteoarthritis

Osteoarthritis (OA) is a common and disabling problem. Worldwide estimates of OA indicate that one in ten men and one in five women aged over 60 years have symptomatic OA (1): these will increase further with our ageing and increasingly obese society. OA generally refers to a clinical syndrome of joint pain, functional loss, and reduced quality of life. It is classically characterized by focal loss of articular cartilage, degradation of subchondral bone, and the development of osteophytes. While OA was previously considered to be a disease of the articular cartilage and bone, it is now recognized that OA is a whole-joint organ disease (2, 3) and the aetiology and progression of OA may be because of any of the tissues of the affected organ, including the subchondral bone, synovium, capsule, periarticular muscles, sensory nerve endings, ligaments, and, if present, menisci (4).

Pathogenesis and risk factors

Risk factors thought to contribute to OA include genetic predisposition (5), obesity (6, 7), diminished bone mineral density (8), female sex (7), and insufficient nutrition (9). Localized joint or direct mechanical influences include ongoing joint overloading (including occupational [10] and sporting participation [11]), joint malalignment (7, 12, 13), previous joint trauma (14), and existing joint pathology, such as ligament damage (15) and irregular bone shape (16). Every presentation of OA will be the result of interactions between one or more risk factors.

Clinical features

Pain is considered to be the most important symptom with OA and is the major reason that people seek treatment (17). Pain in OA, however, is complex, and the severity and impact varies enormously with each individual but generally occurs during weightbearing: nocturnal pain, however, has also been noted, particularly in more severe OA (18). Whilst able to exist independently of one another, typically pain and decreased physical activity occur concurrently (19).

OA rarely presents in only one joint and it is important to note that the impact of OA, particularly foot OA, is exponentially increased when it occurs in combination with other joints (20): consideration of the impact of other sites of OA is essential when planning treatment.

Traditionally, much was made of the radiographic appearance of OA, which was thought to be related to pain. This has been challenged, with evidence to suggest that 50% of people in the general population who have radiographic evidence of OA report no pain (21) and over half of those with suspected pain thought to be associated with OA had no definite radiographic evidence of the disease (22). The use of magnetic resonance imaging (MRI) has enabled a new approach to evaluation of the tissues involved in OA, including cartilage, bone, synovium, ligaments, and menisci. Studies have demonstrated the importance of bone marrow lesions, not only associated with pain (16), but also predicting disease progression (23). Furthermore, the inflammatory nature of OA has also been described—with inflammatory mediators released by cartilage, bone, and synovium (24). Synovitis is now considered to be a feature of OA and offers the potential for new treatment targets.

While much attention has been placed on the physical aspects of OA, it is important to note that patients with OA have been found to have higher levels of depression and anxiety, which is associated with decreased physical ability (25).

Management

The National Institute for Health and Care Excellence (NICE) highlight the importance of a holistic approach in the management of OA (26) and recommend that healthcare professionals should assess the effect of OA on the individual's function, quality of life, occupation, mood, relationships, and leisure activities. NICE has produced a list of prompts when assessing people with OA (Figure 4.1).

While many of the recommendations are based on hip and knee OA evidence, the principles for the foot are similar and the following core treatments should be offered to those with foot OA:

1. Access to information that will promote education and facilitate self-management.
2. Activity and exercise, which includes muscle strengthening and general cardiovascular fitness.
3. Weight loss if the person is overweight or obese.
4. Footwear with shock absorptive properties for OA of the lower limb.

Many of the non-pharmacological management strategies for OA have some, albeit not definitive, evidence. Thermotherapy, electrotherapy, bracing, and assistive devices (such as walking sticks) should be considered as adjunct therapy; however, there is no evidence to support the use of nutraceuticals (such as glucosamine or chondroitin products) and acupuncture in the management of OA (26).

Previously considered the first line of OA management, the use of paracetamol has been shown to be ineffective (27) and non-steroidal anti-inflammatory drugs (NSAIDs) are now considered the first line of pharmacological treatment of OA, ahead of highly selective NSAID (COX-2)s or opioids. Topical NSAIDs should be tried before oral medication. NICE recommends that NSAIDs should be used at the lowest effective dose for the shortest period of time, and co-prescribed with a proton pump inhibitor. Further, although NSAIDs have analgesic effects of a similar magnitude, they vary in their potential gastrointestinal, liver, and cardiorenal toxicity. Therefore, when choosing the agent and dose, individual patient risk factors, including age, should be considered. When prescribing these drugs, consideration should also be given to appropriate assessment and/or ongoing monitoring of these risk factors (26). Referral for surgical assessment should be undertaken only if core and adjunct treatments have been unsuccessful and with consideration of the circumstances of the individual.

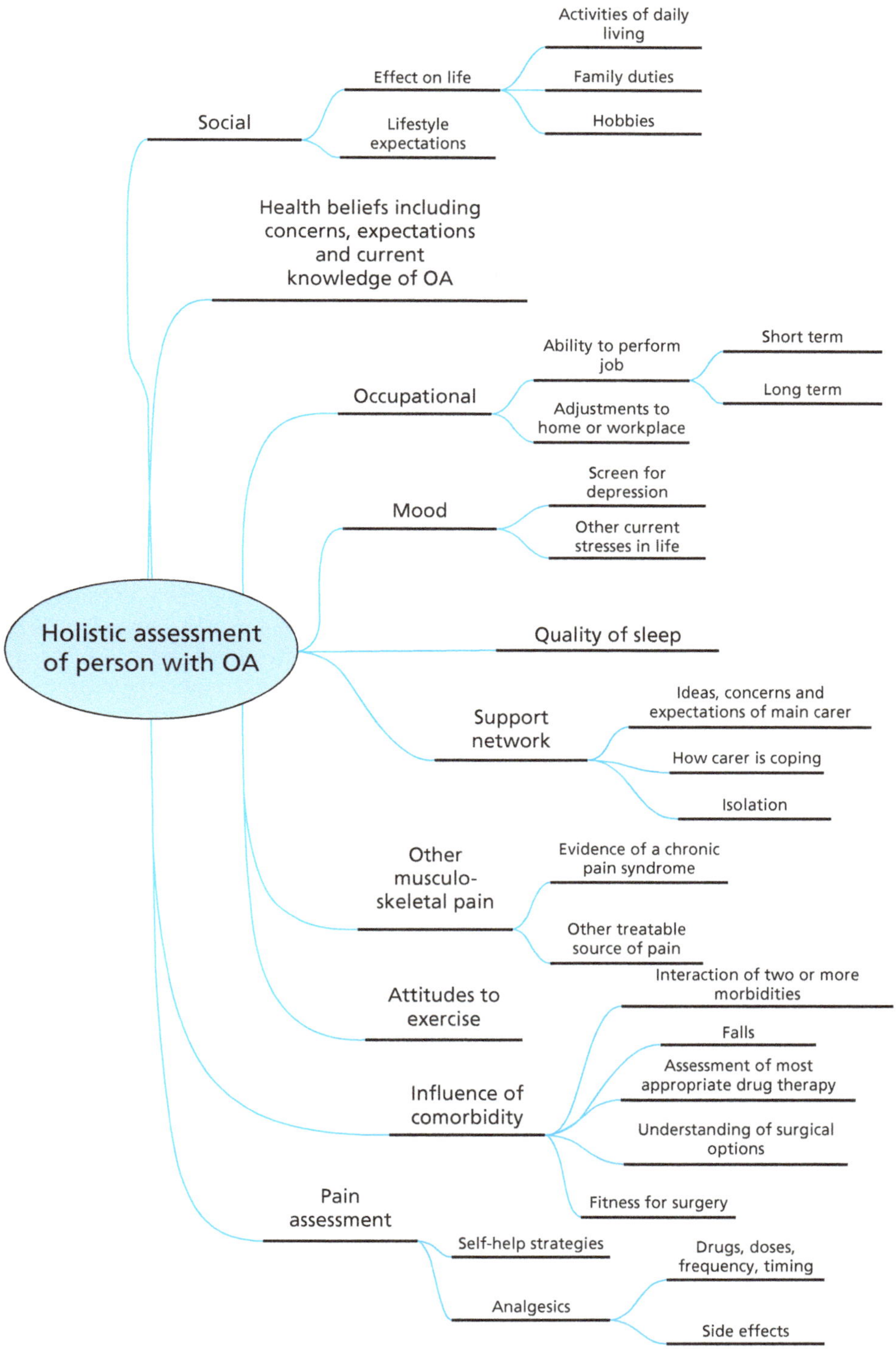

Figure 4.1 Key topics to assess in the holistic management of those with osteoarthritis (OA) taken from the National Institute for Health and Care Excellence (NICE) Guidelines.

Osteoarthritis of the foot and ankle

Prevalence and impact of foot disease

OA of the foot is highly prevalent. Population-based studies of adults aged 50 years or older show that the prevalence of symptomatic radiographic OA of the foot is 17%. The most commonly affected joint of the foot is the first metatarsophalangeal (MTP) joint (prevalence 8%) but OA of the midfoot (first cuneiform metatarsal joint; second cuneiform metatarsal joint, navicular cuneiform joint and/or talonavicular joint) is also very common (prevalence 12%) (28). Overall, symptomatic foot OA is more common in women (19% versus 14%) and is more likely in people with a history of working in routine and manual occupations relative to managerial and professional occupations (28). There is a paucity of reliable data regarding the prevalence of OA of the rearfoot (subtalar and tibiotalar joints). However, symptomatic rearfoot OA is relatively uncommon (29, 30). Emerging evidence indicates that hallux abducto valgus has pathological features that include OA (31). However, it will not be included in this review as its aetiology, presentation, and management are different from classical first MTP joint OA.

Symptoms of OA are typically pain and stiffness at the affected joint that increase with activity, as well as a progressive limitation in range of motion of the joint. People with foot OA may present with pain in other areas of their foot or lower limb related to altered gait patterns as they attempt to reduce load in the affected joint(s). Upon physical examination, the joint will typically be tender to palpate. Passive range of motion will reveal restricted motion, particularly in advanced disease, and create pain at or near the extreme of motion (especially with dorsiflexion in first MTP joint OA). Crepitus is variable. There is likely to be an enlargement of the affected joint, owing to the development of osteophytes at the periarticular regions, especially in more advanced disease (32). Although imaging is not necessary to diagnose OA (32), radiographic assessment has commonly been used to confirm the presence of this condition; the classical features of OA are joint space narrowing and osteophytes (33). Modern imaging techniques have shed new light on the pathogenesis of OA: ultrasound, for example (Figure 4.2), can highlight the synovitis and inflammation that is often present with OA; MRI has highlighted the importance of bone marrow oedema and lesions (Figure 4.3).

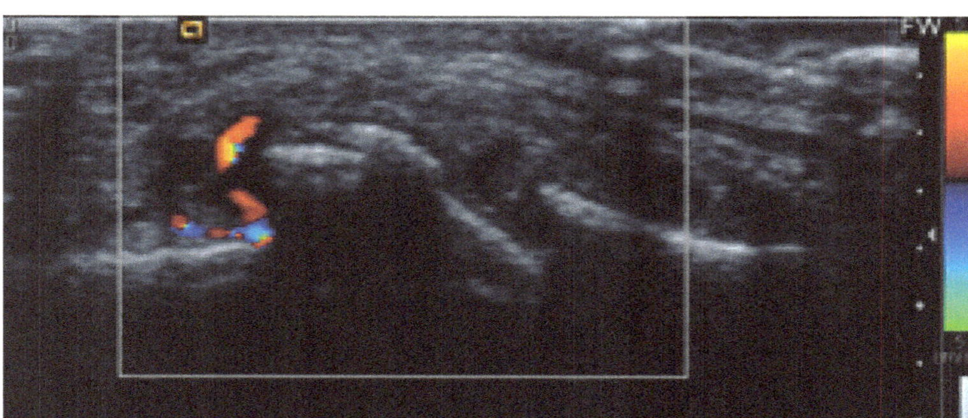

Figure 4.2 Ultrasound image of first metatarsophalangeal joint inflammation with power Doppler demonstrates effusion and associated synovitis, which are the red and yellow areas.

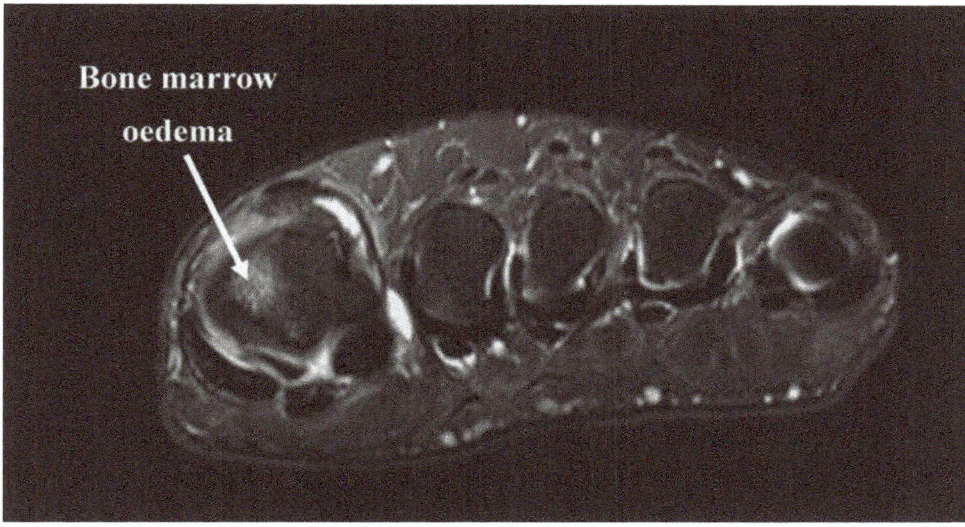

Figure 4.3 Magnetic resonance imaging with bone marrow oedema for the first metatarsophalangeal joint highlighted. (TR 3770 ms, TE 80 ms, TI 130 ms, 173 × 320 mm, 3-mm slice thickness with 0.9-mm gap. Siemens Avanto 1.5T scanner). TE, Echo time; TI, inversion time; TR, repetition time.

Source: Carole Burnett, NIHR Leeds Biomedical Research Centre.

Forefoot disease

The first MTP joint plays a critical role in the transfer of the body during the propulsive phase of gait, so people with first MTP joint OA will often adopt an inefficient walking pattern (34, 35). In addition, first MTP joint OA is associated with reduced health-related quality of life, especially in those activities related to physical functioning (36, 37). In a cross-sectional study by Bergin et al. (38), symptomatic first MTP joint OA was associated with increased foot pain, impaired foot function, and greater difficulties with obtaining suitable footwear (measured using the Foot Health Status Questionnaire), as well as impaired physical function (measured using the SF-36 questionnaire).

Midfoot disease

Midfoot OA is becoming increasingly recognized as a significant cause of foot pain in the community. A survey of 525 community-based adults aged 50 years or older showed that symptomatic midfoot OA was associated with physical impairment using the SF-36 questionnaire (39). Further, midfoot OA was a major contributor to healthcare utilization, with up to 25% of those affected with midfoot OA seeking professional healthcare for their symptoms.

Rearfoot disease

Although OA of the subtalar and tibiotalar joints is relatively uncommon (40), these joints are critical for transferring motion between the lower leg and foot during gait. Consequently, the presence of OA at these joints has the potential to impact significantly on physical performance (41). This has been supported by McDaniel et al. (41), where the presence of radiographic OA of the subtalar joint, but not the tibiotalar joint, was associated with impaired balance.

Foot-specific management

Non-pharmacological management

While there is no shortage of opinions on non-pharmacological treatments for OA of the foot, there is a disappointing lack of evidence to support such treatments. Physical treatments will often be used when there is a mechanical loading of a painful joint, including orthoses and footwear, and will be targeted to that particular joint. Rocker bottom shoes and foot orthoses with a first ray cut out (Figure 4.4), for example, are used in an attempt to offload a painful first MTP joint, both of which have proven to be equally effective in reducing pain (42). Initial evidence also suggests that insoles that stiffen the shoe, thereby reducing movement at the first MTP joint, are also effective (43). There is less evidence of effective treatment with midfoot OA: while a recently published feasibility study suggested that contoured, prefabricated devices may reduce midfoot OA pain (44), more work is needed in this area. There is little evidence to suggest that either mobilization or splinting, often used with hallux abducto valgus, has any benefit.

Pharmacological

Topical therapies

Topical therapies are preferred over systemic treatments for the initial pharmacological treatment for OA, particularly when a small number of peripheral joints are affected such as the foot (45). Topical NSAIDs are the most widely used topical therapy for pain relief in OA and exert anti-inflammatory and analgesic effects via reduction of prostaglandin synthesis. Topical NSAIDs are recommended over oral NSAIDs as there is significantly less absorption of the agent than consumption of the oral equivalent (46). Consequently, the risks of systemic adverse events (such as gastrointestinal effects) caused by their use are minimized. The available evidence for OA shows that the effectiveness of topical NSAIDs is equivalent to oral NSAIDs (45).

Intra-articular injection therapies (corticosteroids and hyaluronic acid)

Intra-articular injections of corticosteroids and hyaluronic acid are recommended as adjunctive therapies for OA. Corticosteroids are used to create long-lasting (months) symptom-modifying effects in OA by suppression of joint inflammation (47). Corticosteroids recommended for intra-articular injection include short-acting (e.g., hydrocortisone acetate), intermediate-acting (e.g., triamcinolone acetonide), and long-acting (e.g., betamethasone sodium phosphate and acetate) products (47) that can be coadministered with local anaesthetic for additional short-term

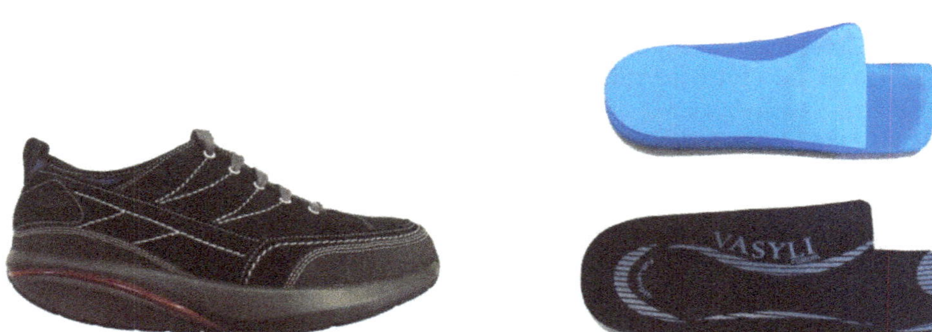

Figure 4.4 Rocker bottom shoes and orthoses with first ray cut out.

analgesia. The use of ultrasound or fluoroscopy for guidance is recommended to facilitate the accurate placement of the needle (48). The maximum frequency of corticosteroid injections is not evidence-based, but a limit of three to four injections in 1 year, allowing 3–4 months between injections, is recommended as there is concern that repeated corticosteroid injections may accelerate atrophy of articular cartilage and associated soft tissues (49).

Hyaluronan

Hyaluronan therapy, also known as viscosupplementation, involves the introduction of hyaluronic acid into a joint with the goal of restoring the viscoelastic properties of synovial joint fluid, as well as providing long-term effects of changing the disease process of the joint through stimulation of endogenous hyaluronic acid production by synovium, suppression of inflammation, and protection of articular cartilage (50). Several hyaluronan products are approved for the treatment of OA, including Hyalgan®, Supartz®, Synvisc®, Orthovisc®, and Euflexxa®. These products differ in their molecular weight (which range from 0.6 to 6 kDa) and in their concentration of hyaluronan and subsequent viscoelastic properties, but it is unclear if this influences their relative effectiveness. Hyaluronan injections are recommended to be administered as a series of weekly injections given over 3–5 weeks (50).

Evidence for the effectiveness of intra-articular injections for foot and ankle osteoarthritis

The therapeutic response to intra-articular injections is variable (47). Few randomized controlled studies have investigated the effectiveness of intra-articular injections for foot or tibiotalar joint OA (51). The existing studies will be reviewed below.

Forefoot osteoarthritis In a participant-blinded randomized controlled trial by Pons et al. (52), 37 participants with mild first MTP joint OA were randomized to receive a single injection of sodium hyaluronate (Ostenil® mini) or corticosteroid (triamcinolone acetonide). In both groups, there was a clinically meaningful improvement in symptoms over the 12-week study period. However, there were few significant differences between the two groups. Additionally, the positive effects of these treatments did not last beyond 12 weeks, as nearly half of the participants required surgery at 12 months. A subsequent participant- and assessor-blinded placebo-controlled trial by Munteanu et al. (53) compared the effectiveness of a single intra-articular injection of hyaluronic acid (Synvisc®, Hylan G-F20) to placebo (saline) in 151 people with first MTP joint OA. Participants were evaluated for 6 months following treatment. In both groups, foot pain and foot-reported disability (assessed using the Foot Health Status Questionnaire) improved over time, but there were no differences between groups.

Midfoot osteoarthritis There is a paucity of high-quality trials investigating the effectiveness of injection therapy for midfoot OA. A retrospective case-series study by Drakonaki et al. (54) investigated the outcomes of ultrasound-guided corticosteroid combined with local anaesthetic (methylprednisolone acetate and bupivacaine hydrochloride) injections in 59 participants with midfoot OA. At 2 weeks, 78% of participants experienced pain relief (better or no pain), but the number reporting improvement declined over time; pain relief occurred in 58% at 3 months, and in less than 15% after 3 months.

Rearfoot osteoarthritis In a small (n=20) double-blind (participant and assessor) randomized controlled trial, Salk et al. (55) evaluated the effectiveness of five weekly injections of hyaluronan (Hyalgan®) compared to normal saline (placebo) for OA of the tibiotalar joint over 26 weeks. Symptoms improved in both groups during the study, and there were trends in favour of hyaluronan treatment. However, there were no significant differences between groups for the primary outcome measure (Ankle Osteoarthritis Score).

Surgery

Surgery is indicated in the management of OA when non-surgical management is unable to sufficiently reduce symptoms of pain and disability (56). Several surgical procedures for foot and tibiotalar joint OA have been described and the choice of the most appropriate procedure is determined by considering the risks and expected benefits of each procedure, taking into consideration factors such as the joint(s) affected, the patient's age, general health, expectations, and ability to cooperate in any treatment plan (57).

First metatarsophalangeal joint osteoarthritis surgery

Numerous surgical procedures have been recommended for first MTP joint OA, and there are no clear surgical treatment algorithms (56). Generally, the severity of the OA disease is an important factor in determining the choice of surgical procedure; joint-preserving techniques such as cheilectomy and osteotomies are recommended for mild and moderate first MTP joint OA, and arthroplasty and arthrodesis recommended for more severe forms of the disease, or when joint-preserving techniques fail (56). Some of the more commonly used surgical procedures are described below.

Cheilectomy is recommended for mild or moderate first MTP joint OA (56). The focus is on restoring the mechanics of the joint and removing any excess bone that may interfere with normal joint function. Typical cheilectomy involves resection of up to 30% of the dorsal articular surface of the first metatarsal head. Osteophytes on the medial and lateral aspects of the metatarsal head and the dorsal aspect of the proximal phalanx are also removed (57). This procedure leaves the joint intact, which keeps most future surgical options open should the joint degeneration progress (56).

Arthroplasty is used for more severe cases of first MTP joint OA, or in cases of failed cheilectomy. The Keller procedure is a widely recognized technique, traditionally involving resection of the proximal one-third of the proximal phalanx. However, because of the long-term complications, including impaired function of the first MTP joint and difficulty in salvaging failures, this technique is less commonly used (56). Modifications to the Keller procedure, including interpositioning of the first MTP joint with a mechanical implant or biologic spacer and attachment of the flexor tendons to the remainder of the proximal phalanx, have led to improved outcomes (58). Despite this, Keller procedures are still only recommended as an alternative to arthrodesis in older patients (aged greater than 70 years), those who are less active, and when a shorter and less complex recovery is desired (56).

Arthrodesis (joint fusion) is a reliable and effective pain-relieving procedure recommended for severe cases of first MTP joint OA (or in cases of failed cheilectomy) (59). A typical arthrodesis involves removal of periarticular osteophytes, removal of the articular cartilage and subchondral bone from the opposing joint surfaces through mechanical means such as drilling and scaling, and then fixating the hallux into a position of 15–25° of dorsiflexion (59, 60).

Midfoot and rearfoot osteoarthritis surgery

Surgical management of midfoot and rearfoot OA generally involves arthrodesis of the affected joints (61, 62). However, arthroscopic treatment may be attempted prior to resorting to arthrodesis of the subtalar and tibiotalar joints (63, 64). Further, implant arthroplasty of the tibiotalar joint has also been used. Case-series studies have reported that arthrodesis is effective for pain reduction in OA of the midfoot and rearfoot with high rates of fusion (64–67). Complications of arthrodesis procedures include pain from implants and non-union but occur in less than 10% of patients (65, 68). Additionally, joint rigidity from arthrodesis can cause impaired foot function and development of secondary disorders such as OA in adjacent joints and overloading of plantar foot structures (65, 69–72).

Clinical trials investigating the effectiveness of surgery for foot and ankle osteoarthritis

Although several case-series and non-randomized studies have been reported for surgery of the foot and tibiotalar joint in OA, only five randomized controlled trials have been reported; four of these have focused on the first MTP joint and one focused on the tibiotalar joint. Sherman et al. (73) investigated the benefit of Kirschner-wire distraction following a Keller's arthroplasty in eight patients. Kirschner-wire distraction provided no additional benefit at 12 months in terms of first MTP joint motion and patient satisfaction. O'Doherty et al. (74) compared Keller's arthroplasty to arthrodesis. At a minimum follow-up of 2 years, the procedures were equally successful at relieving first MTP joint pain, improving walking distance, and reducing problems with footwear. Gibson et al. (75) compared arthrodesis to implant arthroplasty for first MTP joint OA (77 feet) and reported better outcomes in the arthrodesis group. At 24 months, the arthrodesis group reported significantly greater pain relief and fewer complications. In contrast, Baumhauer et al. (76) recently compared a synthetic cartilage bone implant to arthrodesis for first MTP joint and showed equivalent outcomes for pain and function at 1 and 2 years. In the only randomized controlled trial for tibiotalar joint OA, Wood et al. (77) compared two types of tibiotalar joint implant devices (Buechel-Pappas versus the Scandinavian Total Ankle Replacement [STAR™] in 200 tibiotalar joints) and reported pain relief and function improvement to be similar for the two groups (mean follow-up of 54 months). However, the Buechel-Pappas implant has been withdrawn from the market.

Research agenda

For an area that has long been the poor relation in rheumatology research, there are several exciting developments for improving treatment outcomes in OA. The importance of bone marrow oedema and bone marrow lesions has been highlighted with developments in MRI techniques: understanding the bone stress, adaptation, and the development of these lesions will be pivotal in establishing treatments to prevent OA progression, including novel cellular and regenerative therapies and more reliable surgical outcomes. There will be an emphasis on targeted and stratified treatments, including managing multi-joint presentations of OA. Finally, given the projected prevalence and impact of OA with the ever-ageing and ever-more obese population, the influence of multi-morbidities and their impact on living with OA will become a key area.

A review of the World Health Organization International Clinical Trials Registry Platform has identified that there are a number of trials that are planned, being conducted, or have completed that are investigating the effectiveness of interventions for foot OA. Such trials will provide clinicians with increased confidence to manage this condition effectively. These trials include:

- Shoe-stiffening inserts for first MTP joint OA (trial registration ID: ACTRN12616000552482). The effectiveness of shoe-stiffening inserts for first MTP joint OA is being evaluated in a randomized trial at La Trobe University, Melbourne, Australia. The trial is planned for completion in 2018.
- Multi-faceted intervention podiatry treatment for first MTP joint OA (trial registration ID: ACTRN12616001290482). The effectiveness of a multi-modal intervention (consisting of foot orthotics, foot and ankle exercises, as well as advice concerning appropriate footwear,

analgesia, weight management, and general physical activity) for first MTP joint OA is being evaluated in a pilot randomized trial at Melbourne University, Melbourne, Australia. The anticipated date of completion of data collection is February 2017.

- Rocker-sole shoes for ankle OA (trial registration ID: ISRCTN85568283). The effectiveness of rocker-sole shoes for ankle OA is currently being evaluated in a crossover study at University Medical Centre Groningen, Netherlands. Recruitment has been completed.

However, it must be highlighted that the number of trials for OA of the foot is relatively small compared to other regions of the body (such as the knee and hip). Therefore, greater funding is desperately required to support research in this area.

References

1. **Woolf AD, Pfleger B.** Burden of major musculoskeletal conditions. *Bull WHO.* 2003;**81**(9):646–56.
2. **Pelletier JP, Martel-Pelletier J, Abramson SB.** Osteoarthritis, an inflammatory disease: potential implication for the selection of new therapeutic targets. *Arthritis Rheum.* 2001;**44**(6):1237–47.
3. **Rogers J, Shepstone L, Dieppe P.** Is osteoarthritis a systemic disorder of bone? *Arthritis Rheum.* 2004;**50**(2):452–7.
4. **Brandt KD, Radin EL, Dieppe PA, van de Putte L.** Yet more evidence that osteoarthritis is not a cartilage disease. *Ann Rheum Dis.* 2006;**65**(10):1261–4.
5. **Spector TD, Cicuttini F, Baker J, et al.** Genetic influences on osteoarthritis in women: a twin study. *BMJ.* 1996;**312**(7036):940–3.
6. **Lau EC, Cooper C, Lam D, et al.** Factors associated with osteoarthritis of the hip and knee in Hong Kong Chinese: obesity, joint injury, and occupational activities. *Am J Epidemiol.* 2000;**152**(9):855–62.
7. **Sharma L, Cahue S, Song J, Hayes K, Pai YC, Dunlop D.** Physical functioning over three years in knee osteoarthritis: role of psychosocial, local mechanical, and neuromuscular factors. *Arthritis Rheum.* 2003;**48**(12):3359–70.
8. **Hannan MT, Anderson JJ, Zhang Y, et al.** Bone mineral density and knee osteoarthritis in elderly men and women. The Framingham Study. *Arthritis Rheum.* 1993;**36**(12):1671–80.
9. **Felson D, Lawrence R, Dieppe P, et al.** Osteoarthritis: new insights. Part 1: The disease and its risk factors. *Ann Intern Med.* 2000;**133**(8):635–46.
10. **Felson DT, Hannan MT, Naimark A, et al.** Occupational physical demands, knee bending, and knee osteoarthritis: results from the Framingham Study. *J Rheumatol.* 1991;**18**(10):1587–92.
11. **Buckwalter JA, Lane NE, Buckwalter JA, Lane NE.** Athletics and osteoarthritis. *Am J Sports Med.* 1997;**25**(6):873–81.
12. **Sharma L, Hurwitz DE, Thonar EJ, et al.** Knee adduction moment, serum hyaluronan level, and disease severity in medial tibiofemoral osteoarthritis. *Arthritis Rheum.* 1998;**41**(7):1233–40.
13. **Brouwer GM, van Tol AW, Bergin AP, et al.** Association between valgus and varus alignment and the development and progression of radiographic osteoarthritis of the knee. *Arthritis Rheum.* 2007;**56**(4):1204–11.
14. **Honkonen SE, Honkonen SE.** Degenerative arthritis after tibial plateau fractures. *J Orthop Trauma.* 1995;**9**(4):273–7.
15. **Tan AL, Grainger AJ, Tanner SF, et al.** High-resolution magnetic resonance imaging for the assessment of hand osteoarthritis. *Arthritis Rheum.* 2005;**52**(8):2355–65.
16. **Barr AJ, Campbell TM, Hopkinson D, Kingsbury SR, Bowes MA, Conaghan PG.** A systematic review of the relationship between subchondral bone features, pain and structural pathology in peripheral joint osteoarthritis. *Arthritis Res Ther.* 2015;**17**:228.
17. **Dominick KL, Ahern FM, Gold CH, Heller DA.** Health-related quality of life and health service use among older adults with osteoarthritis. *Arthritis Rheum.* 2004;**51**(3):326–31.

18. **Sasaki E, Tsuda E, Yamamoto Y, et al.** Nocturnal knee pain increases with the severity of knee osteoarthritis, disturbing patient sleep quality. *Arthritis Care Res (Hoboken).* 2014;**66**(7):1027–32.
19. **O'Malley KJ, Suarez-Almazor M, Aniol J, et al.** Joint specific multidimensional assessment of pain (J-MAP): factor structure, reliability, validity and responsiveness in patients with knee osteoarthritis. *J Rheumatol.* 2002;**30**:534–43.
20. **Petchell A, Keenan A-M, Landorf K.** *Clinical Guidelines for Orthotic Therapy Provided by Podiatrists.* Victoria: Australian Podiatry Council; 1998.
21. **Birrell F, Croft P, Cooper C, et al.** Health impact of pain in the hip region with and without radiographic evidence of osteoarthritis: a study of new attenders to primary care. The PCR Hip Study Group. *Ann Rheum Dis.* 2000;**59**(11):857–63.
22. **McAlindon TE, Snow S, Cooper C, Dieppe PA.** Radiographic patterns of osteoarthritis of the knee joint in the community: the importance of the patellofemoral joint. *Ann Rheum Dis.* 1992;**51**(7):844–9.
23. **Edwards MH, Parsons C, Bruyere O, et al.** High Kellgren-Lawrence grade and bone marrow lesions predict worsening rates of radiographic joint space narrowing; The SEKOIA Study. *J Rheumatol.* 2016;**43**(3):657–65.
24. **Berenbaum F.** Osteoarthritis as an inflammatory disease (osteoarthritis is not osteoarthrosis!). *Osteoarthritis Cartilage.* 2013;**21**(1):16–21.
25. **Axford J, Butt A, Heron C, et al.** Prevalence of anxiety and depression in osteoarthritis: use of the Hospital Anxiety and Depression Scale as a screening tool. *Clin Rheumatol.* 2010;**29**(11):1277–83.
26. **National Institute for Care and Clinical Excellence.** *Osteoarthritis: Care and Management.* London: National Institute for Care and Clinical Excellence; 2014.
27. **da Costa BR, Reichenbach S, Keller N, et al.** Effectiveness of non-steroidal anti-inflammatory drugs for the treatment of pain in knee and hip osteoarthritis: a network meta-analysis. *Lancet.* 2016;**387**(10033):2093–105.
28. **Roddy E, Thomas MJ, Marshall M, et al.** The population prevalence of symptomatic radiographic foot osteoarthritis in community-dwelling older adults: cross-sectional findings from the Clinical Assessment Study of the Foot. *Ann Rheum Dis.* 2015;**74**(1):156–63.
29. **Buckwalter JA, Saltzman C, Brown T.** The impact of osteoarthritis: implications for research. *Clin Orthop Relat Res.* **2004**(427 Suppl.):S6–15.
30. **Goldberg AJ, MacGregor A, Dawson J, et al.** The demand incidence of symptomatic ankle osteoarthritis presenting to foot & ankle surgeons in the United Kingdom. *Foot (Edinb).* 2012;**22**(3):163–6.
31. **D'Arcangelo PR, Landorf KB, Munteanu SE, Zammit GV, Menz HB.** Radiographic correlates of hallux valgus severity in older people. *J Foot Ankle Res.* 2010;**3**:20.
32. **Zammit GV, Munteanu SE, Menz HB.** Development of a diagnostic rule for identifying radiographic osteoarthritis in people with first metatarsophalangeal joint pain. *Osteoarthritis Cartilage.* 2011;**19**(8):939–45.
33. **Menz HB, Munteanu SE, Landorf KB, Zammit GV, Cicuttini FM.** Radiographic classification of osteoarthritis in commonly affected joints of the foot. *Osteoarthritis Cartilage.* 2007;**15**(11):1333–8.
34. **Canseco K, Long J, Marks R, Khazzam M, Harris G.** Quantitative characterization of gait kinematics in patients with hallux rigidus using the Milwaukee foot model. *J Orthop Res.* 2008;**26**(4):419–27.
35. **Zammit GV, Menz HB, Munteanu SE, Landorf KB.** Plantar pressure distribution in older people with osteoarthritis of the first metatarsophalangeal joint (hallux limitus/rigidus). *J Orthop Res.* 2008;**26**(12):1665–9.
36. **Abhishek A, Roddy E, Zhang W, Doherty M.** Are hallux valgus and big toe pain associated with impaired quality of life? A cross-sectional study. *Osteoarthritis Cartilage.* 2010;**18**:923–6.
37. **Bergin SM, Munteanu SE, Zammit GV, Nikolopoulos N, Menz HB.** Impact of first metatarsophalangeal joint osteoarthritis on health-related quality of life. *Arthritis Care Res (Hoboken).* 2012;**64**(11):1691–8.

38. **Bergin SM, Munteanu SE, Zammit GV, Nikolopoulos N, Menz HB.** Impact of first metatarsophalangeal joint osteoarthritis on health-related quality of life. *Arthritis Care Res (Hoboken).* 2012;**64**(11):1691–8.
39. **Thomas MJ, Peat G, Rathod T, et al.** The epidemiology of symptomatic midfoot osteoarthritis in community-dwelling older adults: cross-sectional findings from the Clinical Assessment Study of the Foot. *Arthritis Res Ther.* 2015;**17**:178.
40. **Daniels T, Thomas R.** Etiology and biomechanics of ankle arthritis. *Foot Ankle Clin.* 2008;**13**(3):341–52.
41. **McDaniel G, Renner JB, Sloane R, Kraus VB.** Association of knee and ankle osteoarthritis with physical performance. *Osteoarthritis Cartilage.* 2011;**19**(6):634–8.
42. **Menz HB, Auhl M, Tan JM, Levinger P, Roddy E, Munteanu SE.** Effectiveness of foot orthoses versus rocker-sole footwear for first metatarsophalangeal joint osteoarthritis: randomized trial. *Arthritis Care Res.* 2016;**68**(5):581–9.
43. **Jerilyn TX, Menz HB, Murley GS, Munteanu SE.** Effectiveness of shoe stiffening inserts for first metatarsophalangeal joint osteoarthritis: a proof-of-concept study. *Am J Phys Med Rehab.* 2016;**95**(2):103–11.
44. **Halstead J, Chapman GJ, Gray JC, et al.** Foot orthoses in the treatment of symptomatic midfoot osteoarthritis using clinical and biomechanical outcomes: a randomised feasibility study. *Clin Rheumatol.* 2016;**35**(4):987–96.
45. **Zhang W, Doherty M, Leeb BF, et al.** EULAR evidence based recommendations for the management of hand osteoarthritis: report of a Task Force of the EULAR Standing Committee for International Clinical Studies Including Therapeutics (ESCISIT). *Ann Rheum Dis.* 2007;**66**(3):377–88.
46. **Sawynok J.** Topical and peripherally acting analgesics. *Pharmacol Rev.* 2003;**55**(1):1–20.
47. **Cardone DA, Tallia AF.** Joint and soft tissue injection. *Am Fam Physician.* 2002;**66**(2):283–9.
48. **Sofka CM, Adler RS.** Ultrasound-guided interventions in the foot and ankle. *Semin Musculoskelet Radiol.* 2002;**6**(2):163–8.
49. **Pekarek B, Osher L, Buck S, Bowen M.** Intra-articular corticosteroid injections: a critical literature review with up-to-date findings. *Foot (Edinb).* 2011;**21**(2):66–70.
50. **Grogan KA, Chang TJ, Salk RS.** Update on viscosupplementation in the treatment of osteoarthritis of the foot and ankle. *Clin Podiatr Med Surg.* 2009;**26**(2):199–204.
51. **Peterson C, Hodler J.** Evidence-based radiology (part 2): is there sufficient research to support the use of therapeutic injections into the peripheral joints? *Skeletal Radiol.* 2010;**39**(1):11–18.
52. **Pons M, Alvarez F, Solana J, Viladot R, Varela L.** Sodium hyaluronate in the treatment of hallux rigidus. A single-blind, randomized study. *Foot Ankle Int.* 2007;**28**(1):38–42.
53. **Munteanu SE, Menz HB, Zammit GV, et al.** Efficacy of intra-articular hyaluronan (Synvisc®) for the treatment of osteoarthritis affecting the first metatarsophalangeal joint of the foot (hallux limitus): study protocol for a randomised placebo controlled trial. *J Foot Ankle Res.* 2009;**2**:2.
54. **Drakonaki E, Kho JB, Sharp R, Ostlere S.** Efficacy of ultrasound-guided steroid injections for pain management of midfoot joint degenerative disease. *Skeletal Radiol.* 2011;**40**(8):1001–6.
55. **Salk RS, Chang TJ, D'Costa WF, Soomekh DJ, Grogan KA.** Sodium hyaluronate in the treatment of osteoarthritis of the ankle: a controlled, randomized, double-blind pilot study. *J Bone Joint Surg Am.* 2006;**88**(2):295–302.
56. **Perler AD, Nwosu V, Christie D, Higgins K.** End-stage osteoarthritis of the great toe/hallux rigidus: a review of the alternatives to arthrodesis: implant versus osteotomies and arthroplasty techniques. *Clin Podiatr Med Surg.* 2013;**30**(3):351–95.
57. **Moskowitz RW, Altman RD, Hochberg MC, Buckwalter JA, Goldberg VM.** *Osteoarthritis: Diagnosis and Medical/Surgical Management,* 4th edn. Philadelphia, USA: Lippincott Williams & Wilkins; 2007.
58. **Lombardo MA.** The improved Keller arthroplasty. *Clin Podiatr Med Surg.* 1989;**6**(1):133–48.

59. **Little JB.** First metatarsophalangeal joint arthrodesis in the treatment of hallux valgus. *Clin Podiatr Med Surg.* 2014;**31**(2):281–9.

60. **Treadwell JR.** First metatarsophalangeal joint arthrodesis; what is the best fixation option? A critical review of the literature. *Clin Podiatr Med Surg.* 2013;**30**(3):327–49.

61. **Patel A, Rao S, Nawoczenski D, Flemister AS, DiGiovanni B, Baumhauer JF.** Midfoot arthritis. *J Am Acad Orthop Surg.* 2010;**18**(7):417–25.

62. **Jordan RW, Chahal GS, Chapman A.** Is end-stage ankle arthrosis best managed with total ankle replacement or arthrodesis? A systematic review. *Adv Orthop.* 2014;**2014**:986285.

63. **Lopez R, Singh T, Banga S, Hasan N.** Subtalar joint arthrodesis. *Clin Podiatr Med Surg.* 2012;**29**(1):67–75.

64. **Choi WJ, Choi GW, Kwon HM, Lee JW.** Arthroscopic treatment in mild to moderate osteoarthritis of the ankle. *Knee Surg Sports Traumatol Arthrosc.* 2013;**21**(6):1338–44.

65. **Joveniaux P, Harisboure A, Ohl X, Dehoux E.** Long-term results of *in situ* subtalar arthrodesis. *Int Orthop.* 2010;**34**(8):1199–205.

66. **Huang PJ, Chen SK, Chen YW, Cheng YM, Lin SY, Hsu CY.** Subtalar arthrodesis for subtalar arthritis. *Kaohsiung J Med Sci.* 1997;**13**(11):677–81.

67. **Glanzmann MC, Sanhueza-Hernandez R.** Arthroscopic subtalar arthrodesis for symptomatic osteoarthritis of the hindfoot: a prospective study of 41 cases. *Foot Ankle Int.* 2007;**28**(1):2–7.

68. **Rao S, Nawoczenski DA, Baumhauer JF.** Midfoot arthritis: nonoperative options and decision making for fusion. *Tech Foot Ankle Surg.* 2008;**7**(3):188–95.

69. **Mann RA, Prieskorn D, Sobel M.** Mid-tarsal and tarsometatarsal arthrodesis for primary degenerative osteoarthrosis or osteoarthrosis after trauma. *J Bone Joint Surg Am.* 1996;**78**(9):1376–85.

70. **Komenda GA, Myerson MS, Biddinger KR.** Results of arthrodesis of the tarsometatarsal joints after traumatic injury. *J Bone Joint Surg Am.* 1996;**78**(11):1665–76.

71. **Jung HG, Myerson MS, Schon LC.** Spectrum of operative treatments and clinical outcomes for atraumatic osteoarthritis of the tarsometatarsal joints. *Foot Ankle Int.* 2007;**28**(4):482–9.

72. **Coester LM, Saltzman CL, Leupold J, Pontarelli W.** Long-term results following ankle arthrodesis for post-traumatic arthritis. *J Bone Joint Surg Am.* 2001;**83-a**(2):219–28.

73. **Sherman K, Douglas D, Benson M.** Keller's arthroplasty: is distraction useful? A prospective trial. *J Bone Joint Surg Br.* 1984;**66-B**(5):765–9.

74. **O'Doherty DP, Lowrie IG, Magnussen PA, Gregg PJ.** The management of the painful first metatarsophalangeal joint in the older patient. Arthrodesis or Keller's arthroplasty? *J Bone Joint Surg Br.* 1990;**72**(5):839–42.

75. **Gibson JN, Thomson CE.** Arthrodesis or total replacement arthroplasty for hallux rigidus: a randomized controlled trial. *Foot Ankle Int.* 2005;**26**(9):680–90.

76. **Baumhauer JF, Singh D, Glazebrook M, et al.** Prospective, randomized, multi-centered clinical trial assessing safety and efficacy of a synthetic cartilage implant versus first metatarsophalangeal arthrodesis in advanced hallux rigidus. *Foot Ankle Int.* 2016;**37**(5):457–69.

77. **Wood PL, Sutton C, Mishra V, Suneja R.** A randomised, controlled trial of two mobile-bearing total ankle replacements. *J Bone Joint Surg Br.* 2009;**91**(1):69–74.

Chapter 5

Crystal arthritis

Keith Rome and Edward Roddy

General introduction

Many different crystal types can form in the body and potentially cause acute synovitis, chronic arthropathy, or periarticular syndromes. The most common and clinically relevant crystals are monosodium urate (MSU), the causative agent in gout, and calcium pyrophosphate (CPP), both of which commonly affect the foot and ankle. Foot involvement, particularly the first metatarsophalangeal (MTP) joint, is the clinical hallmark of gout.

Gout

Introduction

Gout is the most prevalent form of inflammatory arthritis in men older than 40 years of age and has significant functional, social, and financial impacts (1, 2). The rising prevalence and incidence, high and increasing hospital admission rates, combined with the burden of comorbidities, are a significant current and future issue for healthcare systems across the world (3–5). Recent prevalence estimates are 3.9% in the USA (3), 2.4% in the UK (4), and in New Zealand, 3.2% and 6.1% in European and Maori people, respectively (5).

Gout is a disorder of purine metabolism, the biological precursor being hyperuricaemia, a serum urate level above the physiological saturation threshold of urate in body tissues (approximately 380 μmol/L). During the course of the disease the presence of MSU crystals can clinically manifest as acute attacks of peripheral synovitis, degenerative joint damage, synovial hypertrophy, bone erosions, and it can alter tendon and ligament structure and function (6).

Progression of gout and presentation over time

Definitive diagnosis of gout is confirmed by the identification of MSU crystals in aspirates of synovial fluid or tophus deposits (6). Aspirates can be taken from symptomatic and asymptomatic joints (7). Diagnostic criteria are used to guide clinical care, whereas classification criteria are used to identify cohorts of people for research purposes (8). The universal tool for the classification of gout is the American College of Rheumatology (ACR) preliminary criteria for the classification of the acute arthritis of primary gout (9). However, more recently, new classification criteria for gout have been published (10).

People with gout often have multiple comorbid conditions, such as hypertension, cardiovascular disease (CVD), renal impairment, diabetes mellitus, obesity, hyperlipidaemia, which in combination are known as metabolic syndrome (11). The relationships between these comorbidities and gout are complex, but their presence contributes to overall excessive cardiovascular mortality and morbidity due to myocardial infarction and peripheral arterial disease (12).

The natural history of gout is composed of three periods: asymptomatic hyperuricaemia, episodes of acute attacks of gout interspersed with asymptomatic intercritical periods, and then a chronic phase which involves structural changes to joints and tissues (1). The time course for disease progression from asymptomatic hyperuricaemia to chronic gouty arthropathy varies widely, from 3 to 42 years, and is correlated with the severity and duration of hyperuricaemia (1). Figure 5.1 illustrates the progression of gout over time.

Asymptomatic hyperuricaemia

Asymptomatic hyperuricaemia is defined as an abnormally high serum urate concentration (410 μmol/L) in the absence of clinical symptoms. The prevalence of hyperuricaemia is higher than the prevalence of gout, with an estimated prevalence of 21.4% in the US population (3). Reflecting the sex differences in gout, hyperuricaemia is more prevalent in males, with an estimated 21.6% prevalence compared to 8.6% in women in China (13).

Despite this absence of symptoms, MSU crystals have been visualized under light microscopy in synovial fluid aspirated from lower limb joints of people with asymptomatic hyperuricaemia (14). Furthermore, tophaceous deposits within tendons, joints, and along articular cartilage have also been observed using ultrasound in asymptomatic people with hyperuricaemia (15).

Acute gouty arthritis

The development of gout is correlated with the level and duration of hyperuricaemia. Population studies report a 12% incidence of gout after 14 years in those with serum urate levels between 420 μmol/L and 470 μmol/L (16), while the 5-year incidence of gout in those with serum urate levels above 590 μmol/L is reported to be 30% (17).

Acute gout is characterized by a sudden onset of severe pain, often during the night, waking the patient from sleep (18). This pain reaches its maximum in 6–24 hours and, without treatment, usually resolves in 7–10 days (19). The pain is accompanied by erythema, swelling, and limited motion of the affected joint. Inflammation of the periarticular tissue is also evident and concurrent systemic features, although rare, may be present (19). As the inflammatory process begins to subside, extensive exfoliation of skin overlying the affected joint may occur (20).

Although 90% of first attacks are monoarticular, oligoarticular and polyarticular involvement can occur, particularly in elderly patients (21). Joints in the lower limbs and feet, especially the first MTP joint, are the most commonly involved in an initial attack (20). Acute attacks of the ankle, midfoot, and knee, as well as periarticular structures such as tendons, can also occur (19).

Intercritical gout

Many people with uncontrolled hyperuricaemia will go on to experience subsequent attacks (22). Intercritical gout is the asymptomatic phase between acute gout attacks and may range from a few months to several years. The more advanced the disease, the shorter the intercritical periods and the more frequent, prolonged, and disabling the attacks (23). Studies have shown, through synovial fluid aspiration and ultrasound, that, despite the lack of symptoms during the intercritical period, MSU crystal deposition and low-grade inflammation continue (7, 24–26).

Chronic gouty arthropathy and tophaceous gout

Chronic gouty arthropathy involves more frequent attacks with destructive polyarticular involvement and persistent pain (1). Twelve per cent of patients will develop chronic tophaceous gout after 5 years of untreated disease, and 55% after 20 years due to deposits of aggregated MSU crystals (Figure 5.2) (9). Tophi are the result of a chronic inflammatory tissue response to MSU crystals. Microscopically they appear as a central MSU crystalline core encased in a corona zone

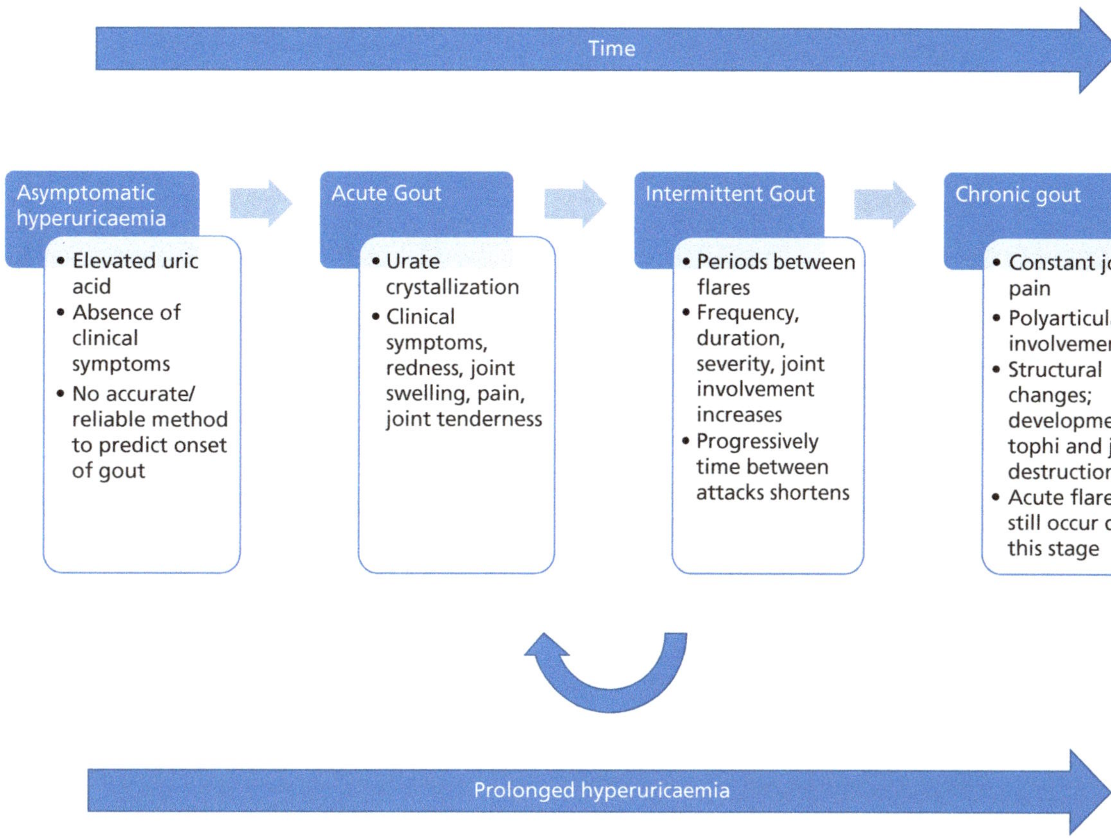

Figure 5.1 Progression of gout over time.

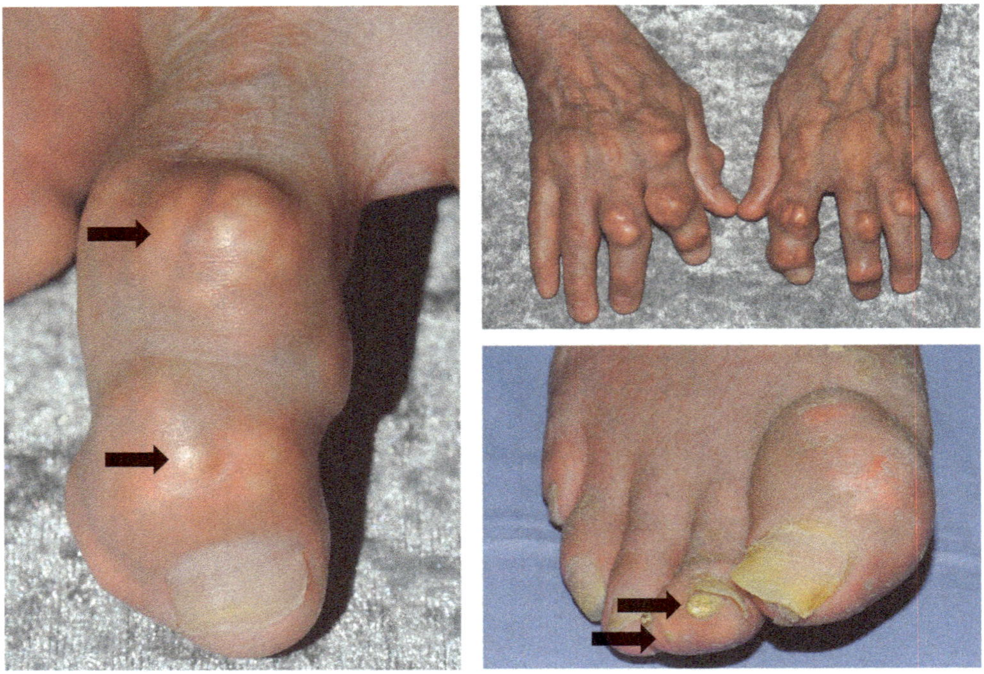

Figure 5.2 Tophaceous gout affecting the right great toe, right second toe and finger interphalangeal joints. Note the asymmetrical swelling and yellow-white discoloration (black arrows).

containing mono- and multi-nucleated immune cells and surrounded by dense fibrovascular tissue (27).

Tophi can form anywhere in the body and typically progress insidiously, but their rate of formation correlates with the degree and duration of hyperuricaemia. Tophi are frequently seen around the knees, over the olecranon process at the elbow, the Achilles tendon (Figure 5.3), and within and around the toe and finger joints—particularly over osteoarthritic Heberden's or Bouchard's nodes (28). They can also form intradermally, appearing as white or yellowish deposits beneath taut overlying skin (Figure 5.2) (29). Although tophi are asymptomatic and acute symptoms during attacks may be adequately controlled, tophaceous gout results in prominent joint damage and musculoskeletal disability (30), causing functional impairment and reduced health-related quality of life (31).

Gout in the foot and ankle

Gout has a predilection for the lower limb, with the first MTP joint and midtarsal joints most commonly affected (32–34). A recent study using dual-energy computed tomography found the first metatarsal head was the site most commonly affected by MSU deposition (38%), followed by the lateral malleolus (25%) and proximal calcaneus (25%) (32). MSU crystal deposition was also observed in the lesser (second to fifth) metatarsals, medial malleolus, talus, navicular, cuboid, and cuneiforms, and Achilles and peroneal tendons.

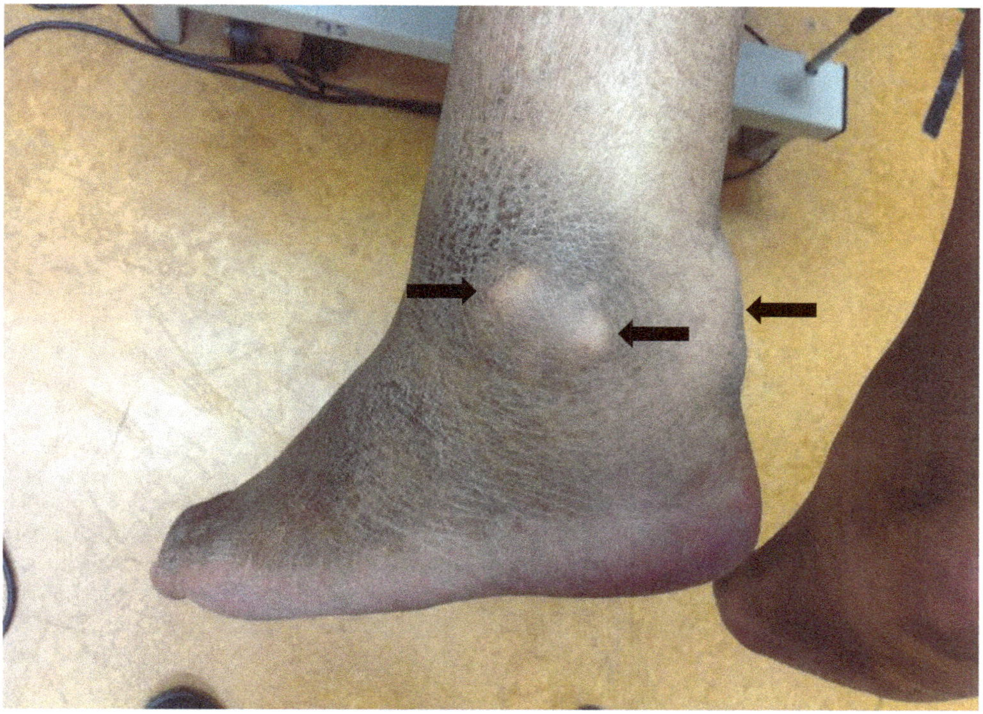

Figure 5.3 Tophaceous deposits in the Achilles tendon and overlying the lateral malleolus (black arrows).

Reproduced from Stewart S, Dalbeth N, Rome K. The impact of gout on the foot: a review. *Gout and Hyperuricaemia*. 2016;**3**:1–8 with permission from *Gout and Hyperuricemia*.

Patients with gout report significant foot pain, impairment, and disability during acute attacks, which cause severe restrictions in activities related to daily living and recreation (35). Importantly, although foot pain reduces by 73% once the attacks resolve, more than half of patients still reported moderate foot-related problems (35). The presence of moderate foot pain during intercritical periods is corroborated by the same authors in additional studies in which patients also reported high-to-severe levels of foot impairment and disability in the absence of acute attack (36, 37). People with gout also had a significantly reduced walking speed compared to healthy controls (36). Difficulty with everyday tasks such as walking has been rated very highly by people with gout as a discriminatory feature of the disease, which emphasizes the extent of foot-related functional disability (38).

Although the physical size of tophi located on the foot and ankle is not as large as those in other areas, such as the elbow (39, 40), in the absence of treatment or with the progression of severe deformity, surgery may occasionally be indicated if associated with mechanical problems (41). However, the mainstay of treatment to shrink and eradicate tophi is pharmacological urate-lowering therapy. Tophaceous gout involving the foot may also interfere with the wearing of properly fitting shoes (42). In fact, gout patients report they give up sport and take days off work because they cannot tolerate shoes or because they cannot walk (2, 43). A study of 50 patients with chronic gouty arthropathy reported that 54% wore shoes that were too narrow to accommodate the foot adequately (37). Over half of the shoes had been worn for more than 12 months and the majority lacked cushioning. Furthermore, their shoes displayed poor motion-control properties, which the authors proposed may contribute to instability and the foot problems seen in people with gout. Generally, tophi are painless, but when in close proximity to joints or when involving tendons they may impair joint function and reduce tendon strength. Tophaceous deposits have been observed to occur frequently in the Achilles and peroneal tendons (Figure 5.3) (32).

Structures involved in the foot and ankle

First metatarsophalangeal joint

The first MTP joint is the most commonly affected site in gout and is regarded as a discriminatory diagnostic feature (38, 44). Between 56% and 78% of first acute attacks occur at the first MTP joint (45), while 59–89% of people will experience a flare in the joint at some point (44, 46). Both chronic first MTP joint pain (16% versus 6%) and hallux valgus (41% versus 25%) are reported more frequently by people with gout than by age- and sex-matched controls without gout (47). A more recent community-based cross-sectional study aimed to determine the prevalence and associations of foot problems in people with gout and to assess the frequency with which they lead to consultation with healthcare professionals (48). The findings reported that hallux valgus (36%), foot pain (23%), and related disability (15%) are common in people with gout and frequently lead to healthcare consultation. Hallux valgus has similar associations to those seen in the general population, whereas foot pain is more common in the obese and those who have had oligoarticular or polyarticular attacks, and disabling foot pain associates with obesity and comorbidity.

The predilection of gout for the first MTP joint is still to be fully explained (34). Despite a similar level of urate supersaturation throughout the body, deposited MSU crystals demonstrate a restricted distribution in joints and other soft tissues (49). The first MTP joint in particular appears to be a frequent target for MSU crystals in both patients with gout (50, 51) and also in people with asymptomatic hyperuricaemia (14, 15). Factors other than hyperuricaemia must contribute to the predilection for gout flares to target this joint and these include temperature, physical trauma, hydrostatic pressure, biomechanical stress, and osteoarthritis (34). A recent New Zealand study reported that people with gout demonstrated first MTP joint-specific changes indicative of subclinical inflammation, even in the absence of acute arthritis (52). People with asymptomatic hyperuricaemia, who exhibit no features or symptoms of gout, also report high levels of foot- and lower limb-related pain and disability (52).

Achilles tendon

A small number of studies have examined the structural, functional, and biomechanical changes in the Achilles tendon resulting from tophaceous gout. Almost one in four people with tophaceous gout have evidence of MSU crystal deposition within the Achilles tendon using dual-energy computed tomography: 38% of these had only non-entheseal involvement, 40% had both entheseal and non-entheseal involvement, and 22% had only entheseal involvement (32). The authors postulate that deposition of MSU crystals in the Achilles tendon may be as a result of increased biomechanical strain. A small observational study found higher serum urate levels in people presenting with Achilles tendon rupture than age- and sex-matched controls (53). The authors postulated that a raised serum urate level may affect tendon nutrition through an effect of proteoglycan metabolism. Fibrillar echotexture of tendons on ultrasound has been shown to be completely deranged by the presence of intratendinous tophus deposits (54).

Disease-specific management and imaging strategies

Major advances have been made in treatment strategies, new therapeutic agents, and the publication of management guidelines by the British Society for Rheumatology (55), European League Against Rheumatism (EULAR) (56), and ACR (57, 58). The fundamental strategy in pharmacological management is long-term urate lowering therapy to achieve MSU crystal dissolution. The ACR guidelines recommend that, for most people with gout, the target serum urate concentration is <6 mg/dL (360 μmol/L). However, a lower target serum urate of <5 mg/dL (300 μmol/L) has been proposed for people with tophi to improve the signs and symptoms of disease (55). The first-line urate-lowering agent is usually allopurinol, followed by febuxostat or a uricosuric drug such as sulfinpyrazone, probenecid, or benzbromarone. In conjunction with intensive urate-lowering therapy, effective anti-inflammatory medications such low-dose colchicine or non-steroidal anti-inflammatory drugs (NSAIDs) to both prevent and treat gout attacks are required in people with tophaceous gout.

Non-pharmacological recommendations center on providing patient education surrounding the role of uric acid in gout, long-term urate treatment targets, dietary, and lifestyle factors (57). Dietary recommendations include avoidance of high purine-containing meats, high fructose beverages or foods, and excessive alcohol. People with gout are encouraged to limit serving sizes of meats and seafood, table sugar, salt, and alcohol, and increase consumption of low-fat or non-fat dairy foods and vegetables (57). Recommendations also include that all people with gout have a clinical examination to evaluate disease activity and burden, with attention to modifiable secondary causes of hyperuricaemia such as comorbidities and medications (57). Ice has been recommended for acute flares (59), and recent research suggests that walking shoes with good cushioning and motion control may reduce foot pain and disability (52). A recent study found that multiple, small areas of ulceration are typical of foot ulceration in gout, particularly chronic tophaceous polyarticular gout (60). Debriding tophi, good wound care management, and advice on good footwear are required to reduce the incidence of foot ulceration in people with gout.

Ultrasound research in crystal arthropathies is still in its infancy (61). The main practical advantages of ultrasound over the other imaging techniques in assessing microcrystal arthropathies include the following: high sensitivity that allows the recognition of crystal aggregates at histological resolution (0.1 mm); non-invasive, quick examination of multiple anatomical areas, allowing a detailed mapping of topography of crystal deposition; safe and reliable guide to aspirate even minimal fluid collection suitable for microscopic analysis at anatomical sites otherwise difficult to reach; short-term therapy monitoring of gouty arthritis; and monitoring of crystal dissolution and tophi reduction induced by urate-lowering therapy at both joint and tendon levels (61).

Recent ultrasound studies have reported that urate crystal deposition is present in some asymptomatic individuals with hyperuricaemia, suggesting that subclinical urate deposition occurs prior to presentation with symptomatic disease (14, 15, 62). Dalbeth et al. (63) reported that it is currently unclear why some hyperuricaemic individuals with urate deposits on advanced imaging do not develop symptomatic gout. Sites of deposition may play a role; for example, periarticular deposition may not lead to clinically apparent disease.

Calcium pyrophosphate crystal deposition

Introduction

Deposition of CPP crystals in articular cartilage, particularly fibrocartilage, is a common age-related phenomenon. CPP crystal deposition (CPPD) can present clinically in four different ways: asymptomatic radiographic cartilage calcification (chondrocalcinosis [CC]), acute attacks

Table 5.1 Revised European League Against Rheumatism terminology for calcium pyrophosphate crystal deposition

Term	Definition	Additional information
Calcium pyrophosphate (CPP) crystals	Simplified name for calcium pyrophosphate dihydrate crystals	
Calcium pyrophosphate deposition (CPPD)	Umbrella term for all instances of CPP crystal occurrence	
Chondrocalcinosis (CC)	Cartilage calcification, identified by imaging or histological identification	Commonly but not always due to CPPD
Clinical presentations associated with CPPD		
Asymptomatic CPPD	CPPD with no apparent clinical consequence	May be either isolated CC or OA with CPPD
Osteoarthritis (OA) with CPPD	CPPD in a joint which also shows changes of OA on imaging or histological examination	
Acute CPP crystal arthritis	Acute onset, self-limiting synovitis with CPPD	Replaces the term 'acute pseudogout'
Chronic CPP crystal inflammatory arthritis	Chronic inflammatory arthritis associated with CPPD	

EULAR, European League Against Rheumatism.

Reproduced from Zhang W, Doherty M, Bardin T et al. European League Against Rheumatism recommendations for calcium pyrophosphate deposition. Part I: terminology and diagnosis. Ann Rheum Dis 2011; **70**:563–570 with permission from the British Medical Journal.

of self-limiting peripheral joint synovitis (acute CPP crystal arthritis), co-occurrence of CPPD with structural changes of osteoarthritis (osteoarthritis with CPPD), and chronic CPP crystal inflammatory arthritis. In 2011, EULAR proposed a revised terminology for CPPD (Table 5.1) (64).

Radiographic CC most commonly occurs at the knee, followed by the wrist (65, 66). The crude community prevalence of radiographic CC at the knee in older adults ranges from 7.0% to 10.4% in studies from the UK, USA, Spain, Italy, and Sweden, with one UK study estimating an age, sex, and knee pain standardized prevalence of 4.5% in those aged 40 years and over (65, 67–70). There was disagreement over the association of CC with sex, with some studies showing no difference between the genders (67, 68) and other studies showing a female preponderance (65, 69, 70). The risk of radiographic CC increases markedly with age, doubling with every 10-year increase in age between 45 and 85 years of age (71). Whilst age is the most important factor predisposing to CPPD, rarely it occurs secondary to metabolic diseases, for example, hereditary haemochromatosis, hypomagnesaemia, hyperparathyroidism, and hypophosphatasia (72). Similar to gout, definitive diagnosis of CPPD requires identification of CPP crystals in synovial fluid aspirates (64).

How calcium pyrophosphate crystal deposition presents in the foot and ankle and structures involved

Acute CPP crystal arthritis presents similarly to acute gout, with sudden onset of severe joint pain that reaches peak intensity within 12–24 hours. Signs of synovitis (joint swelling, erythema, tenderness to touch, and local heat) are usually present. The ankle joint is the third most commonly affected site after the knee and wrist, particularly in men (73). Acute Achilles tendonitis secondary to CPPD is also described (74). The most important differential diagnoses of acute CPP crystal arthritis are acute gout and septic arthritis.

Osteoarthritis with CPPD presents similarly to osteoarthritis, with chronic pain, stiffness, and impaired function. It mainly affects elderly women. Similar to acute CPP crystal arthritis, the ankle is one of the most commonly affected sites after the knee, along with the wrist and shoulder (73). Patients may also experience superimposed attacks of acute CPP crystal arthritis. Physical signs of osteoarthritis such as bony swelling, crepitus, restricted movement, and deformity are usually present, and there may also be evidence of synovitis. Although osteoarthritis with CPPD can resemble uncomplicated osteoarthritis, ankle involvement (which is uncommon in primary osteoarthritis), superimposed acute attacks, or the presence of signs of inflammation are clues to a diagnosis of osteoarthritis with CPPD. Chronic CPP crystal inflammatory arthritis most commonly presents with monoarticular/oligoarticular involvement. Presenting features include pain, morning stiffness, synovitis, and, occasionally, systemic upset, and may resemble rheumatoid arthritis or polymyalgia rheumatica.

Progression of calcium pyrophosphate crystal deposition and presentation over time

Although some patients experience recurrent attacks, the proportion of people with incident acute CPP crystal arthritis who experience a second attack is not known. Recurrent attacks appear to be more common in men than women (73).

The prognosis of osteoarthritis with CPPD appears to be good. In one study, only one-quarter of participants reported symptomatic decline over a mean follow-up period of 4.6 years (75). Although progressive arthropathy was observed at the knee, hip, and shoulder and progressive CC at the knee and wrist, these were infrequent findings and neither arthropathy nor CC appeared to progress at the ankle.

Specific management and imaging strategies

CC is the cardinal radiographic feature of CPPD and is most frequently seen at the knee, wrist, and symphysis pubis. Fine linear calcification may be seen within the Achilles tendon. Although CC is most commonly due to CPPD, other crystals, particularly basic calcium phosphates, can also lead to CC. Furthermore, small CPP crystal deposits may not be visible on radiographs. Hence, definitive diagnosis of CPPD requires identification of CPP crystals in aspirated synovial fluid (64). The radiographic appearances of osteoarthritis with CPPD are CC and radiographic features of osteoarthritis, namely, cartilage loss (joint space narrowing), subchondral cysts and sclerosis, and osteophytes. Osteophytes may have a hypertrophic appearance. In patients with chronic CPP crystal inflammatory arthritis, the absence of marginal erosions is helpful to distinguish from rheumatoid arthritis.

As with gout, there has been much recent interest in using ultrasound to evaluate CPPD. Ultrasound appearances include thin hyperechoic bands, a 'punctuate' pattern consisting of several thin hyperechoic spots, and homogeneous hyperechoic nodular/oval deposits localized in bursae and articular recesses (76). There has also been interest in the 'double contour' sign, hyperechoic enhancement of the superficial margin of articular cartilage, which has been said to be specific to gout (25). However, one recent study suggests that this is a common feature in CPPD also, and, although sensitive and specific for crystal arthritis, distinguishes gout and CPPD less well (77).

Similar to acute gout, treatment of the acute attack aims to provide rapid relief of the pain and inflammation, typically using NSAIDs, colchicine, or corticosteroids (78). There is no long-term definitive pharmacological treatment (akin to allopurinol) for CPPD. Long-term management consists of treating associated osteoarthritis with a combination of pharmacological (for example, paracetamol and topical NSAIDs) and non-pharmacological measures, and treating superimposed attacks of acute CPP crystal arthritis as they arise. Non-pharmacological treatment includes education, weight loss, where appropriate, and local quadriceps strengthening and generalized aerobic fitness exercises. Occasionally, joint replacement surgery is required.

Research agenda and future directions

Despite the common recognition of frequent involvement of the foot and ankle in crystal arthritis, particularly gout, there has been relatively little research specifically into the extent of involvement and how it should be treated. Future research is needed to quantify foot and ankle involvement and the burden it poses and to investigate standardized assessment approaches when investigating patient-reported outcomes specifically relating to the foot in crystal arthritis. Further investigation utilizing advanced imaging techniques should determine the structural characteristics of the joint in relation to clinical features, particularly how the foot and Achilles tendon involvement affects patient-reported outcomes and the ability to carry out daily activities such as walking, and may help to explain the biomechanical role of the first MTP joint in the frequent occurrence of gout at this joint. Assessments of the clinical and cost-effectiveness of non-pharmacological interventions that are specifically aimed at the foot in people with crystal arthritis are much needed.

Recent guidelines for the management of both gout and CPPD provide a roadmap for clinicians for both non-pharmacological and pharmacological management (55–58, 78). Yet, despite these clear guidelines, there are widespread reports of suboptimal management of these conditions (79). Furthermore, these guidelines almost exclusively omit to make specific recommendations about management of foot and ankle problems, which are common in both conditions. The role of customized or off-the-shelf foot orthoses and footwear interventions for both conditions should be considered as future directions because previous studies in gout have found poor footwear to be an issue. Reduced foot and ankle muscle strength associates with foot pain and disability in gout. Future studies should therefore employ advanced imaging methods to explore the relationships between muscle strength and tophi in lower limb and foot musculoskeletal structures and evaluate strengthening exercises and non-pharmacological interventions that specifically target ankle plantar flexion, inversion, and eversion musculature.

References

1. **Brook R, Forsythe A, Smeeding J, et al.** Chronic gout: epidemiology, disease progression, treatment and disease burden. *Curr Med Res Opin*. 2010;**26**:2813–21.
2. **Lindsay K, Gow P, Vanderpyl J, et al.** The experience and impact of living with gout: a study of men with chronic gout using a qualitative grounded theory approach. *J Clin Rheumatol*. 2011;**17**:1–6.
3. **Zhu Y, Pandya BJ, Choi HK.** Prevalence of gout and hyperuricaemia in the US general population: the National Health and Nutrition Examination Survey 2007–2008. *Arthritis Rheum*. 2011;**63**:3136–41.
4. **Kuo C, Grainge M, Mallen C, et al.** Rising burden of gout in the UK but continuing suboptimal management: a nationwide population study. *Ann Rheum Dis*. 2014;**74**:661–7.
5. **Winnard D, Wright C, Taylor WJ, et al.** National prevalence of gout derived from administrative health data in Aotearoa New Zealand. *Rheumatology*. 2012;**51**:901–9.
6. **Zhang W, Doherty M, Bardin T, et al.** EULAR evidence based recommendations for gout. Part I: Diagnosis. Report of a task force of the Standing Committee for International Clinical Studies Including Therapeutics (ESCISIT). *Ann Rheum Dis*. 2006;**65**(10):1301–11.

7. **Pascual E, Batlle-Gualda E, Martínez A, et al.** Synovial fluid analysis for diagnosis of intercritical gout. *Ann Int Med.* 1999;**131**:756–9.
8. **Taylor WJ, Fransen J, Jansen TL, et al.** Study for updated gout classification criteria (SUGAR): identification of features to classify gout. *Arthritis Care Res.* 2015;doi:10.1002/acr.22585
9. **Wallace S, Singer JZ.** Therapy in gout. *Rheum Dis Clin North Am.* 1988;**14**:441–57.
10. **Neogi T, Jansen TL, Dalbeth N, et al.** 2015 Gout classification criteria: an American College of Rheumatology/European League against Rheumatism collaborative initiative. *Ann Rheum Dis.* 2015;**74**:1789–98.
11. **Choi H, Ford ES, Li C, Curhan G.** Prevalence of the metabolic syndrome in patients with gout: the Third National Health and Nutrition Examination Survey. *Arthritis Rheum.* 2007;**57**:109–15.
12. **Krishnan E, Pandya BJ, Lingala B, et al.** Hyperuricaemia and untreated gout are poor prognostic markers among those with a recent acute myocardial infarction. *Arthritis Res Ther.* 2012;**14**:R10.
13. **Liu B, Wang T, Zhao H, et al.** The prevalence of hyperuricaemia in China: a meta-analysis. *BMC Public Health.* 2011;**11**:832.
14. **De Miguel E, Puig JG, Castillo C, et al.** Diagnosis of gout in patients with asymptomatic hyperuricaemia: a pilot ultrasound study. *Ann Rheum Dis.* 2012;**71**:157–8.
15. **Pineda C, Amezcua-Guerra L, Solano C, et al.** Joint and tendon subclinical involvement suggestive of gouty arthritis in asymptomatic hyperuricaemia: an ultrasound controlled study. *Arthritis Res Ther.* 2011;**13**:R4.
16. **Langford H, Blaufax M, Barhani N.** Is thiazide-produced uric acid elevation harmful? Analysis of data from the Hypertension Detection and Follow-up Program. *Arch Int Med.* 1987;**147**:645–9.
17. **Campion EW, Glynn RJ, DeLabry LO.** Asymptomatic hyperuricemia. Risks and consequences in the Normative Aging Study. *Am J Med.* 1987;**82**:421–6.
18. **Doherty M.** New insights into the epidemiology of gout. *Rheumatology.* 2009;**48**:Sii2–ii8.
19. **Grassi W, Angelis R.** Clinical features of gout. *Reumatismo.* 2011;**63**:238–45.
20. **Richette P, Bardin T.** Gout. *Lancet.* 2010;**375**:318–28.
21. **De Leonardis F, Govoni M, Colina M, et al.** Elderly-onset gout: a review. *Rheumatol Int.* 2007;**28**:1–6.
22. **Shoji A, Yamanaka H, Kamatani N.** A retrospective study of the relationship between serum urate level and recurrent attacks of gouty arthritis: evidence for reduction of recurrent gouty arthritis with antihyperuricemic therapy. *Arthritis Rheum.* 2004;**51**:321–5.
23. **Teng G, Nair R, Saag K.** Pathophysiology, clinical presentation and treatment of gout. *Drugs.* 2006;**66**:1547.
24. **Thiele RG, Schlesinger N.** Diagnosis of gout by ultrasound. *Rheumatology.* 2007;**46**:1116–21.
25. **Wright SA, Filippucci E, McVeigh C, et al.** High-resolution ultrasonography of the first metatarsal phalangeal joint in gout: a controlled study. *Ann Rheum Dis.* 2007;**66**:859–64.
26. **Roddy E, Menon A, Hall A, et al.** Polyarticular sonographic assessment of gout: a hospital-based cross-sectional study. *Joint Bone Spine.* 2013;**80**:295–300.
27. **Dalbeth N, Pool B, Gamble G, et al.** Cellular characterization of the gouty tophus: a quantitative analysis. *Arthritis Rheum.* 2010;**62**:1549–56.
28. **De Souza A, Fernandes V, Ferrari, A.** Female gout: clinical and laboratory features. *J Rheumatol.* 2005;**32**:2186–8.
29. **Chopra K, Grossman M.** Images in clinical medicine. Finger-pad tophi. *The New England Journal of Medicine.* 2002;**346**:1714.
30. **Alvarez-Nemegyei J, Cen-Pisté JC, Medina-Escobedo M, et al.** Factors associated with musculoskeletal disability and chronic renal failure in clinically diagnosed primary gout. *J Rheumatol.* 2005;**32**:1923–7.
31. **Chandratre P, Roddy E, Clarson L, Richardson J, Hider SL, Mallen CD.** Health-related quality of life in gout: a systematic review. *Rheumatology.* 2013;**52**:2031–40.
32. **Dalbeth N, Kalluru R, Aati O, et al.** Tendon involvement in the feet of patients with gout: a dual-energy CT study. *Ann Rheum Dis.* 2013;**72**:1545–8.

33. **Grahame R, Scott J.** Clinical survey of 354 patients with gout. *Ann Rheum Dis.* 1970;**29**:461–8.
34. **Roddy E.** Revisiting the pathogenesis of podagra: why does gout target the foot? *J Foot Ankle Res.* 2011;**4**:13.
35. **Rome K, Frecklington M, McNair P, et al.** Foot pain, impairment, and disability in patients with acute gout flares: a prospective observational study. *Arthritis Care Res.* 2012;**64**:384–8.
36. **Rome K, Survepalli D, Sanders A, et al.** Functional and biomechanical characteristics of foot disease in chronic gout: a case-control study. *Clin Biomech.* 2011a;**26**:90–4.
37. **Rome K, Frecklington M, McNair P, et al.** Footwear characteristics and factors influencing footwear choice in patients with gout. *Arthritis Care Res.* 2011b;**63**:1599–604.
38. **Prowse RL, Dalbeth N, Kavanaugh A, et al.** A Delphi exercise to identify characteristic features of gout: opinions from patients and physicians, the first stage in developing new classification criteria. *J Rheumatol.* 2013;**40**:1–9.
39. **Schumacher H, Becker M, Palo W, et al.** Tophaceous gout: quantitative evaluation by direct physical measurement. *J Rheumatol.* 2005;**32**:2368–72.
40. **Schumacher H, Becker M, Edwards N, et al.** Magnetic resonance imaging in the quantitative assessment of gouty tophi. *Int J Clin Pract.* 2006;**60**:408–14.
41. **Kumar S, Gow P.** A survey of indications, results and complications of surgery for tophaceous gout. *NZ Med J.* 2002;**115**:1–4.
42. **Stewart S, Vandal AV, Gow P, et al.** The effect of good and poor walking shoe characteristics on plantar pressure and gait in people with gout. *Clin Biomech.* 2014;**29**:1158–63.
43. **Martini N, Bryant L, Karu L, et al.** Living with gout in New Zealand: an exploratory study into people's knowledge about the disease and its treatment. *J Clin Rheumatol.* 2012;**18**:125–30.
44. **Peláez-Ballestas I, Hernández Cuevas C, Burgos-Vargas R, et al.** Diagnosis of chronic gout: evaluating the American College of Rheumatology proposal, European league against rheumatism recommendations, and clinical judgment. *J Rheumatol.* 2010;**37**:1743–8.
45. **Johnson P, Fayad L, Fishman E.** CT of the foot: selected inflammatory arthridites. *J Computer Assist Tomogr.* 2007;**31**:961–9.
46. **Roddy E, Zhang W, Doherty M.** Are joints affected by gout also affected by osteoarthritis? *Ann Rheum Dis.* 2007a;**66**:1374–7.
47. **Roddy E, Zhang W, Doherty M.** Gout and nodal osteoarthritis: a case-control study. *Rheumatology.* 2008;**47**:732–3.
48. **Roddy E, Muller S, Rome K, et al.** Foot problems in people with gout in primary care: baseline findings from a prospective cohort study. *J Foot Ankle Res.* 2015b;**8**:31.
49. **McGill N, Dieppe P.** Evidence for a promoter of urate crystal formation in gouty synovial fluid. *Ann Rheum Dis.* 1991;**50**:558–61.
50. **Choi H, Al-Arfaj A, Eftekhari A, et al.** Dual energy computed tomography in tophaceous gout. *Ann Rheum Dis.* 2009;**68**:1609–12.
51. **Kim SK, Lee H, Kim JH, et al.** Potential interest of dual-energy computed tomography in gout: focus on anatomical distribution and clinical association. *Rheumatology.* 2013;**52**:402–3.
52. **Stewart S, Dalbeth N, Vandal AC, Rome K.** Characteristics of the first metatarsophalangeal joint in gout and asymptomatic hyperuricaemia: a cross-sectional study. *J Foot Ankle Res.* 2015;**8**:41.
53. **Dodds W, Burry, H.** The relationship between Achilles tendon rupture and serum uric acid level. *Injury.* 1984;**16**:94–5.
54. **Grassi W, Meenagh G, Pascual E, et al.** 'Crystal clear': sonographic assessment of gout and calcium pyrophosphate deposition disease. *Sem Arthritis Rheum.* 2006;**36**:197–202.
55. **Hui M, Carr A, Cameron S, et al.** The British Society for Rheumatology Guideline for the Management of Gout. *Rheumatology (Oxford).* 2017;**56**(7):1056–9.

56. **Richette P, Doherty M, Pascual E, et al.** 2016 updated EULAR evidence-based recommendations for the management of gout. *Ann Rheum Dis.* 2017;**76**(1):29–42.
57. **Khanna D, Fitzgerald JD, Khanna PP, et al.** 2012 American College of Rheumatology guidelines for management of gout. Part 1: systematic non-pharmacologic and pharmacologic therapeutic approaches to hyperuricemia. *Arthritis Care Res.* 2012a;**64**:1431–46.
58. **Khanna D, Khanna PP, Fitzgerald JD, et al.** 2012 American College of Rheumatology guidelines for management of gout. Part 2: therapy and anti-inflammatory prophylaxis of acute gouty arthritis. *Arthritis Care Res.* 2012b;**64**:1447–61.
59. **Schlesinger N, Detry MA, Holland BK, et al.** Local ice therapy during bouts of acute gouty arthritis. *J Rheumatol.* 2002;**29**:331–4.
60. **Rome K, Erikson K, Otene C, Sahid H, Sangster K, Gow P.** Clinical characteristics of foot ulceration in people with chronic gout. *Int Wound J.* 2016;**13**:209–15.
61. **Grassi W, Okanoa T, Filippuccia E.** Use of ultrasound for diagnosis and monitoring of outcomes in crystal arthropathies. *Curr Opin Rheumatol.* 2015;**27**:147–55.
62. **Kimura-Hayama E, Criales-Vera S, Nicolaou S, et al.** A pilot study on dual-energy computed tomography for detection of urate deposits in renal transplant patients with asymptomatic hyperuricaemia. *J Clin Rheumatol.* 2014;**20**:306–9.
63. **Dalbeth N, House M, Aati O, et al.** Urate crystal deposition in asymptomatic hyperuricaemia and symptomatic gout: a dual energy CT study. *Ann Rheum Dis.* 2015;**74**:908–11.
64. **Zhang W, Doherty M, Bardin T, et al.** European League Against Rheumatism recommendations for calcium pyrophosphate deposition. Part I: terminology and diagnosis. *Ann Rheum Dis.* 2011;**70**:563–70.
65. **Bergstrom G, Bjelle A, Sundh V, Svanborg A.** Joint disorders at ages 70, 75 and 79 years: a cross-sectional comparison. *Br J Rheumatol.* 1986;**25**:333–41.
66. **Zhang Y, Terkeltaub R, Nevitt M, et al.** Lower prevalence of chondrocalcinosis in Chinese subjects in Beijing than in white subjects in the United States: the Beijing Osteoarthritis Study. *Arthritis Rheum.* 2006;**54**:3508–12.
67. **Neame RL, Carr AJ, Muir K, Doherty M.** UK community prevalence of knee chondrocalcinosis: evidence that correlation with osteoarthritis is through a shared association with osteophyte. *Ann Rheum Dis.* 2003;**62**:513–18.
68. **Felson DT, Anderson JJ, Naimark A, Kannel W, Meenan RF.** The prevalence of chondrocalcinosis in the elderly and its association with knee osteoarthritis: the Framingham Study. *J Rheumatol.* 1989;**16**:1241–5.
69. **Sanmarti R, Panella D, Brancos MA, et al.** Prevalence of articular chondrocalcinosis in elderly subjects in a rural area of Catalonia. *Ann Rheum Dis.* 1993;**52**:418–22.
70. **Ramonda R, Musacchio E, Perissinotto E, et al.** Prevalence of chondrocalcinosis in Italian subjects from northeastern Italy. The Pro.V.A. (PROgetto Veneto Anziani) study. *Clin Exp Rheumatol.* 2009;**27**:981–4.
71. **Zhang W, Neame R, Doherty S, Doherty M.** Relative risk of knee chondrocalcinosis in siblings of index cases with pyrophosphate arthropathy. *Ann Rheum Dis.* 2004;**63**:969–73.
72. **Richette P, Bardin T, Doherty M.** An update on the epidemiology of calcium pyrophosphate dihydrate crystal deposition disease. *Rheumatology.* 2009;**48**:711–15.
73. **Dieppe PA, Alexander GJ, Jones HE, et al.** Pyrophosphate arthropathy: a clinical and radiological study of 105 cases. *Ann Rheum Dis.* 1982;**41**:371–6.
74. **Gerster JC, Lagier R, Boivin G.** Achilles tendinitis associated with chondrocalcinosis. *J Rheumatol.* 1980;**7**:82–8.
75. **Doherty M, Dieppe P, Watt I.** Pyrophosphate arthropathy: a prospective study. *Br J Rheumatol.* 1993;**32**:189–96.

76. **Frediani B, Filippou G, Falsetti P, et al.** Diagnosis of calcium pyrophosphate dihydrate crystal deposition disease: ultrasonographic criteria proposed. *Ann Rheum Dis.* 2005;**64**:638–40.
77. **Löffler C, Sattler H, Peters L, et al.** Distinguishing gouty arthritis from calcium pyrophosphate disease and other arthritides. *J Rheumatol.* 2015;**42**:513–20.
78. **Zhang W, Doherty M, Pascual E, et al.** EULAR recommendations for calcium pyrophosphate deposition. Part II: management. *Ann Rheum Dis.* 2011;**70**:571–5.
79. **Stamp L, Merrimen T, Barclay M, et al.** Impaired response or insufficient dosage? Examining the potential causes of 'inadequate response' to allopurinol in the treatment of gout. *Sem Arthritis Rheum.* 2014;**44**:170–4.

Chapter 6

Rheumatoid arthritis

Mike Backhouse and Heidi Siddle

Rheumatoid arthritis (RA) is the most common autoimmune inflammatory arthropathy (1, 2). It is a chronic, progressive disorder with synovial inflammation typically producing a symmetrical arthropathy and progressive joint destruction if left untreated (3, 4). Whilst there is marked heterogeneity in disease outcomes, disability, surgery, and increased mortality result in considerable personal, social, and economic impact (3, 5–10).

Epidemiology

Rheumatoid arthritis is a global disease, with between 0.5% and 1% of the world's adult population affected. This varies between populations, with a lower prevalence reported in rural sub-Saharan Africa and high prevalence in specific native American tribes (1, 2). As is the case with most autoimmune diseases, RA affects women more frequently than men, with a female to male ratio of 2.7:1 and prevalence of 1.16% and 0.44% in the UK, respectively (11).

The disease can occur at any age, with the peak onset being between the third and fourth decade in life (3). Although the prevalence increases with age in both sexes, the difference between the sexes decreases in older patients, which can be explained by the decreasing incidence in postmenopausal women (12).

Aetiology

Although the exact cause of RA remains elusive, genetic and environmental factors play a role throughout the disease course (Figure 6.1) (1, 13).

Genetic factors are important in susceptibility to RA. Family studies demonstrate that first-degree relatives of people with RA develop the disease at a higher rate than the general population, and twin studies have revealed 15% disease concordance in monozygotic twins compared to 4% in dizygotic twins (14).

The fact that RA concordance is not 100% in monozygotic twins indicates that non-genetic factors must play a role. Smoking is an important environmental factor and has long been associated with an increased risk of developing seropositive disease, especially in men. A large population-based case control-study (858 cases, 1048 controls) showed a striking gene–environment interaction between smoking and HLA-DRB1 genotypes (Table 6.1) (15). The genetic risk factor of shared epitope homozygosity conveyed a relative risk of developing seropositive RA of 4.2, which was then dramatically increased to 15.7 in current smokers. Smoking also diminishes response to biologic therapies, with current heavy smokers having the poorest response (16, 17). Other environmental factors, such as infectious agents (e.g., Epstein–Barr virus and cytomegalovirus), bacteria

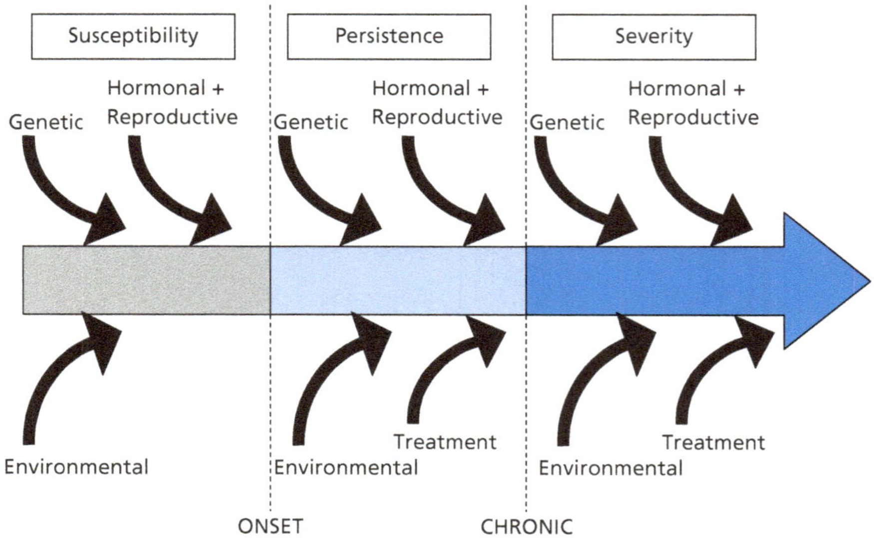

Figure 6.1 Contributory factors to the three phases of the natural history of rheumatoid arthritis.

Adapted from Symmons, D.P.M., Epidemiology of rheumatoid arthritis: determinants of onset, persistence and outcome. *Best Practice & Research in Clinical Rheumatology*, 2002. **16**(5): p. 707–22 with permission from Elsevier.

in periodontal disease (e.g., *Porphyromonas gingivalis*), and the gastrointestinal microbiome, are also gaining evidence as potential contributory factors (18, 19).

An increased prevalence amongst women, which is almost halved amongst those who have ever taken the oral contraceptive pill, suggests that female hormones play a role in developing the disease (1). Sex also plays a role in disease course, with a number of studies reporting increased functional disability, poorer outcome, and increased likelihood of requiring orthopaedic surgery in women (1, 6, 20).

Table 6.1 Relative risk of developing seropositive rheumatoid arthritis according to smoking and presence of shared epitope genes

Smoking status	SE genotype	Relative risk	95% CI
Never	Any SE	2.8	1.6–4.8
Never	Double SE	4.2	2.1–8.3
Current	No	2.4	1.3–4.6
Current	Any SE	7.5	4.2–13.1
Current	Double SE	15.7	7.2–34.2

CI, Confidence interval; SE, shared epitope.

Reproduced from Padyukov, L., et al., A gene–environment interaction between smoking and shared epitope genes in HLA-DR provides a high risk of seropositive rheumatoid arthritis. *Arthritis & Rheumatism*, 2004. **50**(10): p. 3085–92 with permission from Wiley.

Pathogenesis of rheumatoid arthritis

Insights into the pathogenesis of RA have transformed care. New knowledge has led to the development of targeted pharmacological therapies that have transformed patient outcomes.

RA is an autoimmune disease where recognition of 'self' antigens is abnormal and this loss of 'self' tolerance leads to the inflammation and joint destruction. Despite being a disease primarily of synovium, it increasingly appears that the initial loss of self-tolerance starts in barrier tissues such as the lungs and gastrointestinal tract. Here, environmental stressors (e.g., smoking, silica, changes in microbiome) lead to post-transformational modifications and citrullination of mucosal proteins (19). Loss of immune tolerance to these neoepitopes then elicits production of anticitrullinated protein antibodies (ACPA) detectable with a diagnostic anti-cyclic citrullinated peptide (CCP) assay (21). We now know that much of this occurs before the onset of joint symptoms, but it is not clear exactly how a sustained inflammatory response then develops within the joint. This probably occurs through a poorly understood mechanism involving microvascular, neurologic, biomechanical, or other tissue-specific pathways (19).

Synovitis is caused when a plethora of cells enters the synovium via activated endothelial cells expressing adhesion molecules (13). Within the synovium, antigens are presented to T cells (primarily CD4+ T cells) by antigen-presenting cells (APCs) such as dendritic cells, macrophages, or activated B cells (3). These activated T cells stimulate monocytes, macrophages, and synovial fibroblasts to secrete key inflammatory cytokines such as interleukin-1 (IL-1), IL-6, tumour necrosis factor-α (TNF-α), and matrix metalloproteinases (MMPs) (22).

Activated T cells also stimulate B cells to produce various cell-surface molecules such as CD20 and CD22 and differentiate into autoantibody-producing cells, which secrete rheumatoid factor and further anti-CCP antibodies (13). Activated B cells in turn act as APCs, leading to T cell activation and a self-perpetuation of the autoimmune response (23).

Histological changes in joints in rheumatoid arthritis

The changes in the inflamed synovium of patients with RA are histologically striking (2). In the early stages of the disease, the most evident feature is tissue inflammation and oedema, which manifests clinically as joint swelling and pain. Within a short period the usually thin synovial lining becomes hyperplastic and commonly thickens to become 10 or more cells deep (24). Concurrent cellular infiltration consisting primarily of mononuclear cells, and blood vessel generation (angiogenesis) and proliferation is also observed (Figure 7.2).

The formation of locally invasive pannus is a distinctive feature of RA and is histologically separate from other regions of synovium (25). Pannus is rich in macrophages and fibroblast-like synoviocytes, which produce large amounts of destructive protease enzymes called MMPs (22). Together with receptor activator of nuclear factor kappa-B ligand (RANKL)-enhanced osteoclast activity, these MMPs play a key role in bone destruction, leading to the hallmark periarticular osteoporosis and focal erosions seen in RA (26, 27). The osteoclastogenic effect of RANKL is in turn further enhanced via proinflammatory cytokines such as TNF, IL-1, IL-6, and IL-17 (28).

Clinical features of rheumatoid arthritis

As with most diseases, the clinical presentation of RA is driven by the underlying pathophysiology. In addition to the classic symmetrical articular symptoms of swelling, pain, stiffness, and deformity, extra-articular symptoms in the cardiovascular, pulmonary, endocrine, neurological, and wider skeletal systems are increasingly recognized (19).

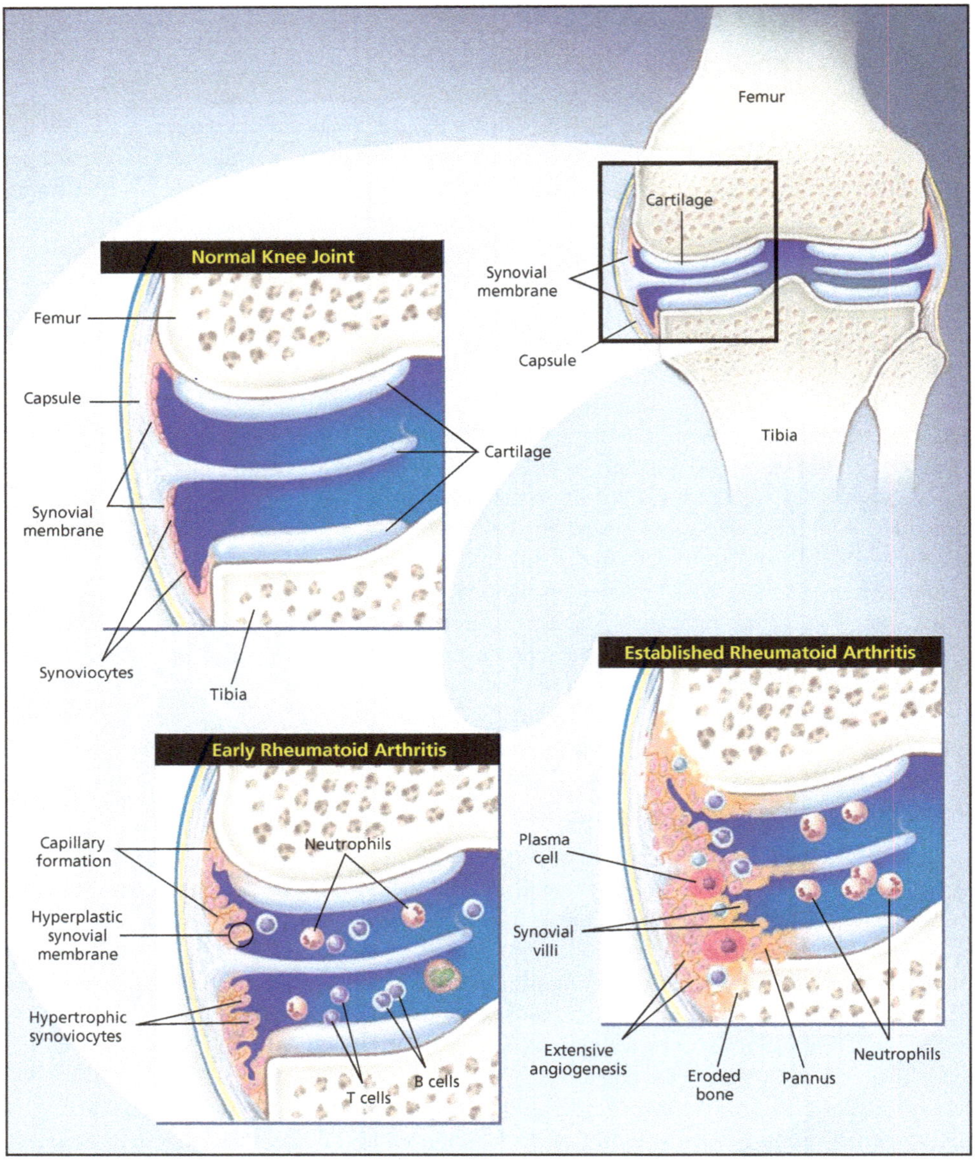

Figure 6.2 Progression of histological changes of joints in rheumatoid arthritis.

Reproduced from Choy, E.H. and G.S. Panayi, Cytokine pathways and joint inflammation in rheumatoid arthritis. *N Engl J Med*, 2001. **344**(12): p. 907–16 © 2001 Massachusetts Medical Society. Reprinted with permission from Massachusetts Medical Society.

However, the course of RA and the initial presentation can be highly variable between people. Although some patients present with rapid onset of the disease with symptoms such as fever and polyarthritis, a gradual and insidious onset is more common. Disease severity, rate of progression, and extent of joint damage are equally heterogeneous between people and, of course, fluctuate within individual patients over time (29, 30).

The foot and ankle at disease onset

The classic symptom at disease onset is joint pain and those with more dramatic onset may present with fever. Typically, the disease will present in symmetrical swelling of the proximal interphalangeal (PIP) joints, metacarpophalangeal (MCP) joints, the wrists, or metatarsophalangeal (MTP) joints. However, those with a more insidious onset may present with an oligoarthritis or monoarthritis. Joints with inflammation are painful, swollen, and stiff to move, and patients often describe a classic 'morning stiffness', which eases as the day progresses. Other common symptoms include fatigue and loss of energy.

Increasing emphasis is placed on the early diagnosis of people with RA to enable timely initiation of effective therapies and prevention of subsequent disease progression. Indeed, delays at this stage can have a marked impact on the long-term outcome of people with RA, yet delays are frequent and widespread (31).

With foot involvement as the second most common site of disease onset and foot involvement described as a 'hallmark of early RA' (32, 33), people with new undiagnosed inflammatory arthritis often present to services such as podiatry. Therefore all clinicians treating foot and ankle problems should be able to recognize symptoms of early inflammatory arthritis, and know local routes for onward referral to enable prompt diagnosis and treatment (33). Current guidelines (34, 35) differ slightly but are clear that clinicians should rapidly refer patients to a rheumatologist in the event of *clinical suspicion of RA*, which may be supported by the following:

- Three or more swollen joints
- MTP/MCP joint involvement
- Squeeze test positive pressure applied across the MTP or MCP joints simultaneously
- Morning stiffness of ≥30 minutes.

It should be noted that normal blood tests and X-rays may be normal in the early stages of disease and should not preclude referral (35).

Many readers will be familiar with the 1987 American College of Rheumatology (ACR) criteria for RA (36). These became the benchmark for defining RA but were limited in that they were developed to discriminate those with established RA from people with other rheumatological diagnoses. They were therefore not helpful in identifying those with early disease and were criticized for being insensitive in this population. As treatment paradigms progressed, a new classification criteria for RA was developed by ACR and the European League Against Rheumatism (EULAR) in 2010 (Table 6.2) (37).

The 2010 criteria are now the internationally recognized standard and are widely used. However, it should be noted that the authors were at pains to point out that these are 'classification criteria' rather than 'diagnostic criteria' and are designed to be used on a population level (37). They do not remove the onus from individual rheumatologists of reaching a diagnosis on individual patients, some of whom will present in atypical ways. Perhaps, more importantly in the context of this book, the 2010 criteria should not be used by clinicians to consider which patients to refer to a rheumatologist. Instead, clinicians should follow the guidelines for referral.

Disease-disability pathway

When considering the concept of disability and disease impact, it is important to consider it in the context of the biopsychosocial model of health rather than the older medical model of disease. Perhaps the best explanation of this lies within the World Health Organization's (WHO) International Classification of Functioning, Disability and Health (ICF) whereby the ICF recognizes that a person's functional ability is determined by the interaction between features of

Table 6.2 The 2010 American College of Rheumatology/European League Against Rheumatism classification criteria for rheumatoid arthritis

	Score
Target population (who should be tested?). Patients who: 1) With at least 1 joint with definite clinical synovitis (swelling) 2) With synovitis not better explained by another disease	
Classification criteria for RA (score-based algorithm: add score of categories A–D: a score of ≥6/10 is needed for classification of a patient as having definite RA	
A. Joint involvement	
1 large joint	0
2–10 large joints	1
1–3 small joints (with or without involvement of large joints)	2
4–10 small joints (with or without large joints)	3
>10 joints (at least 1 small joint)	5
B. Serology (at least 1 test result is needed for classification)	
Negative RF *and* negative ACPA	0
Low positive RF *or* low positive ACPA	2
High positive *or* high positive ACPA	3
C. Acute-phase reactants (at least 1 test is needed for classification)	
Normal CRP *and* normal ESR	0
Abnormal CRP *or* normal ESR	1
D. Duration of symptoms	
<6 weeks	0
≥6 weeks	1

ACPA, Anticitrullinated protein antibodies; CRP, C-reactive protein; ESR, erythrocyte sedimentation rate; RA, rheumatoid arthritis; RF, rheumatoid factor.

Reprinted from Aletaha, D., et al., 2010. Rheumatoid arthritis classification criteria: an American College of Rheumatology/European League Against Rheumatism collaborative initiative. *Arthritis and Rheumatism*, 2010. **62**(9): p. 2569–81 with permission from Wiley.

the person (biopsycho) and the overall context in which the person lives (social) (38, 39). Indeed, within the ICF, functional ability is viewed as the outcome of bidirectional interactions between 'health condition' and 'contextual factors', which encompass *environmental* and *personal* factors. Environmental factors make up the physical, social, and attitudinal environment in which people live and conduct their lives (40). Finally, personal factors refer to the individual person, and include factors such as age, sex, social status, and life experiences (41).

With its hallmark joint pain, swelling, and destruction, it is well recognized that RA can cause significant functional impairment, and this is expanded upon in Chapter 11. Observational studies have identified that even at the point of diagnosis 57% of people with RA report walking disability (42). Van der Leeden et al. noted that, after the first year, the prevalence of walking disability, as reported by the walking subscale of the Health Assessment Questionnaire (HAQ), dropped to approximately 40% and stayed relatively stable around that point for the 8-year follow-up period.

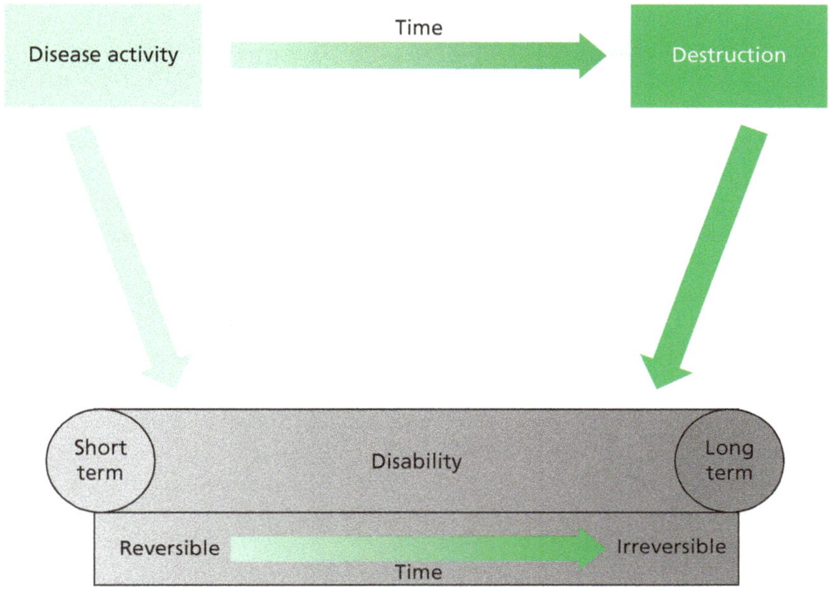

Figure 6.3 The disease disability pathway showing relationship between disease activity, joint destruction, and the reversible and irreversible components of disability.

Adapted from *The Lancet*, 370(9602), Smolen, J.S., et al., New therapies for treatment of rheumatoid arthritis, p. 1861–74, Copyright (2007), with permission from Elsevier.

However, the severity of walking disability continued to increase, slowly, amongst those affected. These data raise several important points, and perhaps one of the most striking is the ~17% reduction in reported walking disability within the first year following diagnosis. Why does this reduction occur? To answer this question, we must consider how RA affects joints.

In the early stages of RA functional impairment is largely influenced by joint pain, swelling, and the consequences of RA such as fatigue and depression, and is thought to be driven by active inflammation. Effective pharmacological control can suppress the inflammation and lead to a reduction in symptoms and therefore restoration of function: hence the ~17% reduction in walking disability reported by van der Leeden et al. (42). In other words, inflammation is the main driver of disability in the early stages of RA, whereas accrued damage dominates later in the disease course (Figure 6.3). Potential factors contributing to the irreversible component of functional limitation include joint destruction, deformity, tendon damage, and comorbidities linked to RA (such as cardiovascular disease). Other studies have found similar results, but it is important to note that at any one time there is a reversible and irreversible component to a person's functional limitation, and that the ability to reverse functional limitation reduces over time (43).

Systemic treatment of rheumatoid arthritis

Advances in the understanding of the pathophysiological processes involved in RA have led to a revolution in pharmacological treatment and subsequent patient outcomes. Whereas a few years ago treatment was largely palliative, now, treatment paradigms focus on early identification of patients with inflammatory arthritis and initiation of treatment within a 3-month window of opportunity. Rapid induction of remission or low disease activity through escalation of therapies and an ongoing 'treat to target' approach guided by imaging, clinical assessment, and serological tests aims to suppress inflammation and maintain patients' quality of life.

Conventional synthetic disease-modifying antirheumatic drugs (DMARDs) such as methotrexate remain the cornerstone of disease management and are recommended as first-line agents, either in combination or as monotherapy where combination therapy is contraindicated (35, 44). Biologic drugs are much larger molecules designed to inhibit specific cytokine activity or deplete specific immune cells, and are produced in genetically modified bacteria. These have been available for over a decade now but molecules aimed at new targets continue to be developed. Their use is still largely limited to second-line therapies within guidelines, but recent studies have suggested that they may be more potent if used as a first-line therapy (45, 46).

Following the end of patent restrictions, particularly for some of the original TNF inhibitors, new biosimilar molecules are increasingly available and at considerably lower cost. As such, the use of biosimilars is increasing rapidly in practice in parallel with efforts to capture long-term safety and effectiveness data. Other new pharmacological therapies include a renewed focus on small molecules that target specific intracellular pathway (e.g., JAK-STAT) (47, 48). Unlike the large biologic molecules these much smaller, synthetic molecules can be taken orally, which avoids the need for injections or infusions. Some of these have already received approval for use from regulatory bodies and have shown promise in early studies (49).

Despite the ongoing revolution in the pharmacological management of RA, it is clear that sustained remission does not occur in the majority of people with RA, and that foot disease continues to impact upon people's lives. RA affects multiple organ systems and many facets of a person's life, so effective holistic, patient-centred therapy requires input from a coordinated multidisciplinary team (MDT).

Rheumatoid arthritis and foot disease

It is widely understood that the development and severity of foot problems in patients with RA increases with the duration of active inflammation (50–55). As well as the contribution of synovitis the most important factor leading to bone damage and deformity is likely to be mechanical stresses as a result of weightbearing. The foot has multiple soft-tissue structures such as ligaments, joint capsules, and tendons which play an important part in supporting the alignment of the foot. Active inflammation weakens these and, together with the mechanical stresses of weightbearing and ambulation, this results in foot pain and pathomechanical deformities.

Prevalence of foot disease

RA is predominantly a disease of the peripheral joints. During the past 40 years cross-sectional studies of patient-reported foot involvement have continually demonstrated symptoms at the start of their disease (42, 56–60), almost as frequently as initial symptoms reported in the hands. Forefoot involvement has been identified in up to 45% of the patients at the start of their disease; this is in comparison to only 17% of patients complaining of rearfoot or ankle involvement (57). The forefoot is described as the most common site of symptoms in the foot and ankle of patients with RA, with pain across the MTP joints being identified as the most frequent cause (42, 52, 57, 59, 61).

In a UK cohort of 585 people with RA, 93.5% of people had experienced foot pain during the course of their disease, with 62.1% reporting current foot pain (59). Despite the introduction of more aggressive therapies such as TNF inhibitors, the prevalence of foot pain and foot joint involvement does not appear to be diminishing (57, 62). Recent evidence from a large Dutch cohort study of 848 patients also detected painful and/or swollen MTP joints in a substantial proportion of patients classified as being in disease remission (Disease Activity Score for 28 joints [DAS28] < 2.6 [63]) (64).

The prevalence of erosive foot disease relies on data from radiographic studies, which we know are unlikely to be accurate in current-day rheumatology practice with the use of magnetic resonance imaging (MRI) and ultrasound imaging to detect erosions much earlier in the disease process. Erosions are most frequently seen at the fifth MTP joint at both disease onset and during the course of the disease, and least frequently at the second MTP joint (42, 65). With respect to the rest of the foot, historical radiographic studies have identified the talonavicular joint as the most frequently affected joint (31.5%) (52). Radiographic changes at the ankle joint (tibiotalar joint) and subtalar joint occur in about a quarter of patients with subtalar joint pathology, greatly increasing between 5 and 10 years of disease duration and regularly preceding changes in the ankle joint. However, rearfoot and ankle disease is rarely seen without midtarsal and MTP joint radiographic changes (52, 61, 66).

In summary, in patients with RA the forefoot appears to be involved early in the disease process, with the most destructive disease occurring at the fifth MTP joint. However, the forefoot has been studied in greater detail than the rearfoot and ankle, and therefore a true representation is not likely to have been reported.

Forefoot disease

The forefoot is the most common site of symptoms within the foot, and people with RA frequently present with pain across the MTP joints (42). 'Walking on pebbles/marbles/stones' is a sensation that patients often describe whether they are newly diagnosed and present with no obvious forefoot deformity or have longstanding disease and significant forefoot deformity.

The forefoot sensation described above is typically the result of synovitis of the MTP joints, which is a significant feature of both early and active disease. Synovitis results in localized pain and swelling, and, because of its symmetrical nature, usually affects all the MTP joints, leading to deformities such as hallux valgus, forefoot widening, hammer and claw toes, subluxation and dislocation of the joints, and plantar bursae (51, 58, 67) (Figure 6.4). Proliferation and oedema of the synovium leads to separation of the toes, known as the 'day-light' sign (Figure 6.4a), resulting in stretching and weakening of the joint capsule and loss of integrity of the stabilizing structures such as the collateral ligaments and plantar plate (68, 69). As a consequence, it is proposed that the

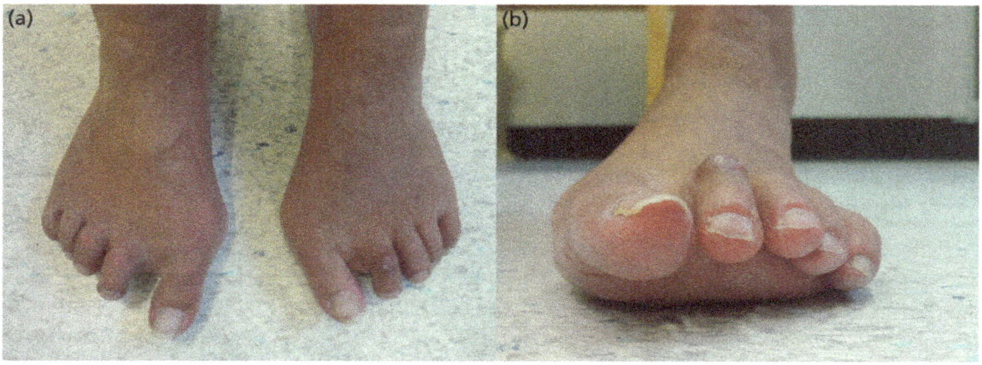

Figure 6.4 (a) Typical hallux valgus deformity with widening of the forefoot in rheumatoid arthritis. (b) Hammered and clawed toes as a result of subluxation and dislocation of the metatarsophalangeal joints, producing separation of the toes, contributing to a broader forefoot.

combination of subluxation and eventual dislocation of the MTP joints occurs together with an imbalance between the intrinsic and extrinsic muscles of the foot, resulting in forefoot deformity, including progressive hammer or claw toes (61). The hallux also loses its capsular integrity and deviates laterally from the long axis of the metatarsal into a valgus position.

Evidence during the past 10 years suggests a relationship between local stresses, joint damage from active disease, and painful symptoms in the forefoot (70, 71). Inflammatory and mechanical factors have a role to play in determining severity of pathology at the MTP joints in patients with RA, with recent evidence supporting the hypothesis of a relationship between biomechanical demands in the foot and inflammatory bone changes (72). MRI studies have demonstrated that damage to plantar structures such as the capsule and plantar plate of the MTP joints is more common at the fifth MTP joint, the most common site of erosions in the painful forefoot of patients with RA (73, 74). Ultimately, further longitudinal follow-up is required to determine the specific mechanism of forefoot pathology in patients with RA.

Midfoot disease

Clinicians will be familiar with patients exclaiming that 'my arch has dropped'. Clinically this is known as flattening of the medial longitudinal arch and is a characteristic change reported in up to half of patients with RA. The pathomechanical process leading to this deformity has not been clearly elucidated in the literature owing to the limited studies conducted and the complex nature of such deformity. Arthritis of the talonavicular and subtalar joints was reported to be much more common in patients with RA and a flattening of the foot. Historically it has been suggested that these changes are not seen in early disease, although admittedly such studies used relatively insensitive X-rays, so it is speculated that arthritis at these joints results from mechanical stresses on weakened and inflamed joints and soft-tissue structures, including the tibialis posterior tendon (52, 68). A more recent study of lateral weightbearing X-rays has suggested two different patterns of flattening of the foot with RA; in the first group there was plantar dislocation of the talar head and subluxation of the subtalar joint, but in the second group the subtalar joint was affected without destruction of the talonavicular joint (75). Again, this study relies on plain film X-ray, which is ultimately a 2D projection of a complex 3D structure. Previous experience has shown that, even in relatively simple structures such as the knee, the story is likely to be more complex when studied in true 3D. Furthermore, studies in osteoarthritis have shown that relying on a single view underestimates the presence of midfoot disease. The tibialis posterior tendon is a significant stabilizer of the midfoot as well as the rearfoot, and pathologies such as tenosynovitis (Figure 6.5) and tendinopathy are associated with the commonly reported flattened foot, also known as pes plano valgus deformity. Recent electromyography studies have highlighted once again that the combination of inflammation and mechanical dysfunction coexists to lead to foot impairment and related disability (76).

Rearfoot and ankle disease

Valgus or an everted deformity of the rearfoot (Figure 6.6) is a typical feature of foot disease in patients with RA. The level of rearfoot valgus deformity has been shown to increase with disease duration, especially in the first 5 years (51, 52, 68, 77). Positive correlations occur between rearfoot pain and progressive valgus deformity (53, 58, 68). Reduced range of motion at the ankle and subtalar joints is also seen in this group of patients with valgus deformity of the rearfoot. Although deformity increases with disease duration, clinical synovitis diminishes after 10 years (51, 53). In the majority of patients the rearfoot valgus deformity is a mobile deformity that can be functionally altered with the use of foot orthoses (see Chapter 14).

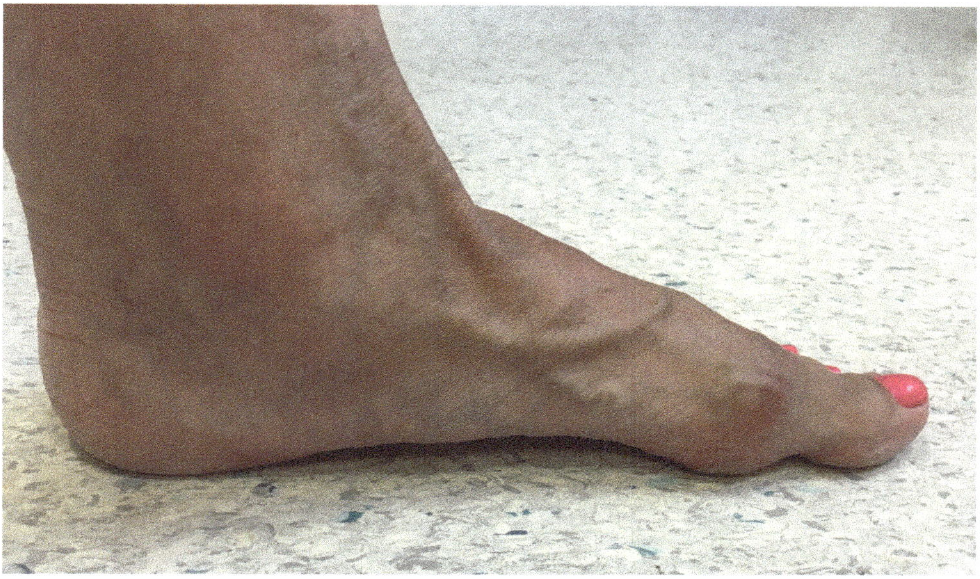

Figure 6.5 Tenosynovitis of the tibialis posterior tendon.

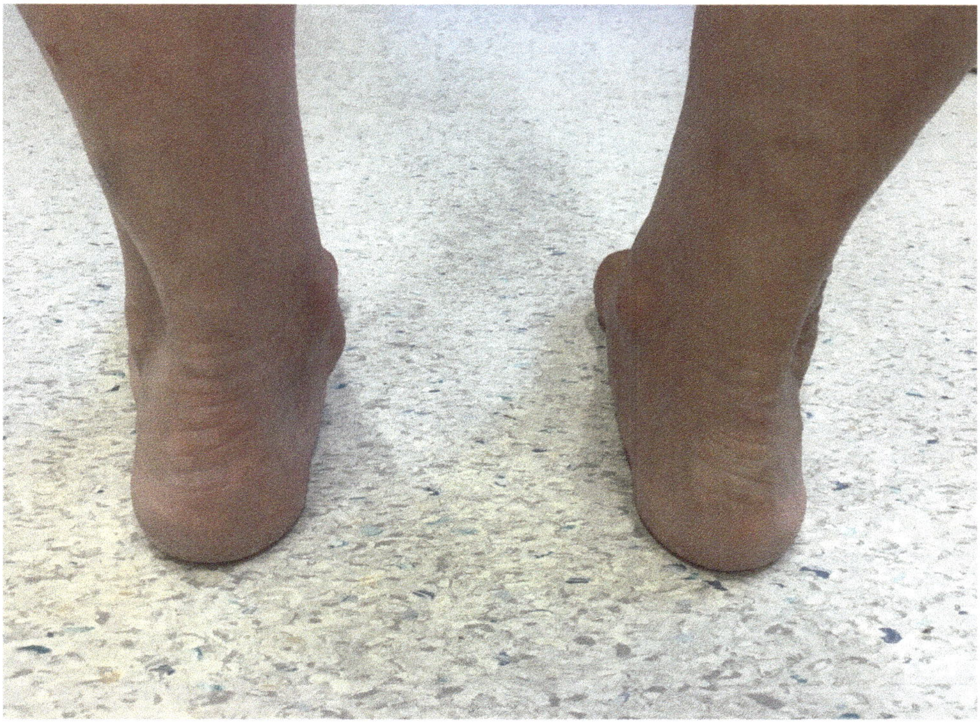

Figure 6.6 Early rearfoot valgus deformity.

Varus deformity is described in up to 16% of patients (52, 61, 78) but often not reported in studies. It has been proposed that patients with persistent forefoot pain and MTP joint synovitis despite systemic disease control walk on the outside of their feet in an attempt to avoid loading the metatarsal heads, resulting in a varus rearfoot deformity (79).

Disease-specific imaging considerations

Modalities for imaging the foot and ankle are covered in more detail in Chapter 12 but here we outline some specific considerations for people with RA.

Conventional radiography (CR) is still an important method for measuring the extent of joint damage at a given time and monitoring progression over time. The ability to take weightbearing images is useful in imaging the foot and ankle to assess the alignment of the joints and extent of deformity, particularly during the planning of any surgical intervention.

Ultrasound allows the clinician to visualize the inflammatory soft-tissue processes in RA as well as the extent of joint damage. High-frequency linear transducers, which have a shorter wavelength, are highly suited to imaging superficial musculoskeletal structures. The 3D capability and power Doppler (PD) to detect blood flow and subsequently identify synovitis in joints and soft tissues have greatly enhanced the role of musculoskeletal ultrasound in inflammatory arthritis. Ultrasound has been shown to be more sensitive than clinical assessment at detecting synovitis in the complex articular and extra-articular structures of the foot and ankle (80). This improved diagnosis of inflammatory lesions has been shown to influence decision-making about whether or not to administer corticosteroid injections to specific sites in the foot and ankle, and improve clinical outcomes, in people with chronic rheumatic disease referred for injection (81).

MRI has been acknowledged as the superior imaging modality for most foot and ankle pathologies but, unlike ultrasound, its use remains limited by cost and availability. MRI studies in early RA demonstrate that imaging findings in the feet are as prevalent as those in the hand, and, furthermore, suggest that MRI of the feet may be useful in detecting disease when CR of the hands and feet do not demonstrate erosions and MRI of the hand is normal (82, 83). However, routine MRI of the feet in early RA is unlikely to occur in current clinical practice.

Developments in MR hardware and imaging sequences over recent years have improved the ability to visualize the small irregular structures in the foot and ankle in greater detail (84).

Tissue viability

Tissue viability is an important consideration for patients with RA if there is an increased risk of tissue breakdown, i.e., as a result of foot deformity or long-term steroid use. This is further exacerbated if the patient is taking immunosuppressive medication such as biologic therapies to manage their systemic disease or there is some loss of sensation in the feet.

Neuropathy, mostly subclinical, is common in patients with RA; sensorimotor type peripheral neuropathy occurs in the foot and ankle (85–87). Estimates of the prevalence of neuropathy vary significantly, and some studies suggest that over half of those with RA may have some neurological deficit in their feet (88, 89). However, the clinical implications of this remain unclear.

The incidence of foot ulceration in patients with RA has been poorly understood until recently. In a cross-sectional multi-centre study of 285 consecutive patients with RA in The Netherlands, authors reported that 13% of patients have had a foot wound since being diagnosed with RA, and 5% had an active ulceration at the time of the study (90). In a much larger prevalence study of foot ulcers in 883 patients in the UK, the overall prevalence of foot ulceration was 9.73%, with a point prevalence of 3.39%, indicating that the incidence of foot ulceration in RA is not uncommon (91).

Recent epidemiological studies and case series have reported that ulceration in RA occurs at multiple sites and usually on the pressure-vulnerable bony sites in the forefoot; these include the dorsal aspect of hammer toes (48%), the plantar aspect of metatarsal heads (32%), and the medial aspect of the first MTP joint in patients with hallux valgus (20%) (91–94).

A recent multi-centre, observational study to determine the predictors of foot ulceration in patients with RA showed that risk of ulceration rose with increasing loss of sensation and foot deformity as well as with vascular insufficiency (95). Although often clinically perceived as the cause, raised plantar pressures did not predict the risk of foot ulceration. Alteration of the foot loading patterns by patients with RA has been widely reported. Off-loading the painful and deformed forefoot is a characteristic feature in this patient cohort (96), which may explain why raised plantar pressures are not associated with the risk of ulceration in this patient group.

The devastation associated with diabetic foot ulceration is well recognized. Masson and colleagues have been the only people to compare the rate of ulceration in a small group of patients with RA to a group of patients with diabetes directly (97). Although the rate of ulceration in the RA group was low, their plantar pressures were equal to or higher than those found in the diabetes group, known to be a significant cause of ulceration in patients with diabetes. Hence, the authors of this early study concluded that high pressure alone was not a direct cause of ulceration, which has been recently confirmed by Firth and colleagues (95). Masson et al. excluded patients with peripheral vascular disease and no information was given on the systemic medical treatments that the patients received, which is very important in current clinical practice for patients taking biologic therapies.

Patients with RA are at an increased risk of infection compared to the general population (98), together with an increased risk of peripheral arterial disease (99). Evidence suggests that the rate of serious skin and soft-tissue infections is increased with the use of anti-TNF biologic therapies (100). Hence, patients with RA and foot deformity are at risk of ulceration and consequently of subsequent infection at the ulcer site, especially if they are taking a biologic therapy.

Clinically, wounds in patients with RA are usually small and superficial (94) but, because of their position over deformed sites, bone can be easily exposed, requiring the urgent need to exclude the presence of osteomyelitis, particularly if the patient is being treated with biologic therapies.

Vasculitis, inflammation of the blood vessels, is associated with resulting ulceration. Previously it has been reported that ulceration located on the dorsum of the foot and the lower leg is likely to be caused by the systemic disease vasculitis (101). However, in recent studies of patients with RA and ulceration only affecting their feet, vasculitis has not been identified in these cohorts of patients (94, 102). Improved systemic disease control in patients with RA is probably the reason for a reduced prevalence in recent years.

Rheumatology foot health services have developed specific wound clinics to address the needs of patients with RA who present with foot ulceration. This ensures that any additional complications associated primarily with their drug treatment can be addressed without the deterioration of their overall systemic disease. Foot health management will be provided in further detail in Chapter 14.

Impact of foot disease and footwear

The wider psychosocial impact of RA and specifically foot disease is increasingly recognized in the literature. Studies have identified the impact of RA on the patient's self-image, sexuality, and personal relationships (103, 104). In addition to visible deformity, weight gain, and changes in gait, emotional effects can also occur, and the impact of fatigue is increasingly recognized as affecting people with RA (105–111).

The visible effects of RA on a person's appearance have often been trivialized but have a clear impact on patients. Joint damage and deformity in visible parts of the body, such as the hand, have long been recognized as important and are a motivating factor for patients to seek hand surgery (112, 113). The appearance of the foot is perhaps more complex and overlooked as feet are often enclosed within footwear, but this varies between climates and cultures. Embarrassment about foot deformity is underrecognized, but patients frequently report wanting to hide their feet and not participating in activities which require them to be exposed. The impact of deformity on participation in valued activities is still poorly understood and patients often feel the need to legitimize its importance (114). Such is the importance of appearance to patients that it has recently been identified as a motivating factor for foot surgery and it has an important role when patients consider the success of their foot surgery (114).

In addition to the psychosocial impact of the disease itself, it is also becoming increasingly clear that there is a secondary psychosocial impact from many of the treatments used. This is particularly so in the lower limb where appliances and especially footwear can adversely affect appearance; this has been shown to have a significant detrimental impact on many facets of patients' lives despite their clinical benefit (105, 115). Unlike other interventions, specialist footwear replaces something that is normally worn: footwear is intrinsically linked with fashion, body image, and sexuality, so loss of choice of footwear has a detrimental psychosocial impact on patients (116). Whereas for men the replacement footwear often resembles the footwear they would normally wear, this is not the case for women; the loss of choice and femininity imposed by the appearance of the footwear impacts many aspects of their lives (115, 117). Female patients report feeling, shame, anger, and sadness when wearing such footwear and this is exacerbated during social activities. Therapeutic footwear has been shown to invoke feelings of sadness, shame, and anger, and it is often seen as a final and symbolic marker of RA on the person's self-perception and their changed life (118). Indeed, people with RA often describe therapeutic footwear as 'improving their mobility but restricting their activities' (117).

Disease-specific management

Foot health management strategies are discussed in more detail in Chapter 14.

Holistic approach by the clinician

A multidisciplinary approach to managing the complications associated with RA is widely advocated. The National Institute for Health and Care Excellence (NICE) recommends that people with RA should have access to a named member of the MDT who is responsible for coordinating their care (35). Unfortunately, the feet remain a forgotten and neglected area by clinicians. This is often because of the lack of knowledge in assessing the foot and ankle, other more urgent systemic conditions that require prioritizing, or, more worryingly, lack of time during clinic appointments. Therefore, it is important that those with responsibility for coordinating the care of people with RA are able to conduct a basic assessment of the foot and ankle and have an understanding of the impact of foot and ankle problems.

The knowledge and expertise of podiatrists in assessing and managing foot and ankle conditions have been acknowledged widely by the rheumatology community; NICE specifically recommend that all people with RA and foot problems should have access to a podiatrist for assessment and periodic review of their foot health needs (35). However, just as we encourage rheumatologists to consider the foot, podiatrists should not consider the foot in isolation of the rest of the person and their systemic disease. It is crucial that podiatrists and other providers of foot care have an understanding of the underlying systemic disease, and that they build links with the local rheumatology MDT to facilitate patient care, particularly in the early stages of the disease and during a flare. Non-medical clinicians who regularly treat people with rheumatic disease should consider developing their knowledge and skills in the management of such conditions through postgraduate rheumatology modules.

Identifying disease activity and differentiating between inflammatory and mechanical disease

Inflammatory and mechanical-related foot pathology has a significant impact on mobility and functional capacity in the majority of patients with RA (118). As discussed earlier in this chapter, despite the revolution in the management of RA, with the introduction of more aggressive drug therapies for the management of systemic disease, reports suggest that the frequency of foot involvement does not appear significantly reduced (57, 62). The current 'treat to target' paradigm of care for managing RA aims to achieve clinical disease remission and targets treatment strategies at individual patients' disease activity (119). However, patients in clinical remission still have evidence of active disease in weightbearing joints (64, 120).

As such, a new paradigm of foot healthcare has been proposed for patients with early disease that promotes the tight control principles but has a focus on local disease in the foot (33). The paradigm promotes the early detection of joint disease utilizing the MTP joint-squeeze test, a combination of targeted therapy at inflammatory lesions and associated mechanically based impairments using ultrasound-guided corticosteroid injections and custom orthoses, 'tight control' of foot arthritis, and disease monitoring using disease measures (DAS), imaging methods, and foot outcome measures. These principles also provide an opportunity to optimize care in patients with established disease and persisting inflammatory foot and ankle involvement.

Region-specific management strategies

One approach to managing foot and ankle disease in patients with RA is typically to direct our interventions at specific regions in the foot, i.e., the forefoot, midfoot, rearfoot and ankle. The forefoot in both early disease when swelling is present and in established disease in the presence of deformity requires accommodation and off-loading approaches. Support for the midfoot is usually needed when the arch begins to collapse, and, although rehabilitating weakened muscles such as tibialis posterior seems sensible, there is little evidence evaluating its effect. In contrast, high-quality randomized controlled trial evidence supports the use of insoles in people with a mobile rearfoot valgus. Here, insoles not only help to reduce the levels of pain and disability but also slow the progression of rearfoot deformity. Patients will typically present with tight calf muscles that reduce ankle dorsiflexion, and therefore stretches and eccentric loading exercises to maintain range of movement at the ankle are essential.

Research agenda

Although our knowledge of foot and ankle problems is more advanced in RA than other rheumatic and musculoskeletal diseases, there is still much we do not know and the continued impact on patients clearly indicates that we need to further improve our treatment strategies. Our knowledge of the epidemiology of foot and ankle problems in RA should be revisited in light of current systemic therapies, and more precise information on specific pathologies is required. The following is by no means an exhaustive list but ultimately the research agenda should be guided by the needs of people with RA.

Patients with RA and persistent foot and ankle symptoms frequently seek help from multiple health professionals on multiple occasions, often with limited success. Pathways of care targeted at those with persistent foot and ankle symptoms should be developed to help clinicians differentiate between inflammatory and mechanical causes, thus enabling the clinician to target their interventions more appropriately.

Across many healthcare systems, there is pressure to improve the cost-effectiveness of treatments, and foot health interventions are not exempt from this. This includes the need to reduce the costs of providing foot orthoses, which remain a key component of treatment packages for people with RA. Although there is some good evidence for the use of foot orthoses in RA, it has been focused on the prescription of bespoke foot orthoses, particularly in early disease (121, 122). Cheaper and more readily available prefabricated orthoses offer the potential to provide adequate support and improve symptoms and therefore rigorous research programmes should be directed toward evaluating their comparative effectiveness. At the other end of the spectrum, developments in technology also offer the opportunity to use a mass customization process, where individualized orthoses can be quickly designed and manufactured from 3D scanning of the feet. This approach offers many potential benefits, and future studies should consider the clinical benefits and cost-effectiveness of this approach.

Another major concern for patients is footwear. This has long been recognized as an important topic for research but, to date, shoes that accommodate foot deformity, are light, provide cushioning, satisfy clinical requirements, and that people with rheumatic and musculoskeletal diseases want to wear, remain elusive for many.

References

1. **Symmons DPM.** Epidemiology of rheumatoid arthritis: determinants of onset persistence and outcome. *Best Pract Res Clin Rheumatol.* 2002;**16**(5):707–22.
2. **Lee DM, Weinblatt ME.** Rheumatoid arthritis. *The Lancet.* 2001;**358**(9285):903–11.
3. **Buch M, Emery P.** The aetiology and pathogenesis of rheumatoid arthritis. *Hospital Pharmacist.* 2002;**9**(1):5–10.
4. **O'Dell JR.** Therapeutic strategies for rheumatoid arthritis. *N Engl J Med.* 2004;**350**(25):2591–602.
5. **Barrett EM, Scott DG, Wiles NJ, et al.** The impact of rheumatoid arthritis on employment status in the early years of disease: a UK community-based study. *Rheumatology.* 2000;**39**(12):1403–9.
6. **James D.** Orthopaedic intervention in early rheumatoid arthritis. Occurrence and predictive factors in an inception cohort of 1064 patients followed for 5 years. *Rheumatology (Oxford).* 2004;**43**(3):369–76.
7. **Kapetanovic MC, Lindqvist E, Saxne T, et al.** Orthopaedic surgery in rheumatoid arthritis patients over 20 years. Prevalence and predictive factors of large joint replacement. *Ann Rheum Dis.* 2008;**67**:1412–16.
8. **Choy EH, Panayi GS.** Cytokine pathways and joint inflammation in rheumatoid arthritis. *N Engl J Med.* 2001;**344**(12):907–16.
9. **Allaire S, et al.** Contemporary prevalence and incidence of work disability associated with rheumatoid arthritis in the US. *Arthritis Rheum.* 2008;**59**(4):474–80.
10. **Kapetanovic MC, et al.** Orthopaedic surgery in rheumatoid arthritis patients over 20 years. Prevalence and predictive factors of large joint replacement. *Ann Rheum Dis.* 2008;**67**:1412–16.
11. **Symmons D, et al.** The prevalence of rheumatoid arthritis in the United Kingdom: new estimates for a new century. *Rheumatology.* 2002;**41**(7):793–800.
12. **Symmons DP, et al.** The incidence of rheumatoid arthritis in the United Kingdom: results from the Norfolk Arthritis Register. *Br J Rheumatol.* 1994;**33**(8):735–9.
13. **Smolen JS, et al.** New therapies for treatment of rheumatoid arthritis. *Lancet.* 2007;**370**(9602):1861–74.
14. **Silman AJ, et al.** Twin concordance rates for rheumatoid arthritis: results from a nationwide study. *Br J Rheumatol.* 1993;**32**(10):903–7.

15. **Padyukov L, et al.** A gene–environment interaction between smoking and shared epitope genes in HLA-DR provides a high risk of seropositive rheumatoid arthritis. *Arthritis Rheum.* 2004;**50**(10):3085–92.
16. **Hyrich KL, et al.** Predictors of response to anti-TNF-alpha therapy among patients with rheumatoid arthritis: results from the British Society for Rheumatology Biologics Register. *Rheumatology (Oxford).* 2006;**45**(12):1558–65.
17. **Soderlin MK, Petersson IF, Geborek P.** The effect of smoking on response and drug survival in rheumatoid arthritis patients treated with their first anti-TNF drug. *Scand J Rheumatol.* 2012;**41**(1):1–9.
18. **Scher JU, Abramson SB.** The microbiome and rheumatoid arthritis. *Nat Rev Rheumatol.* 2011;7(10):569–78.
19. **McInnes IB, Schett G.** The pathogenesis of rheumatoid arthritis. *N Engl J Med.* 2011;**365**(23):2205–19.
20. **Gordon P, et al.** A 10 year prospective follow up of patients with rheumatoid arthritis 1986–96. *J Rheumatol.* 2001;**28**(11):2409–15.
21. **Avouac J, Gossec L, Dougados M.** Diagnostic and predictive value of anti-cyclic citrullinated protein antibodies in rheumatoid arthritis: a systematic literature review. *Ann Rheum Dis.* 2006;**65**(7):845–51.
22. **Choy EHS, Panayi GS.** Cytokine pathways and joint inflammation in rheumatoid arthritis. *N Engl J Med.* 2001;**344**(12):907–16.
23. **Panayi GS.** B cells: a fundamental role in the pathogenesis of rheumatoid arthritis? *Rheumatology.* 2005;**44**(Suppl. 2):ii3–ii7.
24. **Pap T, et al.** Fibroblast biology. Role of synovial fibroblasts in the pathogenesis of rheumatoid arthritis. *Arthritis Res.* 2000;**2**(5):361–7.
25. **Tak P, Bresnihan B.** The pathogenesis and prevention of joint damage in rheumatoid arthritis: advances from synovial biopsy and tissue analysis. *Arthritis Rheum.* 2000;**43**(12):2619–33.
26. **Schett G, et al.** Mechanisms of disease: the link between RANKL and arthritic bone disease. *Nat Clin Pract Rheum.* 2005;**1**(1):47–54.
27. **Schett G.** Cells of the synovium in rheumatoid arthritis. *Arthritis ResTher.* 2007;**9**(1):203–9.
28. **Tracey D, et al.** Tumor necrosis factor antagonist mechanisms of action: a comprehensive review. *Pharmacol Therapeutics.* 2008;**117**(2):244–79.
29. **Emery P, et al.** Clinical identification and treatment of a rapidly progressing disease state in patients with rheumatoid arthritis. *Rheumatology (Oxford).* 2008;**47**(4):392–8.
30. **Gossec L, et al.** Prognostic factors for remission in early rheumatoid arthritis: a multiparameter prospective study. *Ann Rheum Dis.* 2004;**63**(6):675–80.
31. **Pratt AG, et al.** Components of treatment delay in rheumatoid arthritis differ according to autoantibody status: validation of a single-centre observation using national audit data. *Rheumatology (Oxford).* 2016;**55**(10):1843–8.
32. **Mjaavatten MD, et al.** Pattern of joint involvement and other disease characteristics in 634 patients with arthritis of less than 16 weeks' duration. *J Rheumatol.* 2009;**36**(7):1401–6.
33. **Woodburn J, et al.** Looking through the 'window of opportunity': is there a new paradigm of podiatry care on the horizon in early rheumatoid arthritis? *J Foot Ankle Res.* 2010;**3**:8.
34. **Emery P, et al.** Early referral recommendation for newly diagnosed rheumatoid arthritis: evidence based development of a clinical guide. *Ann Rheum Dis.* 2002;**61**(4):290–7.
35. **National Institute for Health and Care Excellence.** *Rheumatoid Arthritis: National Clinical Guideline for Management and Treatment in Adults.* London: National Institute for Health and Care Excellence, 2009.
36. **Arnett FC, et al.** The American Rheumatism Association 1987 revised criteria for the classification of rheumatoid arthritis. *Arthritis Rheum.* 1988;**31**(3):315–24.
37. **Aletaha D, et al.** 2010 Rheumatoid arthritis classification criteria: an American College of Rheumatology/European League Against Rheumatism collaborative initiative. *Arthritis Rheum.* 2010;**62**(9):2569–81.
38. **Weigl M, et al.** The ICF comprehensively covers the spectrum of health problems encountered by health professionals in patients with musculoskeletal conditions. *Rheumatology.* 2006;**45**(10):1247–54.

39. **World Health Organization**. *Towards a Common Language for Functioning Disability and Health: ICF.* Geneva: World Health Organization, 2002.
40. **Boonen A, Maksymowych W.** Measurement: function and mobility (focussing on the ICF framework). *Best Pract Res Clin Rheum.* 2010;**24**(5):605–24.
41. **Stucki G, Grimby G.** Applying the ICF in medicine. *J Rehab Med.* 2004;**44** (Suppl.):5–6.
42. **van der Leeden M, et al.** Prevalence and course of forefoot impairments and walking disability in the first eight years of rheumatoid arthritis. *Arthritis Rheum.* 2008;**59**(11):1596–602.
43. **Aletaha D, Smolen J, Ward MM.** Measuring function in rheumatoid arthritis: identifying reversible and irreversible components. *Arthritis Rheum.* 2006;**54**(9):2784–92.
44. **Smolen JS, et al.** EULAR recommendations for the management of rheumatoid arthritis with synthetic and biological disease-modifying antirheumatic drugs: 2013 update. *Ann Rheum Dis.* 2014;**73**(3):492–509.
45. **Emery P, et al.** Sustained remission with etanercept tapering in early rheumatoid arthritis. *N Engl J Med.* 2014;**371**(19):1781–92.
46. **Emery P, et al.** Evaluating drug-free remission with abatacept in early rheumatoid arthritis: results from the phase 3b multicentre randomised active-controlled AVERT study of 24 months with a 12-month double-blind treatment period. *Ann Rheum Dis.* 2015;**74**(1):19–26.
47. **O'Shea JJ, et al.** The JAK-STAT pathway: impact on human disease and therapeutic intervention. *Annu Rev Med.* 2015;**66**:311–28.
48. **Schwartz DM, et al.** Type I/II cytokines JAKs and new strategies for treating autoimmune diseases. *Nat Rev Rheumatol.* 2016;**12**(1):25–36.
49. **Bukhari M.** Have we had a paradigm change in the treatment of rheumatoid arthritis after the American Congress of Rheumatology 2015? *Rheumatology (Oxford).* 2016;**55**(9):1531–3.
50. **Vainio K.** The rheumatoid foot; a clinical study with pathological and roentgenological comments. *Ann Chir Gynaecol Fenn Suppl.* 1956;**45**(1):1–107.
51. **Spiegel TM, Spiegel JS.** Rheumatoid arthritis in the foot and ankle—diagnosis pathology and treatment. The relationship between foot and ankle deformity and disease duration in 50 patients. *Foot Ankle.* 1982;**2**(6):318–24.
52. **Bouysset M, et al.** Flattening of the rheumatoid foot in tarsal arthritis on X-ray. *Scand J Rheumatol.* 1987;**16**(2):127–33.
53. **Michelson J, et al.** Foot and ankle problems in rheumatoid arthritis. *Foot Ankle Int.* 1994;**15**(11):608–13.
54. **Shi K, et al.** Foot deformities in rheumatoid arthritis and relevance of disease severity. *J Rheumatol.* 2000;**27**(1):84–9.
55. **Bouysset M, et al.** Rheumatoid flat foot and deformity of the first ray. *J Rheumatol.* 2002;**29**(5):903–5.
56. **Fleming A, Crown JM, Corbett M.** Incidence of joint involvement in early rheumatoid arthritis. *Rheumatol Rehabil.* 1976;**15**(2):92–6.
57. **Grondal L, et al.** The foot: still the most important reason for walking incapacity in rheumatoid arthritis: distribution of symptomatic joints in 1000 RA patients. *Acta Orthop.* 2008;**79**(2):257–61.
58. **Kerry RM, Holt GM, Stockley I.** The foot in chronic rheumatoid arthritis: a continuing problem. *Foot.* 1994;**4**(4):201–3.
59. **Otter SJ, et al.** Foot pain in rheumatoid arthritis prevalence risk factors and management: an epidemiological study. *Clin Rheumatol.* 2010;**29**(3):255–71.
60. **Rydgren L, Fredrikson E.** The development of foot deformities in early rheumatoid arthritis. *Br J Rheumatol.* 1996;**35**(Abstracts Suppl. 1):198.
61. **Vidigal E, et al.** The foot in chronic rheumatoid arthritis. *Ann Rheum Dis.* 1975;**34**(4):292–7.
62. **Otter SJ, et al.** Comparison of foot pain and foot care among rheumatoid arthritis patients taking and not taking anti-TNF alpha therapy: an epidemiological study. *Rheumatol Int.* 2011;**31**(11):1515–19.
63. **Fransen J, Creemers MC, Van Riel PL.** Remission in rheumatoid arthritis: agreement of the disease activity score (DAS28) with the ARA preliminary remission criteria. *Rheumatology.* 2004;**43**(10):1252–5.

64. **van der Leeden M, et al.** Forefoot disease activity in rheumatoid arthritis patients in remission: results of a cohort study. *Arth Res Ther.* 2010;**12**(1):R3.
65. **Hulsmans HM, et al.** The course of radiologic damage during the first six years of rheumatoid arthritis. *Arthritis Rheum.* 2000;**43**(9):1927–40.
66. **Belt EA, et al.** Relationship of ankle joint involvement with subtalar destruction in patients with rheumatoid arthritis. A 20-year follow-up study. *J Bone Spine.* 2001;**68**(2):154–7.
67. **Dixon AS.** Medical aspects of the rheumatoid foot. *Proc R Soc Med.* 1970;**63**(7):677–9.
68. **Keenan MA, et al.** Valgus deformities of the feet and characteristics of gait in patients who have rheumatoid arthritis. *J Bone Joint Surg.* 1991;**73**(2):237–47.
69. **Jaakkola JI, Mann RA.** A review of rheumatoid arthritis affecting the foot and ankle. *Foot Ankle Int.* 2004;**25**(12):866–74.
70. **Davys HJ, et al.** Debridement of plantar callosities in rheumatoid arthritis: a randomized controlled trial. *Rheumatology (Oxford).* 2005;**44**(2):207–10.
71. **Tuna H, et al.** Pedobarography and its relation to radiologic erosion scores in rheumatoid arthritis. *Rheumatol Int.* 2005;**26**(1):42–7.
72. **Siddle HJ, et al.** Anatomical location of erosions at the metatarsophalangeal joints in patients with rheumatoid arthritis. *Rheumatology (Oxford).* 2014;**53**(5):932–6.
73. **Siddle HJ, et al.** Magnetic resonance arthrography of lesser metatarsophalangeal joints in patients with rheumatoid arthritis: relationship to clinical biomechanical and radiographic variables. *J Rheumatol.* 2012;**39**(9):1786–91.
74. **Siddle HJ, et al.** MRI identifies plantar plate pathology in the forefoot of patients with rheumatoid arthritis. *Clin Rheum.* 2012;**31**(4):621–9.
75. **Hattori T, et al.** Radiological study of joint destruction patterns in rheumatoid flatfoot. *Clin Rheumatol.* 2008;**27**(6):733–7.
76. **Barn R, et al.** Tibialis posterior tenosynovitis and associated pes plano valgus in rheumatoid arthritis: electromyography multisegment foot kinematics and ultrasound features. *Arthritis Care Res (Hoboken).* 2013;**65**(4):495–502.
77. **Woodburn J, Helliwell PS.** Relation between heel position and the distribution of forefoot plantar pressures and skin callosities in rheumatoid arthritis. *Ann Rheum Dis.* 1996;**55**(11):806–10.
78. **Bouysset M, et al.** The rheumatoid heel: its relationship to other disorders in the rheumatoid foot. *Clin Rheumatol.* 1989;**8**(2):208–14.
79. **Helliwell P, et al.** *The Foot and Ankle in Rheumatoid Arthritis. A Comprehensive Guide.* London: Churchill Livingstone Elsevier, 2007.
80. **Wakefield RJ, et al.** The optimal assessment of the rheumatoid arthritis hindfoot: a comparative study of clinical examination ultrasound and high field MRI. *Ann Rheum Dis.* 2008;**67**(12):1678–82.
81. **d'Agostino MA, et al.** Impact of ultrasound imaging on local corticosteroid injections of symptomatic ankle hind- and mid-foot in chronic inflammatory diseases. *Arthritis Rheum.* 2005;**53**(2):284–92.
82. **Boutry N, et al.** Magnetic resonance imaging appearance of the hands and feet in patients with early rheumatoid arthritis. *J Rheumatol.* 2003;**30**(4):671–9.
83. **Ostendorf B, et al.** Diagnostic value of magnetic resonance imaging of the forefeet in early rheumatoid arthritis when findings on imaging of the metacarpophalangeal joints of the hands remain normal. *Arthritis Rheum.* 2004;**50**(7):2094–102.
84. **Chhabra A, et al.** Current concepts review: 3T magnetic resonance imaging of the ankle and foot. *Foot Ankle Int.* 2012;**33**(2):164–71.
85. **Lanzillo B, et al.** Subclinical peripheral nerve involvement in patients with rheumatoid arthritis. *Arthritis Rheum.* 1998;**41**(7):1196–202.
86. **Nadkar MY, et al.** Neuropathy in rheumatoid arthritis. *J Assoc Physicians India.* 2001;**49**:217–20.
87. **Agarwal V, et al.** A clinical electrophysiological and pathological study of neuropathy in rheumatoid arthritis. *Clin Rheumatol.* 2008;**27**(7):841–4.

88. **Wilson O, Kirwan JR.** Measuring sensation in the feet of patients with rheumatoid arthritis. *Musculoskeletal Care.* 2006;**4**(1):12–23.
89. **Rosenbaum D, et al.** Plantar sensitivity foot loading and walking pain in rheumatoid arthritis. *Rheumatology (Oxford).* 2006;**45**(2):212–14.
90. **Matricali GA, et al.** The presence of forefoot problems and the role of surgery in patients with rheumatoid arthritis. *Ann Rheum Dis.* 2006;**65**(9):1254–5.
91. **Firth J, et al.** The prevalence of foot ulceration in patients with rheumatoid arthritis. *Arthritis Rheum.* 2008;**59**(2):200–5.
92. **Davys HJ, et al.** Foot ulceration in patients with rheumatic diseases. *Ann Rheum Dis.* 2006;**65**(Abstract Suppl. 2):ii241.
93. **Firth J, et al.** The predictors of foot ulceration in patients with rheumatoid arthritis: a preliminary investigation. *Clin Rheumatol.* 2008;**27**(11):1423–8.
94. **Siddle HJ, et al.** A case series to describe the clinical characteristics of foot ulceration in patients with rheumatoid arthritis. *Clin Rheumatol.* 2012;**31**(3):541–5.
95. **Firth J, et al.** The predictors of foot ulceration in patients with rheumatoid arthritis. *Clin Rheumatol.* 2014;**33**(5):615–21.
96. **Semple R, et al.** Regionalised centre of pressure analysis in patients with rheumatoid arthritis. *Clin Biomech (Bristol Avon).* 2007;**22**(1):127–9.
97. **Masson EA, et al.** Abnormal foot pressures alone may not cause ulceration. *Diabet Med.* 1989;**6**(5):426–8.
98. **Doran MF, et al.** Frequency of infection in patients with rheumatoid arthritis compared with controls: a population-based study. *Arthritis Rheum.* 2002;**46**(9):2287–93.
99. **Alkaabi JK, et al.** Rheumatoid arthritis and macrovascular disease. *Rheumatology (Oxford).* 2003;**42**(2):292–7.
100. **Dixon WG, et al.** Rates of serious infection including site-specific and bacterial intracellular infection in rheumatoid arthritis patients receiving anti-tumor necrosis factor therapy: results from the British Society for Rheumatology Biologics Register. *Arthritis Rheum.* 2006;**54**(8):2368–76.
101. **Cawley MI.** Vasculitis and ulceration in rheumatic diseases of the foot. *Baillieres Clin Rheumatol.* 1987;**1**(2):315–33.
102. **Shanmugam VK, Demaria DM, Attinger CE.** Lower extremity ulcers in rheumatoid arthritis: features and response to immunosuppression. *Clin Rheumatol.* 2011;**30**(6):849–53.
103. **Gutweniger S, et al.** Body image of women with rheumatoid arthritis. *Clin Exp Rheumatol.* 1999;**17**(4):413–17.
104. **Hill J, Bird H, Thorpe R.** Effects of rheumatoid arthritis on sexual activity and relationships. *Rheumatology.* 2003;**42**(2):280–6.
105. **Goodacre LJ, Candy FJ.** 'If I didn't have RA I wouldn't give them house room': the relationship between RA footwear and clothing choices. *Rheumatology.* 2011;**50**(3):513–17.
106. **Hewlett S, et al.** Patients' perceptions of fatigue in rheumatoid arthritis: overwhelming, uncontrollable, ignored. *Arthritis Care Res.* 2005;**53**(5):697–702.
107. **Hewlett S, Hehir M, Kirwan JR.** Measuring fatigue in rheumatoid arthritis: a systematic review of scales in use. *Arthritis Care Res.* 2007;**57**(3):429–39.
108. **Kirwan JR, et al.** Patient perspective: fatigue as a recommended patient centered outcome measure in rheumatoid arthritis. *J Rheumatol.* 2007;**34**(5):1174–7.
109. **Nicklin J, et al.** Measuring fatigue in rheumatoid arthritis: a cross-sectional study to evaluate the Bristol Rheumatoid Arthritis Fatigue Multi-Dimensional questionnaire visual analog scales and numerical rating scales. *Arthritis Care Res.* 2010;**62**(11):1559–68.
110. **Nicklin J, et al.** Collaboration with patients in the design of patient-reported outcome measures: capturing the experience of fatigue in rheumatoid arthritis. *Arthritis Care Res.* 2010;**62**(11):1552–8.

111. **Repping-Wuts H, et al.** Fatigue in patients with rheumatoid arthritis: British and Dutch nurses' knowledge attitudes and management. *J Adv Nurs.* 2009;**65**(4):901–11.

112. **Bogoch ER, Judd MG.** The hand: a second face? *J Rheumatol.* 2002;**29**(12):2477–83.

113. **Vamos M, White GL, Caughey DE.** Body image in rheumatoid arthritis: the relevance of hand appearance to desire for surgery. *Br J Med Psychol.* 1990;**63** (Pt 3):267–77.

114. **Backhouse MR, et al.** Interpreting outcome following foot surgery in people with rheumatoid arthritis. *J Foot Ankle Res.* 2016;**9**:20.

115. **Williams AE, Nester CJ, Ravey MI.** Rheumatoid arthritis patients' experiences of wearing therapeutic footwear—a qualitative investigation. *BMC Musculoskeletal Disord.* 2007;**8**:104.

116. **Williams AE, Nester CJ, Ravey MI.** Rheumatoid arthritis patients' experiences of wearing therapeutic footwear—a qualitative investigation. *BMC Musculoskelet Disord.* 2007;**8**(104):104.

117. **Williams AE, et al.** Women's experiences of wearing therapeutic footwear in three European countries. *J Foot Ankle Res.* 2010;**3**:23.

118. **Wickman AM, et al.** Health-related quality of life for patients with rheumatoid arthritis foot involvement. *Foot Ankle Int.* 2004;**25**(1):19–26.

119. **Smolen JS, et al.** Treating rheumatoid arthritis to target: recommendations of an international task force. *Ann Rheum Dis.* 2010;**69**(4):631–7.

120. **Landewe R, et al.** Twenty-eight-joint counts invalidate the DAS28 remission definition owing to the omission of the lower extremity joints: a comparison with the original DAS remission. *Ann Rheum Dis.* 2006;**65**(5):637–41.

121. **Woodburn J, Barker S, Helliwell PS.** A randomized controlled trial of foot orthoses in rheumatoid arthritis. *J Rheumatol.* 2002;**29**(7):1377–83.

122. **Hennessy K, Woodburn J, Steultjens M.** Custom foot orthoses for rheumatoid arthritis: a systematic review. *Arthritis Care Res.* 2012;**64**(3):311–20.

Chapter 7

Spondyloarthropathies

Deborah Turner and Philip Helliwell

Introduction

Spondyloarthropathy historically was regarded as a form of seronegative rheumatoid arthritis (RA), but the pioneering work of Wright and Moll firmly established the characteristic clinical features (1). What struck these authors was the commonality of clinical features across the diseases identified as belonging to this group (namely, ankylosing spondylitis (AS), psoriatic arthritis (PsA), reactive arthritis, and the arthritis of inflammatory bowel disease). At about the time that Wright and Moll first started to publish in this field, others were 'discovering' a common genetic link, HLA B27 (1, 2). Nowadays, there is a trend to 'lump' all these conditions under one label and call them either peripheral or axial spondyloarthropathy (3, 4). However, others do not agree with this trend, preferring to keep the conditions separate, and only by doing so can further imaging, genetic, and immunopathological studies be performed to inform this debate (5).

The hallmark clinical features (Figures 7.1–7.3) are inflammatory spinal disease, dactylitis, and enthesitis, together with an asymmetrical oligoarthritis. It has been argued that the primary underlying pathological feature is enthesitis (6), yet proof of this concept is still lacking. What is clear is that there are many pathological processes going on in spondyloarthropathy. These include enthesitis, synovitis, tenosynovitis, and osteitis—in other words, a wide spectrum of tissues is involved. Combine these with the skin (psoriasis and psoriaform lesions as seen in keratoderma blenorrhagica), eyes (uveitis), heart (aortitis), and known cardiovascular risks, and the wide spectrum of disease becomes clear.

Clearly, given the wide spectrum of clinical manifestations, assessment of disease is going to be complex. It is not possible merely to assess the joints, such as with the 28-joint count, to have an idea of disease activity. Instruments are now available to measure each of the disease domains, including dactylitis and enthesitis (7, 8), and composite disease activity measures are also now becoming available (9) Table 7.1. It is not absolutely necessary to measure each of the domains outside a clinical trial, but we must at least be mindful of how the disease manifests and take a moment to look for these important aspects of the disease. Otherwise, how can we treat the patient effectively, if we do not know how extensive, and active, their disease is?

Good and accurate data on natural history are hard to come by, as most people with significant disease will present for treatment. Historically, we have indications that, if left untreated, people with AS will ultimately develop ankylosis of their spine. This is particularly true if they have been immobilized. Yet many people with AS do not deteriorate from year to year. In PsA we have good longitudinal data from the Toronto cohort where about a quarter of these patients have low-level, non-progressive disease (10). The question arises: can we identify those patients who are going to do well, and the converse, those who will do badly? Across the spondyloarthropathies a high level of C-reactive protein (or erythrocyte sedimentation rate) will predict a poor outcome. In PsA, in addition, the number of tender and swollen joints, female sex, and previous steroid use are bad prognostic factors (11). In AS florid active disease of the spine, as seen on magnetic resonance

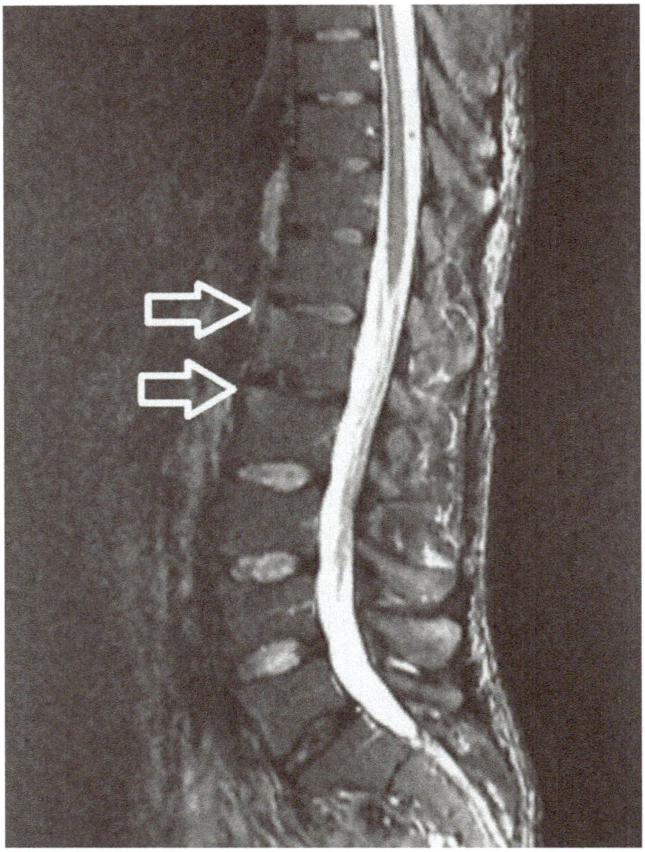

Figure 7.1 Magnetic resonance image scan (short TI inversion recovery sequence) of spine showing bright signal at the vertebral corners (arrows) indicating inflammation.

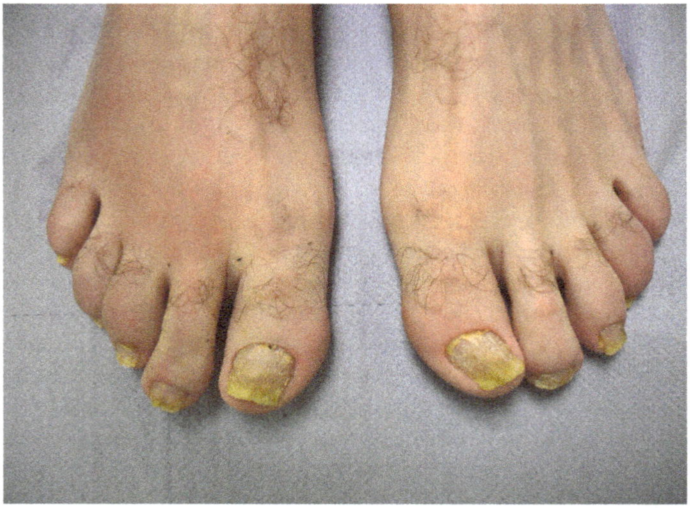

Figure 7.2 Typical dactylitis affecting the right third digit and the left fourth digit.

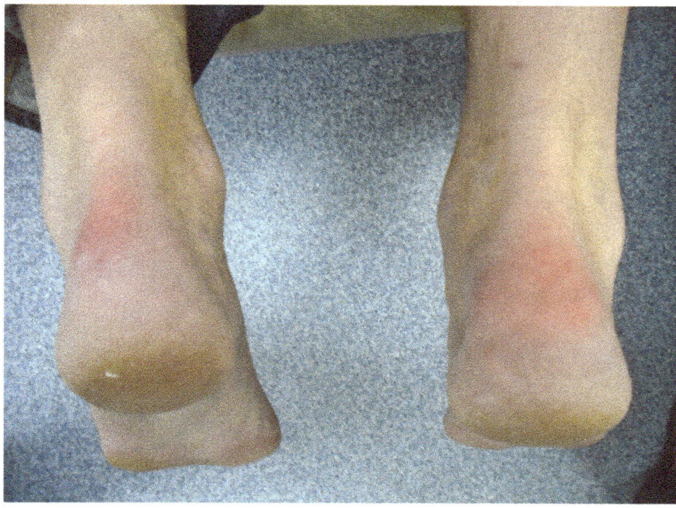

Figure 7.3 Enthesitis at the Achilles insertion.

Table 7.1 Some composite disease activity indices used in spondyloarthropathy

Measure	Components	Comments
Bath Ankylosing Spondylitis Disease Activity Index (BASDAI) (43)	A six-item Likert or VAS patient-completed measure covering fatigue, pain, peripheral joint pain, tender entheseal points, early morning pain, and morning stiffness. Score range 0–10	Quick and easy to complete and score. In psoriatic arthritis may be influenced by peripheral disease activity
Ankylosing Spondylitis Disease Activity Score (ASDAS) (44)	Uses a four-item Likert scale covering pain, morning stiffness, patient global, peripheral joint activity, and the C-reactive protein (CRP) level. Score range 0–10	Easy to collect patient items but need to have concurrent CRP and need a calculator to compute final score
Psoriatic Arthritis Disease Activity Score (PASDAS) (9)	An eight-item scale with a mixture of patient-completed items and physician items. Comprises: patient and physician global scores, the physical function subscore of the SF36, tender and swollen joint counts, enthesitis score, dactylitis score, and the CRP. Score range 0–10	A complex formula requiring a calculator. Need to have a concurrent CRP measurement
Composite Psoriatic Disease Activity Index (CPDAI) (45)	A five-domain scale covering peripheral joints, skin, enthesitis, dactylitis, and the spine. Within each domain a severity score is derived depending on cut-offs. Score range 0–15	Can be completed at the patient visit as no laboratory tests required and no calculator needed. Requires the completion of four patient-reported measures, a tender and swollen joint count, an enthesitis score, and a dactylitis score

VAS, visual analogue scale.

imaging (MRI), is a bad prognostic factor. As yet, a clear marker for arthritis mutilans has not been identified, although patients with this condition are probably more likely to be HLA-B27-positive (and this is a marker for more severe disease in AS). In future, it is likely that there will be a biomarker, or biomarkers, that will enable identification of the worst prognostic patients at presentation, so that treatment can be targeted appropriately.

As befits a disease with such wide clinical manifestations, treatment should encompass all involved domains and be delivered by a multidisciplinary team. In particular, in AS the physician and physiotherapist should work closely, and in PsA the rheumatology and dermatology departments should be closely involved. In recent times, consensus, evidence-based, treatment algorithms have been published for AS and PsA (12–14). From the patient's point of view, one treatment, preferably taken once a day, is favoured to manage all manifestations of disease. Until recently there were very few treatments that fulfilled that promise but, with the advent of biologic drugs, that is now becoming reality. The tumour necrosis factor (TNF) inhibitors are the benchmark drug for efficacy in these disorders, although IL-17 inhibitors are making a good case for equivalent, and, in the case of the skin, better outcomes overall (15). Of course, these drugs are costly and not without risks. Infection is always a concern, particularly mycobacterial infection, which can present in the foot. It is always worth remembering that any focus of infection, an ulcer or a nail, can soon become systemic if biologic drugs are used. There is just one other scenario of note. From time to time cases of paradoxical psoriasis are seen in people treated with TNF inhibitors. These are people who have never had psoriasis previously (they are often having treatment for RA). It is common to present on the palms and soles as a pustular hyperkeratotic rash (Figure 7.4) rather than the classical psoriasis plaques. It is generally a class effect and so switching the biologic within class may not help but other treatments are available to help the patient remain on their drug, particularly if it is working well.

Skin and nails (psoriatic arthritis)

Up to 50% of patients with psoriasis have concurrent nail psoriasis and in those with PsA approximately 80% have nail disease. Therefore, nail involvement is a potentially useful clinical sign

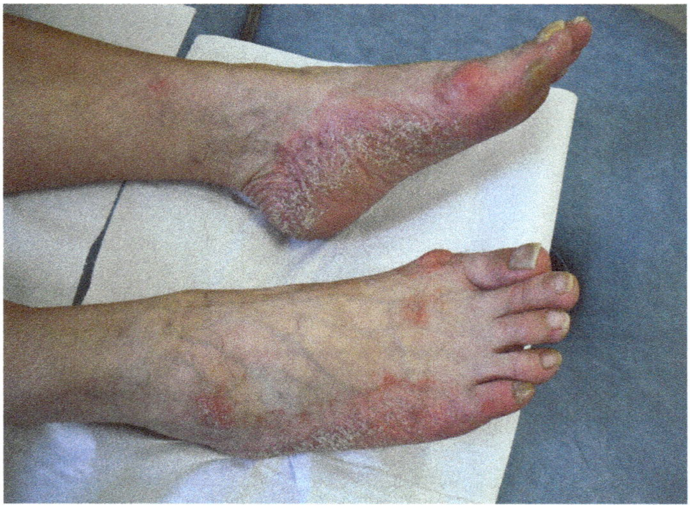

Figure 7.4 Typical pustular psoriasis on the sole.
Picture courtesy of Professor Wolf-Henning Boehncke, Geneva.

when looking/screening for PsA. Psoriaform skin lesions usually precede the symptoms of PsA in approximately 75% of cases (16). Typically, the cutaneous manifestations of the disease develop 10 years prior to the onset of joint symptoms. The severity and progression of skin, joint, and nail symptoms are frequently asynchronous (1), and skin and joint symptoms sometimes do not respond equally or in parallel to systemic or biologic therapeutic agents. Indeed, the pathophysiology of nail dystrophy has been postulated to be more closely associated with joint symptoms than with skin symptoms (17).

There is a great spectrum in the clinical manifestations of nail disease in those with PsA, such as pitting, loosening of the nail bed, splinter haemorrhages, and onycholysis, with the added complexity of secondary infections (bacterial, fungal) aggravating or masking the manifestations. Pitting of the nail is reported to be the most common manifestation of nail involvement in PsA and is a result of lesions in the nail matrix, as are erythema of the lunula, leukonychia (whitening), and crumbling of the nail (dystrophy). However, pitting is rarely seen in the nails of the feet. Involvement at the nail bed presents as 'oil drop' or 'salmon patch' discoloration, splinter haemorrhages, subungual hyperkeratosis, and onycholysis. Onycholysis and hyperkeratosis are the commonest psoriatic nail lesions in the feet (Figures 7.2, 7.5, and 7.6). Onycholysis increases the potential risk of secondary infections, and close monitoring for signs of bacterial infection is recommended, especially in those patients on biologic drug therapies.

To assess the nature and severity of nail involvement and response to therapeutic interventions objectively, reproducible and reliable tools have been developed. The Nail Psoriasis Severity Index (NAPSI) and modified Nail Psoriasis Severity Index (mNAPSI) can be used to score and grade the severity of nail psoriasis, respectively. The NAPSI scores both hands and feet, and the mNAPSI just the hands. The NAPSI assesses each quadrant for the presence/absence/severity of manifestations in the nail matrix and nail bed. The mNAPSI has a complex scoring system, grading pitting, onycholysis, and crumbling in each nail (18). Both measures can be time-consuming and impractical for clinicians in the routine clinic situation, where a simple physician grading (mild, moderate, and severe) may suffice.

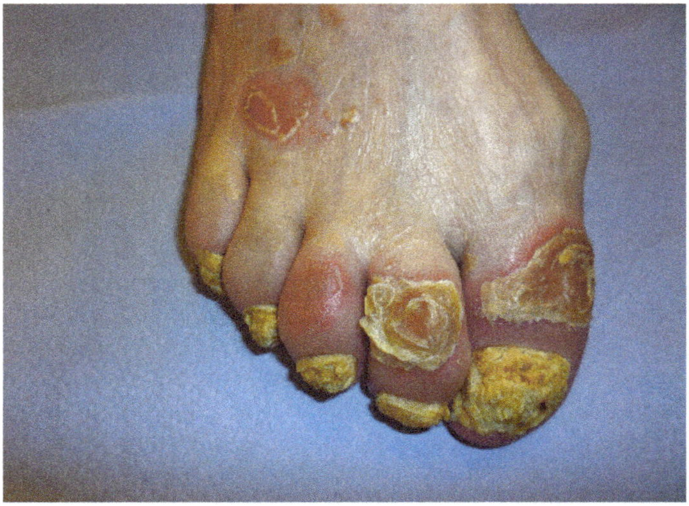

Figure 7.5 Hyperkeratotic nail disease in psoriasis. Note also the psoriasis plaques and dactylitis in the first to third toes.

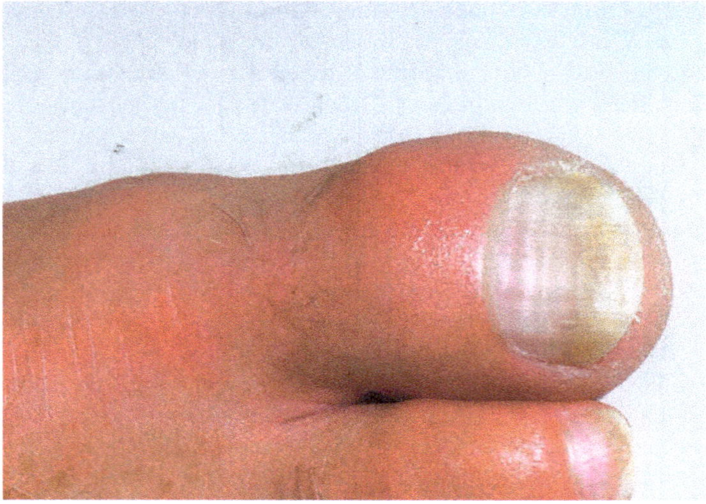

Figure 7.6 The Bauer's digit: psoriatic nail dystrophy and involvement of the interphalangeal joint of the great toe.

Involvement of the toenail may cause problems with pain, infection, and rubbing. Treatment of nail psoriasis should be individualized according to the patient's preferences, severity of nail changes, and presence of skin and/or joint involvement. Careful reduction of the thickness of the nail and removal of the hyperkeratosis may prove beneficial in reducing pain. Topical therapies are safe and effective treatment modalities for nail disease but are often limited by poor adherence and involve a lengthy treatment. Systemic therapy such as oral retinoids and biologic agents may be considered for widespread nail disease causing significant morbidity. In all cases the possibility of fungal infection should be considered and eliminated by appropriate diagnostic methods.

Palmoplantar psoriasis is a disabling variant of psoriasis that is reported to affect approximately 5% of all psoriasis patients (Figure 7.4). It has been shown that patients with palmoplantar psoriasis suffer from greater health-related quality of life impairment than those with moderate-to-severe plaque psoriasis (19) and greater physical disability (20). Palmoplantar psoriasis may occur de novo in patients on TNF inhibitors; this phenomenon may be seen in people who have never previously had clinical signs of psoriasis.

Dactylitis

Dactylitis is the classic presenting feature for spondyloarthropathy and psoriatic arthritis in the foot (Figure 7.2). The presentation is with a uniformly swollen digit, red, painful, and warm in the acute situation. Many early cases are mistaken for infection and treated with antibiotics, and even amputation. The differential diagnosis is infection and acute gout. The distinction between these conditions is a synthesis of clinical, biochemical, and radiographic information. The condition is described as a 'sausage' digit, or a 'chipolata' digit, the latter deriving from a small sausage eaten in France.

MRI has shown that inflammation affects a wide spectrum of tissues in the affected digit: bone, joint, enthesis, tendon, and soft tissue (21). In the acute situation all the tissues are inflamed. Even after the acute inflammation has subsided MRI scans continue to be abnormal. In fact, dactylitis can be considered to be a paradigm of disease, given the extent of inflammation seen on MRI scans.

Dactylitis is more common in the feet than the hands, with the fourth toes most frequently involved (22). The reason for this is undetermined but may involve mechanical factors such as pressure and shear (23). Dactylitis may also occur only in the great toe where, with associated nail dystrophy, it is called onychoperiostitis, or Bauer's digit (Figure 7.6). Dactylitis is an adverse prognostic factor; the presence of any dactylitis is associated with more severe disease and radiological destruction in the affected digit, and generally dactylitis may be a marker for arthritis mutilans. Plain radiography may show typical changes such as erosion of the terminal phalangeal tufts, juxta-articular and entheseal new bone formation, periostitis, and severe osteolysis. As mentioned above, MRI may show inflammation in several tissues, including tenosynovitis, synovitis, enthesitis, and bone oedema.

In terms of treatment, local steroid injections are recommended but lack a good evidence base. Determining a precise location for steroid injection can be difficult, although it is likely that, wherever the steroid is deposited, there will be some diffusion and (beneficial) effect in nearby tissues. Our practice is to inject at the base of the toe, targeting the metatarsophalangeal (MTP) joint. Dactylitis can be difficult to treat and may be the only manifestation of psoriatic arthritis. Although biologic drugs are proven to be effective, national treatment guidelines often make their use difficult. There is currently no specific evidence to support the use of interventions, such as the provision of footwear and orthoses in psoriatic arthritis but, drawing on the combination of evidence for RA and clinical experience, it is reasonable to conclude that the inflammatory and mechanical factors that affect the feet in psoriatic arthritis should be addressed in much the same way as in RA.

Enthesitis

Enthesitis is the striking feature of spondyloarthropathy in the foot, typically at the insertion of the Achilles tendon and origin of the plantar fascia. Achilles enthesitis may precede spinal inflammation in AS and, even in early PsA, the prevalence of plantar fasciitis and Achilles insertional enthesitis has been reported as 12% and 6%, respectively (24). On imaging, enthesitis may also be seen at the attachment of the tibialis posterior tendon and the insertion of peroneus brevis. Other, 'functional' entheses may be involved (see Chapter 2), an example being the peroneus longus tendon as it winds around the cuboid bone. A presentation of isolated, recurrent, or bilateral Achilles enthesitis is very suggestive of a formal diagnosis of spondyloarthropathy. There may be osteitis close to the affected entheses, although this is seldom appreciated clinically, and osteitis may also occur in the sesamoid bones close to the first MTP joint.

Enthesitis is defined as inflammation at tendon, ligament, joint capsule sites, or fascia insertion sites to bone (15). The use of ultrasound and MRI in PsA has increased detection of enthesitis and improved understanding of disease mechanisms. MRI allows visualization of bone marrow oedema and osteitis commonly associated with entheseal disease. In contrast, ultrasound identifies tendon and ligament abnormalities, both structural (tendon thickness, tendon heterogeneity, and new bone formation) and inflammatory (by demonstrating increased blood flow on power Doppler signal) (25). Increased knowledge about the extent of tendon and ligament involvement in spondyloarthritis has prompted the suggestion that enthesitis is the primary event (6).

Clinical assessment of enthesitis is difficult because the inflammation often is not visible and can be hard to distinguish from other forms of joint inflammation. For example, synovial joint inflammation can cause capsule distension with pain and swelling, making clinical differentiation from enthesitis problematic. Also, enthesitis, like synovitis, can be asymptomatic, as evidenced by imaging studies demonstrating enthesopathic changes in the absence of symptoms. It may be difficult to locate the enthesis anatomically if it is deep within surrounding tissue and contiguous with synovium. Further complicating assessment, the location of entheseal sites sometimes overlaps with those of the tender points of fibromyalgia, although none of these occurs in the foot. However, in fibromyalgia, it is not uncommon to find an extremely tender fat pad just inferior to the lateral malleolus, which may cause difficulty in diagnosis and assessment.

Despite the challenges in assessing enthesitis, both the Group for Research and Assessment of Psoriasis and Psoriatic Arthritis (GRAPPA) and the Outcome Measures in Rheumatology (OMERACT) group have identified it as an important domain in the assessment of PsA. GRAPPA determined that any composite tool for the assessment of PsA should include enthesitis to cover the spectrum of psoriatic disease (26). The tool should be able to grade entheseal activity and distinguish it from fibromyalgia. GRAPPA treatment guidelines recognize enthesitis as a discrete manifestation of PsA and propose an algorithmic approach to management (12).

The management of enthesitis is largely empirical, although evidence from randomized clinical trials is emerging. Local steroid injections should be used with extreme caution at entheseal insertions, particularly major insertions such as the Achilles tendon, as rupture can occur. Generally, steroid injections can be used with good effect at the insertions of the peroneus brevis, tibialis posterior, and plantar fascia. The Achilles insertion poses a particular challenge; at this location it is possible to achieve disease control by injecting steroid into the retrocalcaneal bursa, which extends down to, and 'bathes', the Achilles tendon insertion. Other therapies for enthesitis at the Achilles insertion include systemic therapies such as biologic drugs. In cases of isolated, disabling, enthesitis at the heel these drugs can be life-changing, but overcoming regulatory barriers may be a problem. Heel cup raises are often used but are not evidence-based.

Synovitis

Synovitis is mainly seen in peripheral joints. Classically this is an asymmetrical oligoarthritis affecting the large joints of the lower limbs, but in PsA the peripheral joint involvement may predominate. In PsA articular involvement varies, from involvement of a single midfoot or rearfoot joint to a destructive polyarthritis with extensive bone loss, as seen in arthritis mutilans. In established disease, as many as 95% of people with PsA have forefoot involvement, including hallux valgus and claw toes; rearfoot deformity in the form of pes planovalgus has been reported in 65% (24). The presentation may also be as a monoarthritis or oligoarthritis of the rearfoot, sometimes with very prominent synovial hypertrophy without much heat or redness, the so-called hypertrophic synovitis. The natural history and local progression in such cases (a similar presentation may also occur in the knee and elbow) is unclear but clinically it is usually poorly responsive to treatment, both local and systemic.

Synovitis in spondyloarthropathy is typically more vascular, with tortuous vessels visible on the surface of the synovium on arthroscopy. This hypervascularity is likely the cause of the occasional clinical feature of blue discoloration over the joints. The cellular and cytokine profile of spondyloarthropathy differs in several respects from that seen in RA, with increased CD163 and ICAM-1 and a higher number of polymorphonuclear cells. In RA anticitrullinated protein antibodies are found. The paradox of spondyloarthropathy is the coexistence of osteolysis and new bone formation. Osteolysis may also be a feature of RA, and is likely a result of osteoclastic activity, but can be much more severe and prominent in spondyloarthropathy, especially PsA, leading to 'whittled' digits (Figure 7.7). New bone formation is likely a result of osteoblastic activity and is 'driven' by the activity of IL-22. The new bone formation is characteristically seen around the joint margins and may appear 'whiskery', but new bone formation may eventually result in joint fusion (Figure 7.7).

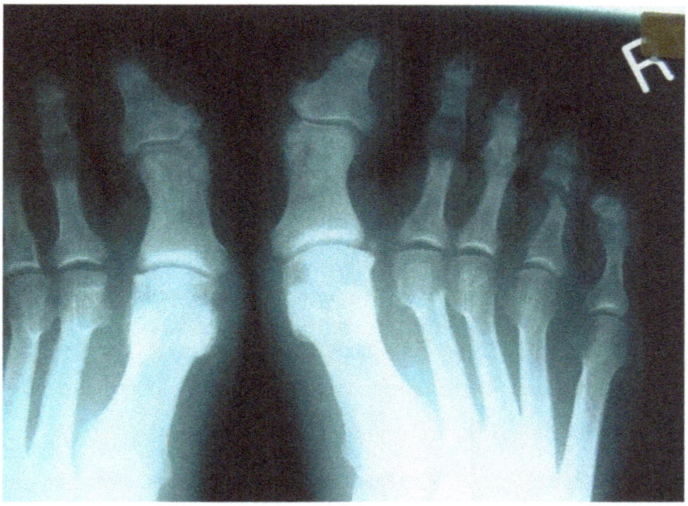

Figure 7.7 Osteolysis and ankylosis in the same foot in psoriatic arthritis.

Clinical synovitis presenting in the foot may therefore be indistinguishable from RA initially but, as noted above, other clinical features may help in differentiation. The synovitis of the small joints is often less profound and may therefore result in an asymmetrical appearance. Sometimes isolated distal interphalangeal joint involvement may be distinguishable clinically, and isolated midfoot and rearfoot involvement may occur. However, even in the foot other clues may be apparent. The appearance of dactylitis and enthesitis are hallmark features, while the presence of skin and nail involvement also provide distinguishing clues. Just casting the glance from the feet to the knees, hands, and elbows will often resolve difficulties in clinical diagnosis.

Tenosynovitis

Whilst enthesitis is a hallmark feature of the spondyloarthropathies, tenosynovitis is not uncommon, and this is frequently seen in the major tendons that cross the ankle joint. A good working knowledge of anatomy is essential to be able to locate and assess the tendons accurately at key sites where they are prone to pathology. This can be driven by mechanical factors, particularly from friction of the tendons as they pass eroded bony surfaces. Both medial and lateral ankle tendons change direction around bony prominences, which occasionally act as pulleys, and these are subject to substantial friction and mechanical stress. Fibrocartilage is usually present on the surface of the bony pulley to prevent the tendon 'sawing' through bone. The presence of fibrocartilage content appears to be a dynamic process as regression of the fibrocartilage has been described with surgical re-routing of tendons (27). As fibrocartilage is typically avascular, distinct avascular zones and changes in the tendon histology have been seen at the anatomical sites shown to be vulnerable to pathology (28, 29).

Similar to the presentation seen in RA, the tendon of tibialis posterior and the peroneal tendons are frequently affected in PsA (24). Inflammation in these tendon sheaths is commonly seen as an extension of the active inflammatory process in adjacent joints, namely the subtalar, talonavicular, and calcaneocuboid joints, with subsequent deterioration of tendon caused by collagenases, released by close inflamed synovial tissue. Furthermore, oedema within bone has been described adjacent to abnormal tendons and this may also be associated with proliferative changes of non-articular bone (30). Erosion at the point of tendon contact with bony prominences, especially those acting as pulleys such as the medial and lateral malleoli, has been described.

The tendons of peroneus longus (PL) and brevis (PB) are generally prone to tenosynovitis and tears in three common locations—the lateral malleolus, the peroneal tubercle on the calcaneus and the undersurface of the cuboid bone (PL), and at the tuberosity at the lateral aspect of the proximal fifth metatarsal bone (PB). Bone marrow oedema has commonly been found at the level of the peroneal tubercle and those with hypertrophy of the tubercle are thought to be predisposed to peroneal tendon tears and tenosynovitis. At the level of the malleolus the peroneal tendons share a common synovial sheath, separating into individual sheaths at the level of the inferior peroneal retinaculum. Distal to the inferior peroneal retinaculum, the PB tendon has a straight course toward its insertion at the base of the fifth metatarsal. The PL tendon crosses the calcaneocuboid joint, courses along the sulcus at the inferolateral aspect of the cuboid bone; as it reaches the cuboid notch, it no longer has a synovial sleeve and is surrounded only by a paratenon. The presence of os peroneum within the PL tendon, typically in close proximity to the cuboid bone, has been presumed to predispose the PL tendon to injury. Once PL enters the cuboid tunnel it continues along the plantar aspect of the forefoot to its insertion sites on the plantar lateral surface of the medial cuneiform bone and the plantar aspect of the first and second metatarsal bases. Given the intimate relationship of the peroneal tendons, it is not surprising that a recent study has shown that pathological features of one tendon correlated strongly with the pathological features of the other tendon, even in an asymptomatic population (31).

Disease of the tibialis posterior (TP) tendon is most common in the medial ankle (32). The tendon passes behind the medial malleolus, where it changes direction and is encased in a sheath beneath the flexor retinaculum to prevent dislocation. There is an area of relative hypovascularity immediately distal to the medial malleolus, which may contribute to the development of degenerative changes and consequent rupture. Indeed, tears in the TP tendon occur most commonly just distal to the medial malleolus, followed by the navicular insertion (33). This occurs more commonly in patients with seronegative arthropathies and RA (approximately 13% and 5% of cases, respectively) (34). The anterior slip of the TP tendon inserts primarily into the tuberosity of the navicular and this is a prime site for pathology in patients with PsA.

Sustained inflammation in the tendon sheaths will eventually lead to deterioration of the collagenous substance of the tendon itself and it may become functionally inadequate; however, as the individual seeks to avoid loading the affected part it can be difficult to determine the level of tendon pathology through clinical examination alone. When assessing patients, it can be very challenging to establish clearly the extent to which tendon damage is being driven predominantly by mechanical and/or inflammatory pathways, therefore it is essential that both are considered, and targeted interventions instigated accordingly.

Management

Gaining an appreciation of the overall current and previous history of disease activity is essential when working with patients who have foot problems related to spondyloarthropathies. The clinician requires accurate and reliable clinical and instrumental assessments of pain, inflammation, disease activity, joint range of motion, functional ability, articular deformity, extra-articular features, and concomitant conditions. With such information, decisions for systemic pharmacological treatment and management of foot problems can be made. Based on GRAPPA treatment guidelines, a management approach is outlined in Figure 7.8. The key to effective management of foot problems is through staged and targeted interventions in early disease, with the ultimate aim of zero tolerance of active disease in the foot through the combination of pharmacological

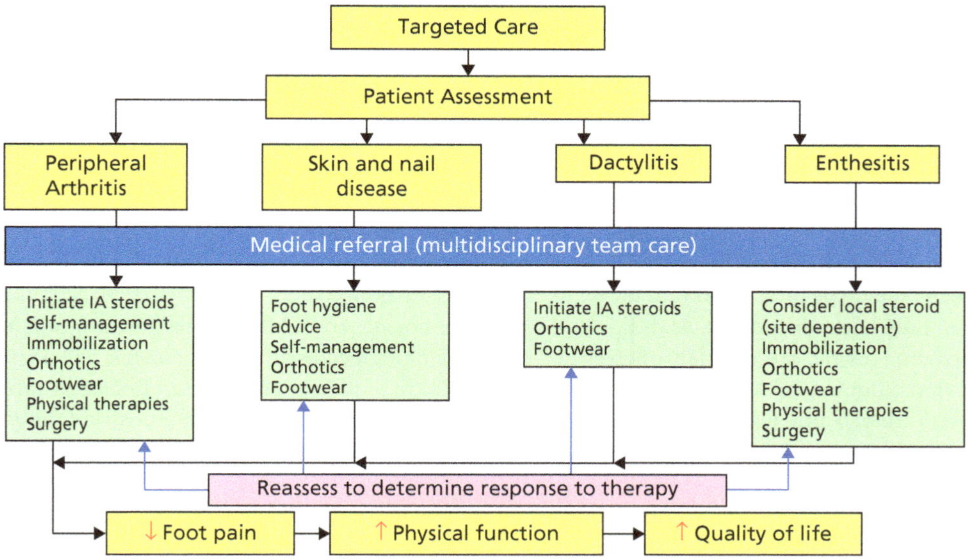

Figure 7.8 A suggested scheme for assessment and treatment of foot problems in patients with psoriatic arthritis based on Group for Research and Assessment of Psoriasis and Psoriatic Arthritis treatment guidelines. IA, Intra-articular.

anti-inflammatory agents, and, ideally, effort should be directed toward preventing and avoiding mechanical articular and peri-articular lesions. In practice, however, there is evidence to suggest that active foot disease persists in many patients despite recent treatment advances and the concept of 'tight control' of disease (21). Furthermore, only a small proportion (20%) of those with moderate to high levels of foot-related impairment and disability will receive foot care (24).

The manifestations of PsA (dystrophic nails, dactylitis, synovitis, bursitis, joint erosions, deformity, callosities) are frequently found in the forefoot (24, 35, 36). Many patients with PsA experience pain under the nails (subungual), as depicted in Figure 7.5. It has been shown that joint disease in the distal interphalangeal joint in PsA is often associated with thickening of the tissues under the nail bed with diffuse inflammation that envelops the nail root and adjacent bone (37). Extra-depth footwear to accommodate any forefoot deformity and to reduce pressures exerted on the subungual tissues should be beneficial in these cases; in conjunction with the provision of help with nail care, if needed, this may prevent onychocryptosis/infections, and this is of paramount importance for those on biologic therapies. It is recognized that the causes of pain at the MTP joint level are complex and can be related to inflammation (36) and increased mechanical pressure over structurally damaged metatarsals (35). Debridement of callus, provision of orthoses and/or extra-depth shoes are all indicated to off-load inflamed/painful MTP joints.

Pes planovalgus deformity has been shown to be relatively common in PsA and, although emerging research suggests benefit in RA, the evidence in PsA is lacking. Whilst the typical deformities in the forefoot and rearfoot appear similar between RA and PsA, it must be recognized that PsA has distinct bone morphology, as noted above, and we need to consider this and adapt mechanical therapies (orthoses, footwear) accordingly. It is reasonable to assume that orthoses designed to attenuate mechanical stresses would be beneficial in joints and soft tissues that are acutely inflamed or in those where disease remains locally persistent. Ideally, we should use corrective functional foot orthoses, aiming to optimize foot function in early disease to provide joint stabilization, correct foot position, rest key anatomical structures, and resist the deforming forces resulting from repeated episodes of inflammation. The aim would be to reduce pain, reduce mechanically driven inflammation, and prevent the development of joint deformity. In cases where the peroneal and TP tendons are affected, an orthotic device that supports the medial longitudinal arch of the foot is thought to be helpful, but controlled trials are lacking in this area. In some cases, patients may have persistent pain/inflammation of the peroneal tendons around the cuboid notch and base of the fifth metatarsal. It is not uncommon for some patients to develop a focus of high pressure around this site and attempts to off-load this site should be made.

In light of the predilection for PsA to affect the Achilles tendon and plantar fascia, specific focus should be directed toward trying to establish normal mechanics in the sagittal plane (ankle joint dorsiflexion and plantar flexion and MTP joint dorsiflexion). Muscle strengthening will be required for the calf muscle weakness that may have developed as a result of antalgic gait adaptations (limited ankle joint movement). The evidence base to support the use of physical therapies (therapeutic ultrasound, laser, extracorporeal shock wave therapy) and eccentric training is lacking in those with spondyloarthropathy as most studies exclude those with inflammatory joint disease.

Local corticosteroid injections are generally considered to have a strong role to play in the treatment of persistent active foot disease, with the exception of the Achilles tendon. This is despite a paucity of good-quality studies to support their use. It must be noted that local corticosteroid injections do not always result in clinical or symptomatic improvement and it has been hypothesized that one reason for a lack of response could be inaccuracy of the injection. In those studies that have examined the effect of accuracy of attempted intra-articular injections on efficacy, the lowest accuracy rates have been reported for joints in the foot/ankle (38, 39). Whilst not specific to spondyloarthropathy populations, ultrasound has been shown in small series to improve the accuracy of needle placement and joint aspiration (40, 41) and to improve the accuracy of joint injection significantly as compared with clinical examination guidance (42). Ultrasound-guided injections should be specifically considered in cases where the anatomy is distorted by the disease process, in cases where previous clinical examination-guided injections have failed to yield a response, and when less-soluble preparations are injected to reduce the likelihood of tissue necrosis and damage to surrounding tissues.

Conclusions and research agenda

The concept of achieving tight control of disease should be applied to the foot; to achieve this goal addressing the core domains recommended by GRAPPA should be included. Through the use of integrated biomechanical and inflammatory measures it should be possible to determine the underlying dominant mechanisms operating in the presentation of the foot impairments and disability in patients with spondyloarthropathy and a personalized targeted approach should be initiated.

There are areas where knowledge is lacking. Much of the treatment administered is based on the, probably correct, assumption that it works elsewhere, and for other diseases, so it must work for psoriatic arthritis. However, it would be ideal if the following areas were investigated:

- Why does dactylitis commonly affect the fourth toe? Is there a biomechanical reason?
- Do mechanical therapies work for enthesitis? Should they be combined with pharmacological therapies such as local steroid injections? These are the underlying assumptions of treatment in RA.
- What influence does skin and nail disease have on the ability to wear orthotics and footwear? Should we be treating the skin (and nails) aggressively for this reason?

References

1. **Wright V, Moll JMH.** *Seronegative Polyarthritis.* Amsterdam: North Holland Publishing Co.; 1976.
2. **Brewerton DA, Caffrey M, Hart FD, James DCO, Nicholls A, Sturrock RD.** Ankylosing spondylitis and HL-A27. *Lancet.* 1973;**1**:904–7.
3. **Rudwaleit M, van der HD, Landewe R, et al.** The development of Assessment of SpondyloArthritis International Society classification criteria for axial spondyloarthritis (part II): validation and final selection. *Ann Rheum Dis.* 2009;**68**(6):777–83.
4. **Rudwaleit M, van der HD, Landewe R, et al.** The Assessment of SpondyloArthritis International Society classification criteria for peripheral spondyloarthritis and for spondyloarthritis in general. *Ann Rheum Dis.* 2011;**70**(1):25–31.
5. **Helliwell P, Wright V.** Epidemiological, environmental and sociological aspects of seronegative arthropathies. *Bailliere's Clin Rheumatol.* 1987;**1**:491–524.
6. **McGonagle D, Gibbon W, Emery P.** Classification of inflammatory arthritis by enthesitis. *Lancet.* 1998;**352**:1137–40.
7. **Healy P, Helliwell PS.** Measuring clinical enthesitis in psoriatic arthritis:assessment of existing measures and development of an instrument specific for psoriatic arthritis. *Arthritis Care Res.* 2008;**59**(5):686–91.
8. **Healy PJ, Helliwell PS.** Measuring dactylitis in clinical trials: which is the best instrument to use?[see comment]. *J Rheumatol.* 2007;**34**(6):1302–6.
9. **Helliwell PS, FitzGerald O, Fransen J, et al.** The development of candidate composite disease activity and responder indices for psoriatic arthritis (GRACE project). *Ann Rheum Dis.* 2013;**72**(6):986–91.
10. **Helliwell PS, Ruderman E.** Natural history, prognosis and socio-economic aspects of psoriatic arthritis. In: Ritchlin C, Fitzgerald O (eds). *Psoriatic and Reactive Arthritis.* Philadelphia: Mosby, 2007: pp. 29–36.
11. **Gladman DD, Farewell VT.** Progression in psoriatic arthritis: role of time varying clinical indicators. *J Rheumatol.* 1999;**26**(11):2409–13.
12. **Coates LC, Kavanaugh A, Mease PJ, et al.** Group for research and assessment of psoriasis and psoriatic arthritis: treatment recommendations for psoriatic arthritis 2015. *Arthritis Rheumatol.* 2016:**68**(5):1060–71.
13. **Gossec L, Smolen JS, Ramiro S, et al.** European League Against Rheumatism (EULAR) recommendations for the management of psoriatic arthritis with pharmacological therapies: 2015 update. *Ann Rheum Dis.* 2016;**75**(3):499–510.
14. **Ward MM, Deodhar A, Akl EA, et al.** American College of Rheumatology/Spondylitis Association of America/Spondyloarthritis Research and Treatment Network 2015 Recommendations for the Treatment of Ankylosing Spondylitis and Nonradiographic Axial Spondyloarthritis. *Arthritis Care Res.* 2016;**68**(2):151–66.
15. **McInnes IB, Mease P, Kirkham B, et al.** Secukinumab, a human anti-interleukin-17A monoclonal antibody, in patients with psoriatic arthritis (FUTURE 2): a randomised, double-blind, placebo-controlled, phase 3 trial. *Lancet.* 2015;**6736**(15):61134–5.
16. **Gladman DD, Shuckett R, Russell ML, Thorne JC, Schachter RK.** Psoriatic arthritis (PSA)—an analysis of 220 patients. *Q J Med.* 1987;**238**:127–41.
17. **Ash Z, Tinazzi I, Kwok C, et al.** Psoriasis patients with nail disease have a greater magnitude of underlying systemic subclinical enthesopathy than those with normal nails. *Ann Rheum Dis.* 2012;**71**(4):553–6.
18. **Cassell SE, Bieber JD, Rich P, et al.** The modified Nail Psoriasis Severity Index: validation of an instrument to assess psoriatic nail involvement in patients with psoriatic arthritis. *J Rheumatol.* 2007;**34**(1):123–9.
19. **Chung J, Callis Duffin K, Takeshita J, et al.** Palmoplantar psoriasis is associated with greater impairment of health-related quality of life compared with moderate to severe plaque psoriasis. *J Am Acad Derm.* 2014;**71**(4):623–32.

20. **Pettey AA, Balkrishnan R, Rapp SR, Fleischer AB, Feldman SR.** Patients with palmoplantar psoriasis have more physical disability and discomfort than patients with other forms of psoriasis: implications for clinical practice. *J Am Acad Derm*. 2003;**49**(2):271–5.
21. **Healy PJ, Groves C, Chandramohan M, Helliwell PS.** MRI changes in psoriatic dactylitis: extent of pathology, relationship to tenderness and correlation with clinical indices. *Rheumatology*. 2008;**47**(1):92–5.
22. **Brockbank JE, Stein M, Schentag CT, Gladman DD.** Dactylitis in psoriatic arthritis: a marker for disease severity? *Ann Rheum Dis*. 2005;**64**(2):188–90.
23. **Wilkins RA, Siddle H, Redmond A, Helliwell P.** The mechanical impact of toe dactylitis in psoriatic arthritis: an exploratory study. *Clin Rheumatol*. 2016;**35**:2333–8.
24. **Hyslop E, McInnes IM, Woodburn J, Turner DE.** Foot problems in psoriatic arthritis: high burden and low care provision. *Ann Rheum Dis*. 2010;**69**(5):928.
25. **Freeston JE, Coates LC, Nam JL, et al.** Is there sub-clinical synovitis in early psoriatic arthritis? A clinical comparison with grey scale and power Doppler ultrasound. *Arthritis Care Res*. 2014;**66**(3):432–9.
26. **Gladman DD, Mease PJ, Strand V, et al.** Consensus on a core set of domains for psoriatic arthritis [6 refs]. *J Rheumatol*. 2007;**34**(5):1167–70.
27. **Sobel M, Geppert M, Hannafin J, Bohne W, Arnoczky S.** Microvascular anatomy of the peroneal tendons. *J Foot Ankle Surg*. 1992;**13**:469–72.
28. **Petersen W, Bobka T, Stein V, Tillmann B.** Blood supply of the peroneal tendons: injection and immunohistochemical studies of cadaver tendons. *Acta Ortho Scand*. 2000;**71**(2):168–74.
29. **Benjamin M, McGonagle D.** The anatomical basis for disease localisation in seronegative spondyloarthropathy at entheses and related sites. *J Anat*. 2001;**199**(Pt 5):503–26.
30. **Morrison WB, Carrino JA, Schweitzer ME, Sanders TG, Raiken DP, Johnson CE.** Subtendinous bone marrow edema patterns on MR images of the ankle: association with symptoms and tendinopathy. *AJR Am J Roentgenol*. 2001;**176**(5):1149–54.
31. **O'Donnell P, Saifuddin A.** Cuboid oedema due to peroneus longus tendinopathy: a report of four cases. *Skel Radiol*. 2005;**34**(7):381–8.
32. **Miller SD, Van Holsbeeck M, Boruta PM, Wu KK, Katcherian DA.** Ultrasound in the diagnosis of posterior tibial tendon pathology. *Foot Ankle Int*. 1996;**17**(9):555–8.
33. **Johnson KA.** Tibialis posterior tendon rupture. *Clin Orthop Rel Res*. 1983;**177**:140–7.
34. **Fessell DP, van Holsbeeck M.** Ultrasound of the foot and ankle. *Sem Musculoskel Radiol*. 1998;**2**(3):271–82.
35. **Turner DE, Hyslop E, Barn R, McInnes IB, Steultjens MP, Woodburn J.** Metatarsophalangeal joint pain in psoriatic arthritis: a cross-sectional study. *Rheumatology (Oxford, England)*. 2014;**53**(4):737–40.
36. **Delle Sedie A, Riente L, Filippucci E, et al.** Ultrasound imaging for the rheumatologist. XXXII. Sonographic assessment of the foot in patients with psoriatic arthritis. *Clin Exp Rheumatol*. 2011;**29**(2):217–22.
37. **McGonagle D.** Enthesitis: an autoinflammatory lesion linking nail and joint involvement in psoriatic disease. *J Eur Acad Derm Venereol:*. 2009;**23**(Suppl. 1):9–13.
38. **Jones A, Regan M, Ledingham J, Pattrick M, Manhire A, Doherty M.** Importance of placement of intra-articular steroid injections. *BMJ (Clinical Research ed)*. 1993;**307**(6915):1329–30.
39. **Eustace JA, Brophy DP, Gibney RP, Bresnihan B, FitzGerald O.** Comparison of the accuracy of steroid placement with clinical outcome in patients with shoulder symptoms. *Ann Rheum Dis*. 1997;**56**(1):59–63.
40. **Balint PV, Kane D, Hunter J, McInnes IB, Field M, Sturrock RD.** Ultrasound guided versus conventional joint and soft tissue fluid aspiration in rheumatology practice: a pilot study. *J Rheumatol*. 2002;**29**(10):2209–13.

41. **Raza K, Lee CY, Pilling D, et al.** Ultrasound guidance allows accurate needle placement and aspiration from small joints in patients with early inflammatory arthritis. *Rheumatology (Oxford, England)*. 2003;**42**(8):976–9.

42. **Cunnington J, Marshall N, Hide G, et al.** A randomized, double-blind, controlled study of ultrasound-guided corticosteroid injection into the joint of patients with inflammatory arthritis. *Arthritis Rheum*. 2010;**62**(7):1862–9.

43. **Garrett S, Jenkinson T, Kennedy LG, Whitelock H, Gaisford P, Calin A.** A new approach to defining disease status in ankylosing spondylitis: the Bath Ankylosing Spondylitis Disease Activity Index. *J Rheumatol*. 1994;**21**(12):2286–91.

44. **Lukas C, Landewe R, Sieper J, et al.** Development of an ASAS-endorsed disease activity score (ASDAS) in patients with ankylosing spondylitis. *Ann Rheum Dis*. 2009;**68**(1):18–24.

45. **Mumtaz A, Gallagher P, Kirby B, et al.** Development of a preliminary composite disease activity index in psoriatic arthritis. *Ann Rheum Dis*. 2011;**70**:272–7.

Chapter 8

Autoimmune connective tissue diseases

Begonya Alcacer-Pitarch, Edward Vital, and Maya Buch

Epidemiology

Systemic sclerosis

Systemic sclerosis (SSc) is a heterogeneous connective tissue disease characterized by vasculopathy, immune activation, and fibrosis (1–3). The prevalence of SSc varies enormously, from 30 to 2280 per 1,000,000 population (4), with geographical variation recorded (5–7). In the UK the prevalence ranges from 31 per million in the West Midlands to 150 per million in South and West London (8–10).

The female-to-male ratio in SSc is approximately 3:1 (ranging from 1 to 14:1) (4, 6, 11, 12). The onset of the disease varies according to ethnic background and sex but usually its peak of incidence is reached at the fifth decade. However, SSc can occur at any age, albeit rare in children and in the very elderly (5, 6, 9, 13, 14).

Systemic lupus erythematosus

Systemic lupus erythematosus (SLE) is a multisystem autoimmune disorder that most commonly affects skin and musculoskeletal systems but can also cause inflammation and damage in any of the major organs. Involvement of the brain, lungs, and kidneys may be fatal, but its greatest impact on mortality is via the long-term effects of disease and glucocorticoid therapy, leading to a 50-fold increase in cardiovascular disease. It usually affects women (9:1 female:male ratio) with onset from the teens to the mid-forties and a relapsing remitting course thereafter. The most severely affected patients are of Afro-Caribbean and East Asian descent and those with paediatric or adolescent onset (15).

Pathophysiology

Systemic sclerosis

SSc is characterized by three pathological features: vasculopathy, immune activation, and fibrosis. These three factors interact in a complex manner, leading to obliterative fibrointimal proliferation of small vessels with vasospastic episodes, resulting in ischaemia; immunological disruption; and activation of resident connective tissue cells with increased deposition of extracellular matrix constituents causing fibrosis (3, 16–18).

Vasculopathy is considered one of the earliest and is a key event in the pathological process of SSc (16, 17, 19), one to which much of the morbidity and mortality in SSc is related. Early on, the disease microvasculopathy can be observed clinically in the form of Raynaud's phenomenon (RP), indicating peripheral vasculopathy. In addition, an uncontrolled fibrosis replaces the normal (controlled) wound healing-associated repair (2), and as the disease progresses the skin lesions become relatively avascular. About 12–18 months after this, there is usually little or no inflammation present but the skin lesions are left sclerotic, i.e., fibrosed, contracted, and scarred (16, 20).

Systemic lupus erythematosus

SLE is predominantly driven by activation of the immune system, affecting the vascular, neurological, renal, musculoskeletal, and integumentary systems. The occurrence of antibodies to DNA in the blood of people many years before the appearance of the disease suggests a link between such antibodies and the disease manifestations. Levels of antibody against DNA are still used as a measure of disease activity. The pathological processes in the end organs are partly driven by antibody/antigen deposition in blood vessels (e.g., glomerulus of kidney), but there are many other nuclear protein targets for antibodies in this disease and some of these lead to disease-specific targets, such as the heart. Other mechanisms of disease pathogenesis include T cellular-driven autoimmunity and cytokine abnormalities.

Lower limb pathology

Scleroderma

SSc is a multi-system disease affecting multiple major organs with distinct and important manifestations in the foot and ankle.

SSc is defined by the presence of skin tightening, and the extent of involvement determines the classification into limited (distal to elbows/knees) or diffuse (proximal to elbows/knees ± chest/trunk) disease (21). Skin changes often start with an oedematous phase (in the papillary and reticular dermis), followed by a firm induration and fibrosis (16). Clinically the oedematous phase can be observed in the form of oedematous feet. Subsequently, the skin becomes thicker and tighter on palpation as it progresses to become sclerotic, contracted, and scarred (Figure 8.1)(16, 18, 22, 23). In the feet, damage to the sebaceous glands can cause hypohidrosis, and substitution of the fat cells with collagen can lead to subcutaneous plantar fat-pad atrophy, which is thought to contribute to the increased plantar foot pressures reported in SSc (24). Initial clinical studies (24) suggest that increased plantar foot pressures and prolonged duration of loading through discrete areas of the foot (Figure 8.2) are associated with pain and functional impairment during walking; this is similar to findings reported in people with rheumatoid arthritis (RA) (25, 26).

As a result of the structural changes within the integumentary system, the foot's normal biological and biomechanical properties are lost. This compromises skin integrity, tissue viability, healing, and the foot's ability to adapt to the increased pressures: for example, the extensibility of the skin is reduced because of fibrosis of the hypodermis (27). The loss of skin extensibility together with the fibrosis of periarticular soft-tissue structures (21, 28) limits range of motion (ROM) at joints, with a subsequent impact on function (24).

The structural and biomechanical changes of the skin, together with tendon and joint pathologies, can lead to the development of flexion contractures. When this happens in the toes, the toes are left in a fixed-flexed position which has a major impact on gait and shoe fit. These deformities not only impair the movement of the affected joints but also contribute to the risk of developing ulcers over the flexed joints and areas of skin tension. Indeed, ulcer aetiology is multifactorial. The skin is exposed to constant stress and shear as a result of external factors such as footwear, and internal factors such as fixed deformities and the skin's inability to adapt to pressure because of the

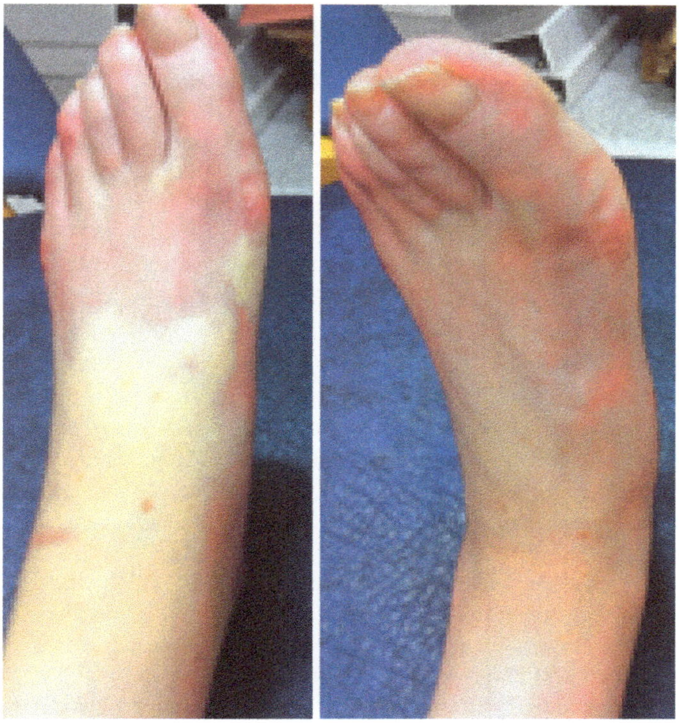

Figure 8.1 Fibrosis affecting the feet, causing capillary compression during normal movement such as ankle plantar flexion.

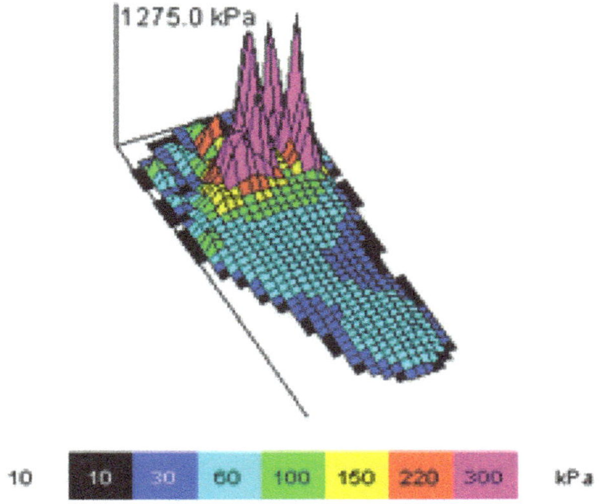

Figure 8.2 Highly elevated plantar foot pressures in the metatarsophalangeal joints of a patient with systemic sclerosis.

Reproduced with kind permission from B. Alcacer-Pitarch.

presence of fibrosis. Combined with vasculopathy this causes the deformed and fibrosed areas to be at high risk of ulceration (29, 30).

Ulceration also occurs in areas without deformity, and particularly on the apex of the toe. The aetiology of ulcers in people with SSc is commonly associated with vasculopathy, presence of calcium deposits, skin fibrosis, and/or hyperkeratosis (31). Once ulcers are present they are extremely painful and have a very slow healing rate, the latter being negatively affected by the amount of skin pathology. The ulcers can become chronic, increasing the risk of amputation (31). Lower limb amputation as a result of refractory ulcers has an incidence of 0.67% (32) in patients with SSc. Even in cases where healing is achieved, the ulcerated area experiences tissue loss and scar tissue formation. Skin scarring, together with the presence of vasculopathy, adds to the impairment of the biomechanical properties of the local skin, leaving the area even more prone to re-ulceration.

Systemic lupus erythematosus

There is very little work on the foot and ankle in SLE. Two patient surveys, one in the UK and one in New Zealand (NZ), have reported a high prevalence of foot complaints in this group—87% in the UK and 77% in NZ (33, 34). The NZ group found that rearfoot and ankle joint pain predominated, but there was a high prevalence of forefoot, especially metatarsophalangeal joint pain, in both groups.

Fifty per cent of both groups of respondents reported significant RP, with about one-fifth reporting foot ulceration at some point. These figures represent a high burden of foot symptoms in SLE, but it must be remembered that these were voluntary respondents and may have self-selected because of their symptoms. In addition, there was no control group with which to compare the frequency of symptoms. One other study has looked at musculoskeletal involvement by performing ultrasound examination of the joints in a small sample—80% of the examined group were found to have grey-scale synovial hypertrophy, although only a minority of these had vascular inflammation (35).

Vascular-related foot pathology in both diseases

One of the first microvascular clinical presentations is RP. It affects between 90% and 98% of patients with SLE and SSc.

The clinical presentation of RP can be divided into three phases. The initial phase is the ischaemic phase, where the digits present with a pallor discoloration (white), reflecting vasospasm; this phase is followed by the deoxygenation phase, where the digits become cyanotic (blue discoloration); in the final phase, the reperfusion phase, the digits become red, expressing the compensatory vasodilation (36–38). These clinical signs are accompanied by symptoms such as cold, paraesthesia, and pain during the duration of the RP attacks (Figure 8.3).

In a study of 100 patients with SSc, 90% were affected by RP in their feet and 31% had necrotizing RP, which is characterized by digital ulcers (9). The reported proportion of patients affected by foot ulcers ranges from 20% to 26% (9, 39).

In SSc, the presence of RP in combination with the microvasculopathy and skin fibrosis can lead to ulcers on the apices of the digits, over the extensor surfaces of the joints, and on the lower leg/malleolus (Figure 8.4) (31, 40, 41). Macrovasculopathy can lead to larger lower limb ulceration and amputation (42). Other risk factors for the development of ulcers in SSc include the presence of calcinosis (Figure 8.4), impaired skin biomechanics due to fibroses or hyperkeratosis (31), and/or neuropathy. The latter, though, lacks a formal body of evidence as it has only been reported in a case study of peripheral sensory neuropathy (43).

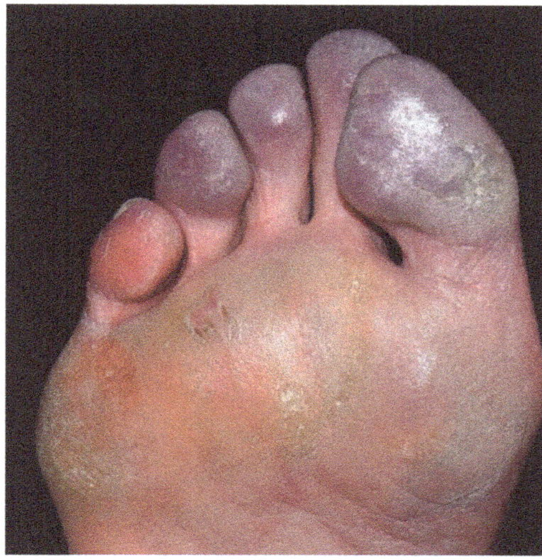

Figure 8.3 The deoxygenation phase in Raynaud's phenomenon.

Ulcers in people with SSc are often extremely painful and can take many months to heal. The mean time-to-heal varies depending on the type of ulcer, ranging from 25 to 281 days, but in some cases it has been reported to be as long as 810 days (31). These lesions are accompanied with pain and functional impairment, and can lead to tissue loss and amputation of fingers and/or toes. All of these factors contribute to a highly negative effect on the patient's quality of life (44, 45).

The development and healing of ulcers in patients with SSc and SLE can be further aggravated by the presence of vasculitis (Figure 8.5). Vasculitis in SSc can lead to severe ischaemia, ulcers, necrosis, and amputations, the latter more commonly seen when the vessels of the digits are involved (46). In some cases, vasculitis can contribute to the pathogenesis of neurological lesions (47, 48) by affecting the arteriae nervorum, causing necrosis of the nerve bundles. Depending on the nerve affected, this can cause peripheral neuropathy (49). Which, clinically, presents as an asymmetric neuropathy or multiple mononeuropathies (49), with diffuse degeneration distal to the lesion area (50). This pattern is characteristic of necrotizing vasculitis (51).

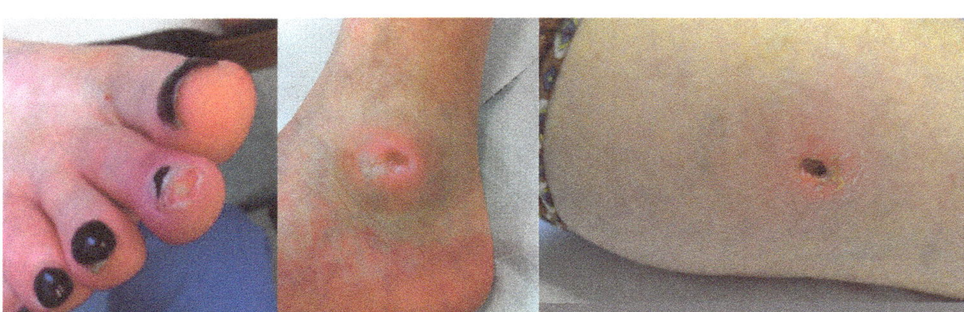

Figure 8.4 (Left) Digital ulcer on the apex of the second toe caused by microvasculopathy. (Middle) Malleolus ulcer caused by skin fibrosis and vasculopathy. (Right) Leg ulcer caused by calcinosis.

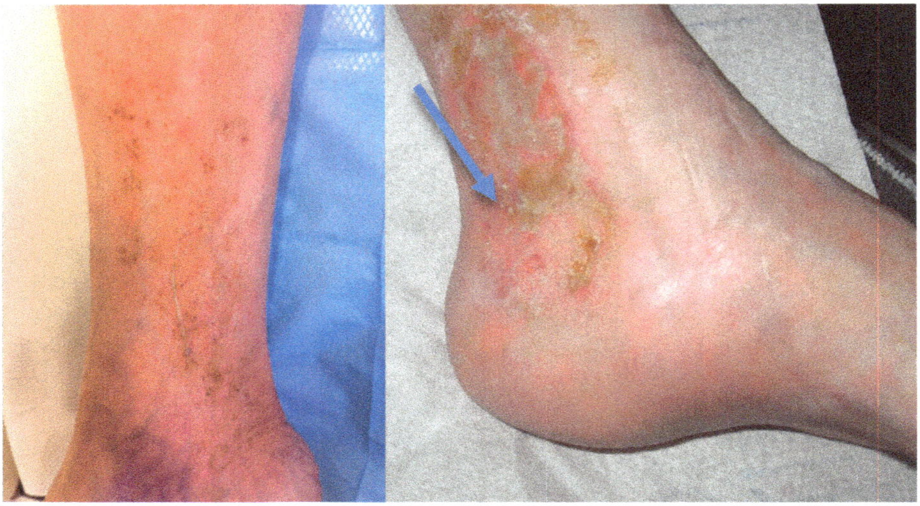

Figure 8.5 (Left) Vasculitis on right leg in an antineutrophil cytoplasmic antibody (ANCA)-positive systemic sclerosis patient, potential precursor for ulceration. (Right) Left leg ulcer with signs of vasculitis in the perilesional skin.

Neurologically related foot pathology

The affected nerve fibres from the autonomic nervous system cause parasympathetic underactivity and sympathetic overdrive (52, 53), which are reflected in the feet as abnormal sympathetic skin responses, RP, and hypohidrosis (52, 54–57). The prevalence of peripheral nervous system abnormalities in SSc varies, but has been reported to be as high as 50% in a small sample (n=14) (54) and as low as 5.6% in a larger cohort (n=125) (58, 59). Patient self-report sensory neuropathy occurred in 16% of a sample of SLE patients in the UK (33). Mononeuritis multiplex, sensorimotor neuropathy, and compression neuropathies are all observed in SLE and SSc. The clinical presentation of peripheral neuropathy is typically distal but with a non-length-dependent pattern to the sensory symptoms, more sensory than motor, and mostly multiple mononeuropathy or asymmetric in involvement (suggesting multifocal pathology) (49, 54). It has also been described to be present with early neurological signs of sensory–motor mononeuropathy, which progresses to a typical distal polyneuropathy in the rest of the body with greater involvement of the lower limbs (60). When sensory symptoms are present they can vary from allodynia, lancinating pains, burning, paraesthesia, and pruritus through to loss of sensation, and these symptoms have been reported to be more prominent in the extremities (54).

Musculoskeletal involvement

Ninety per cent of patients with SLE and SSc report musculoskeletal complaints. These range from intermittent small and large joint arthralgia to chronic polyarthritis (33, 61, 62) and muscle involvement (63, 64). Joint symptoms have been reported to be present in 66% of patients with SSc (65), with muscular symptoms in half of the patients, the latter with a predominance of muscle weakness and myalgia (59). Clinically they may present as a painful, stiff, symmetrical arthropathy, which is clinically indistinguishable from that of RA (61, 65). The arthropathy and joint symptoms are not exclusive to early disease; they can also emerge as the disease progresses, and approximately half of patients with SSc develop arthralgia after diagnosis (65, 66). In the

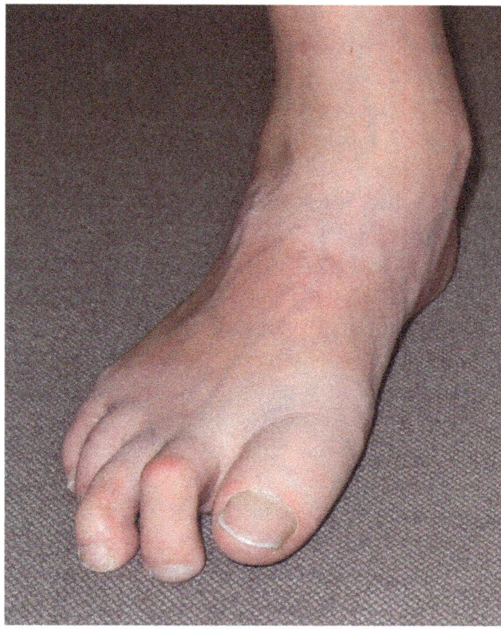

Figure 8.6 Flexion contractures in a patient with systemic sclerosis and acroosteolysis of the hallux's phalanx.

feet the arthropathy presents with a significant degenerative pattern in 18% of patients, fibrotic pattern in 8%, and inflammatory pattern in 7%. In the feet, the toe flexor tendons are affected by tendon contractures (Figure 8.6) and tenosynovitis, while the extensor tendons and the anterior and posterior tibial muscle tendons have been reported to be affected by tendinitis (67) (21, 64). Tendon friction rubs (associated with fibrinous deposits on the tendon sheath) affect the anterior and posterior tibial muscle tendons, toe flexors and extensor tendons, the Achilles' tendon, and the tendons on the dorsum of the foot, but detailed epidemiology data are lacking (21, 64, 68). These three clinical features contribute to the functional impairment of the joints and arthralgia.

Management

Conservative management

There is a lack of evidence regarding the management of disease-specific foot pathologies in patients with SSc and SLE. Instead, clinical management is based on evidence of treating similar pathologies in other diseases.

Careful consideration needs to be taken when clinically assessing and treating foot and ankle problems in patients with SSc and SLE. In relation to foot pathology these patients are considered high-risk patients owing to the severity of the disease, which affects multiple systems, all of which potentially have a direct or indirect effect on foot pathology. For example, impaired lung and heart function in SSc (69–71) will have an effect on the efficacy of soft-tissue oxygenation, therefore contributing to the severe effect that the vasculopathy already has on soft-tissue oxygenation of the limbs. In patients with SLE, renal involvement has been found to be associated with carotid atherosclerosis (72), possibly affecting the vascular tree from the lower limbs, causing peripheral arterial disease (73).

Provision of patient education as a preventative measure to avoid/reduce foot pathology in patients with SSc and SLE is crucial. A recent qualitative study in SLE patients has demonstrated that patients self-report a wide range of foot symptoms but usually self-treat rather than seek medical advice that is often indicated (74). Advice should be given on how to avoid situations that decrease blood flow, such as to minimize RP attacks by avoiding exposure to cold and stress, and smoking cessation. In addition, information should be provided on ulcer care, skin care, nail care, how to avoid increased harmful friction and shear from ill-fitted hosiery and footwear, and on when and how to access foot health services (75–77).

Patients need to be screened on a regular basis for the presence of peripheral neuropathy, as tactile sensitivity has been reported to be impaired in half of patients with SSc (78), and pure sensory and sensory–motor polyneuropathy has been found to be present in 40% of patients with SLE (79). Regular screening is important, as patients are often unaware of the loss of sensitivity, and present with subclinical neuropathy, thus putting them at risk of injury in the presence of harmful stimuli.

Once the skin is affected by fibrosis in SSc it rarely returns to its original form; however, in patients with early diffuse SSc, systemic treatment with methotrexate has been shown to improve skin fibrosis (80). Additionally, skin hypohidrosis can be treated locally with emollients or creams containing a low concentration of urea (5–10%) (81–83). Creams with higher concentrations of urea (i.e., 40%) are recommended in the presence of hyperkeratosis because of the keratolytic effect of urea (84, 85). In addition to using creams with urea, when there is a buildup of hyperkeratosis sharp debridement is recomended. In the case of plantar callosities, the removal of the callus decreases plantar pressures (86, 87). Debridement should also be considered to address high-risk presentations such as extravasated blood or underlying ulceration. Although debridement can alleviate pain, it might be short-lived, as is reported in patients with RA (88).

The treatment of ulcers will vary depending on the aetiology. In SSc and SLE, ischaemic digital ulcers, when active, are treated systemically with calcium channel blockers, angiotensin-converting enzyme inhibitors, losartan, or fluoxetine (89). If ulcers fail to respond, or re-occur, therapy can be escalated to oral sildenafil for 6 weeks, followed by intravenous prostanoids such as iloprost (90, 91). In cases of refractory or progressive ulceration, bosentan can also be used (89). Ulcers in SSc and SLE are extremely painful, so patients should be provided with appropriate pain management, such as a short-term course of opioids (30, 92, 93).

To optimize the healing process in both diseases, systemic treatments should be combined with local ulcer care, treating the wound bed and the perilesional skin (93, 94). For example, vitamin E gel used on the perilesional skin in ulcers of patients with SSc reduces the healing time (95) and debridement of necrotic tissue is recommended to avoid infection and promote healing (93, 94). Ulcer healing can also be impaired by the presence of vasculitis—in these cases systemic treatment with immunosuppressive medication needs to be provided (96).

In ulcers caused by calcinosis, the calcium deposits present on the wound bed (Figure 8.7) should be removed when possible. This is performed either surgically (97) or, as emerging evidence suggests, using carbon dioxide (CO_2) laser (98), as the removal of the calcium may reduce healing time, pain, and infection risk (93).

The presence of disabling foot pain is common in patients with SSc and SLE (76, 99). A multicentre randomized controlled trial in people with plantar foot pain and SSc compared the effectiveness of a simple pressure-relieving insole (Figure 8.8) with an insulating sham insole. The results at 12 weeks demonstrated a systematic improvement in pain in both groups, but the between-group differences were insignificant (100). Neuropathic pain has also been reported in SSc. When lower limb painful neuropathy is present it is commonly treated in the same way as diabetic painful polyneuropathy (101).

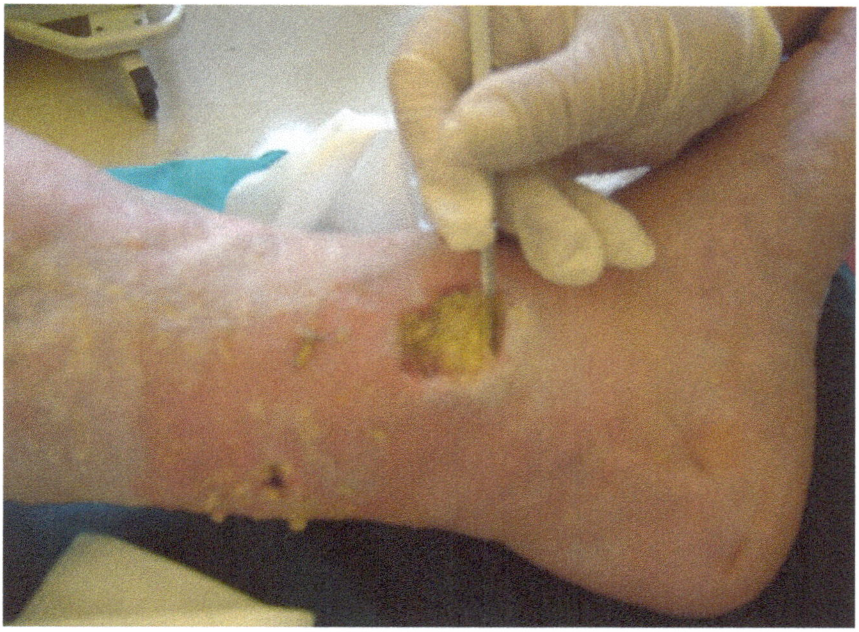

Figure 8.7 A plaque of calcium phosphate (hydroxyapatite) present on the ulcer wound bed of a patient with systemic sclerosis.

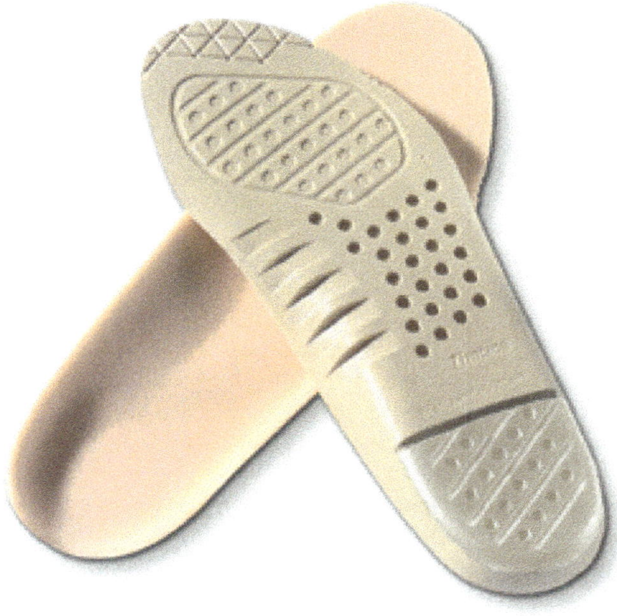

Figure 8.8 Simple pressure-relieving insole used in randomized controlled trial.

Both diseases can present with inflammatory joint pathology and during examination of inflamed joints the clinician needs to bear in mind that, in some cases, pre-existing joint disease and/or treatment with cytotoxic drugs and/or systemic corticosteroids can operate as a predisposing factor for joint infection. This is important because sometimes the progression of symptoms of a chronically abnormal joint can be attributed to underlying inflammatory joint disease, thus delaying the diagnosis of joint infection. Therefore, a monoarticular presentation must be considered as an infection until proven otherwise (102) as the adverse consequences of sepsis increase if left untreated.

Surgical management

Surgical interventions are generally performed as a last resort because of the increased risk of postoperative healing complications as a result of poor tissue viability (98). For example, surgery has been recommended when calcium deposits cause disability owing to the location of the lesion, although it is important to know that after excision further deposits can occur (103). In addition, when severe ischaemia is present, it may be possible to improve the circulation by revascularization of the digits with arterial reconstruction (mainly of large proximal vessels) or regional sympathectomies (77, 104). In cases of recalcitrant ulcers associated with severe ischaemia or widespreading gangrene, surgical amputation might be appropriate (105).

There are no reports of corrective foot and ankle surgery or joint replacement surgery in these diseases and the above considerations about healing would be apposite in this context.

Imaging strategies in systemic sclerosis

Nail fold capillaroscopy is used to aid diagnosis and identify patients at risk of digital ulcerations; ultrasound is used to assess soft-tissue pathologies; ultrasound virtual touch imaging and quantification measures absolute quantification of skin stiffness; and optical coherence tomography is used to assess skin fibrosis.

Nail fold capillaroscopy

This diagnostic imaging technique is used to discriminate primary (idiopathic) RP, affecting 10% of the general population, from secondary (to other disease/condition) RP (36–38). In primary RP normal capillary architecture can be observed, whilst in secondary RP clear abnormalities are recognized; the most well-described changes have been observed in patients with SSc. Structural changes of the skin's capillaries such as haemorrhage, megacapillaries, and loss of capillary density can be observed through the assessment of the nail fold capillaroscopy of the fingers and toes, although the toes seem to be less affected, possibly because of the lesser severity of the RP and skin involvement (106, 107). These capillary changes imply insufficient vasodilatory capacity and also irreparable vascular damage and are associated with the development of digital ulcers (108).

Depending on the nail fold capillaroscopy patterns the presence of an early, active, or late vasculopathy can be determined. These patterns correlate with disease duration and severity and are predictive of future organ prognosis (109–112). The RP and capillary changes manifest on a clinical level prior to the development of fibrosis of the skin, gut, and other internal organs such as lung and myocardial disease. Hence the results from the nail fold capillaroscopy are part of the criteria to diagnose SSc (113).

Touch imaging and quantification

A new ultrasound technology called virtual touch imaging and quantification (VTIQ) has also been applied to assess the skin involvement in SSc. VTIQ is an innovative non-invasive technique that measures the absolute quantification of skin stiffness. A pilot study showed that shear wave velocity (a measure of skin stiffness) was significantly higher in patients with SSc than in controls; it was also strongly correlated with the level of local skin pathology (measured by the modified Rodnan Skin Score) in some anatomical sites and could differentiate between clinically unaffected skin and healthy skin (114). This early study demonstrates the potential of this technology to measure skin involvement in SSc. However, further studies of VTIQ with larger sample size are required to validate this technique.

Optical coherence tomography

Although not yet widely used as a skin assessment tool in SSc, optical coherence tomography is a reliable quantitative outcome measure utilized to assess skin fibrosis in SSc (115, 116). This technology allows the visualization of the loss of the dermal–epidermal junction present in skin fibrosis and a decrease in optical density of the papillary dermis; these are changes associated with a worse modified Rodnan Skin Score. It can also distinguish between affected and healthy skin by a decrease in the optical density pattern on the reticular dermis (116).

Musculoskeletal ultrasound

Ultrasound is widely used in inflammatory musculoskeletal diseases and may be particularly valuable in SLE. Although musculoskeletal disease is one of the most common manifestations of SLE, it may be more difficult to diagnose and treat than other inflammatory arthritis. Recent work has shown that the majority of symptomatic patients do not have clinical synovitis. Of patients with inflammatory symptoms but no clinical synovitis, approximately 40% have ultrasound-detected synovitis, which may indicate the need for more immunosuppressive therapy (117).

Research agenda and future directions

The relative infrequency of these disorders provides a challenge to clinical research. There is a need for studies with large cohorts to evaluate the pathological mechanism of lower limb neurological- and musculoskeletal-related foot pathologies and on the development of tailored clinical interventions for foot pathologies. Since any one centre is unlikely to have a large enough cohort to perform these studies, large multi-centre trials are required, in particular to focus on the development of clinical pathways for the treatment of lower limb pathologies.

References

1. **Johnson SR, et al.** Validation of potential classification criteria for systemic sclerosis. *Arthritis Care Res.* 2012;**64**(3):358–67.
2. **Abraham DJ, Varga J.** Scleroderma: from cell and molecular mechanisms to disease models. *Trends Immunol.* 2005;**26**(11):587–95.
3. **Geyer M, Müller-Ladner U.** The pathogenesis of systemic sclerosis revisited. *Clinic Rev Allerg Immunol.* 2011;**40**:92–103.
4. **Bijlsma JW.** *EULAR Compendium on Rheumatic Diseases.* Canada: BMJ and European League Against Rheumatism, 2009: p. 824.

5. **Ranque B, Mouthon L.** Geoepidemiology of systemic sclerosis. *Autoimmunity Re.v* 2010;**9**:A311–18.
6. **Chifflot H, et al.** *Incidence and Prevalence of Systemic Sclerosis: A Systematic Literature Review.* London: Elsevier, 2008.
7. **Walker UA, et al.** Geographical variation of disease manifestations in systemic sclerosis: a report from the EULAR Scleroderma Trials and Research (EUSTAR) group database. *Ann Rheum Dis.* 2009;**68**(6):856–62.
8. **Silman A, et al.** An epidemiological study of scleroderma in the West Midlands. *Br J Rheumatol.* 1988;**27**(4):286–90.
9. **La Montagna G, et al.** Foot involvement in systemic sclerosis: A longitudinal study of 100 patients Seminars in Arthritis and Rheumatism. 2002;**31**(4):248–55.
10. **Silman A, et al.** Geographical clustering of scleroderma in south and west London. *Br J Rheumatol.* 1990;**29**(2):93–6.
11. **Allcock RJ, et al.** A study of the prevalence of systemic sclerosis in northeast England. *Rheumatology.* 2004;**43**:596–602.
12. **Bijlsma JW.** *EULAR Compendium on Rheumatic Diseases.* London: BMJ Publishing Group Limited, 2009.
13. **Mayes M.** Scleroderma epidemiology. *Rheum Dis Clin N Am.* 2003;**29**(2):239–54.
14. **Robert-Thompson PJ, et al.** Scleroderma in south Australia: further epidemiological observations supporting a stochastic explanation. *Int Med J.* 2006;**36**:489–97.
15. **D'Cruz DP, et al.** Systemic lupus erythematosus. *Lancet.* 2007;**369**:587–96.
16. **Katsumoto TR, et al.** The pathogenesis of systemic sclerosis. *Ann Rev Path: Mech Dis.* 2011;**6**:509–37.
17. **Abraham DJ, et al.** Overview of pathogenesis of systemic sclerosis. *Rheumatology (Oxford).* 2009;**48**(Suppl. 3):iii3–7.
18. **Denton CP, Black CM, Abraham DJ.** Mechanisms and consequences of fibrosis in systemic sclerosis. *Nat Clin Pract Rheumatol.* 2006;**2**(3):134–44.
19. **Guiducci S, Giacomelli R, Cerinic M.** Vascular complications of scleroderma. *Autoimmun Rev.* 2007;**6**(8):520–3.
20. **Krieg T, Takehara K.** Skin disease: a cardinal feature of systemic sclerosis. *Rheumatology.* 2009;**48**(Suppl. 3):iii14–18.
21. **LeRoy EC, et al.** Scleroderma (systemic sclerosis): classification, subsets and pathogenesis. *The Journal of Rheumatology,* 1988;**15**(2):202–205.
22. **Czirjak L, Foeldvari I, Muller-Ladner U.** Skin involvement in systemic sclerosis. *Rheumatology.* 2009;**47**(Suppl. 5):v44–v45.
23. **Claman HN, Giorno RC, Seibold JR.** Endothelial and fibroblastic activation in scleroderma: the myth of the 'uninvolved skin'. *Arthritis Rheum.* 1991;**34**(12):1495–501.
24. **Alcacer-Pitarch B, et al.** Foot problems in SSc a pilot study investigating foot health status and gait (Ab0374). *Ann Rheum Dis.* 2009;**68**(3):748.
25. **Otter SJ, Bowen C, Young A.** Forefoot plantar pressures in rheumatoid arthritis. *J Am Pod Med Ass.* 2004;**94**(3):255–60.
26. **Van der Leeden M, et al.** Forefoot joint damage pain and disability in rheumatoid arthritis patients with foot complaints: the role of plantar pressure and gait characteristics. *Rheumatology.* 2006;**45**:465–9.
27. **Pierard GE, Lapiere Ch M.** Physiopathological variations in the mechanical properties of skin. *Arch Derm Res.* 1977;**260**(3):231–9.
28. **La Montagna G, et al.** The arthropathy of systemic sclerosis: a 12-month prospective clinical and imaging study. *Skel Radiol.* 2005;**34**:35–41.
29. **Guiducci S, Giacomelli R, Matucci Cerinic M.** Vascular complications of scleroderma. *Autoimmunity Rev.* 2007;**6**:520–3.
30. **Chung L, Fiorentino D.** Digital ulcers in patients with systemic sclerosis. *Autoimmunity Rev.* 2006;**5**(2):125–8.

31. **Amanzi L, et al.** Digital ulcers in scleroderma: staging characteristics and sub-setting through observation of 1614 digital lesions. *Rheumatology (Oxford).* 2010;**49**(7):1374–82.
32. **Reidy ME, Steen V, Nicholas JJ.** Lower extremity amputation in scleroderma. *Arch Phys Med Rehabil.* 1992;**73**(9):811–13.
33. **Cherry L, et al.** The prevalence of self-reported lower limb and foot health problems experienced by participants with systemic lupus erythematosus: results of a UK national survey. *Lupus.* 2016; doi: https://doiorg/101177/0961203316670730
34. **Otter S, et al.** Patterns of foot complaints in systemic lupus erythematosus: a cross sectional survey. *J Foot Ankle Res.* 2016;**9**(10): 1–8.
35. **Mukherjee S, et al.** A pilot investigation of the prevalence of US-detectable forefoot joint pathology and reported foot-related disability in participants with systemic lupus erythematosus. *J Foot Ankle Res.* 2016;**9**(27):1–6.
36. **Nitsche A.** Raynaud digital ulcers and calcinosis in scleroderma. *Reumatología Clínica (English Edition).* 2012;**8**(5):270–7.
37. **Herrick A.** Pathogenesis of Raynaud's phenomenon. *Rheumatology (Oxford England).* 2005;**44**(5):587–96.
38. **Belch J.** Raynaud's phenomenon: its relevance to scleroderma. *Ann Rheum Dis.*1991;**50**:839–45.
39. **Sari-Kouzel H, et al.** Foot problems in patients with systemic sclerosis. *Rheumatology (Oxford England).* 2001;**40**(4):410–13.
40. **Hafner J, et al.** Management of leg ulcers in patients with rheumatoid arthritis or systemic sclerosis. *J Vasc Surg.* 2000;**32**:322–9.
41. **Steen V, et al.** Digital ulcers: overt vascular disease in systemic sclerosis. *Rheumatology.* 2009;**48** (Suppl. 3):iii19–24.
42. **Dorevitch M, Clemens L, Webb J.** Lower limb amputation secondary to large vessel involvement in scleroderma. *Br J Rheumatol.* 1988;**27**(5):403–6.
43. **Sant S, Murphy G.** Neurotropic ulceration in systemic sclerosis. *Clin Exp Dermatol.* 1994;**19**(1):65–6.
44. **Mouthon L, et al.** Impact of digital ulcers on disability and health-related quality of life in systemic sclerosis. *Ann Rheum Dis.* 2010;**69**(1):214–17.
45. **Korn JH, et al.** Digital ulcers in systemic sclerosis: prevention by treatment with bosentan an oral endothelin receptor antagonist. *Arthritis Rheum.* 2004;**50**(12):3985–93.
46. **Herrick A, et al.** Vasculitis in patients with systemic sclerosis and severe digital ischaemia requiring amputation. *Ann Rheum Dis.* 1994;**53**(5):323–6.
47. **Herrick A.** Neurological involvement in systemic sclerosis. *Br J Rheumatol.* 1995;**34**(11):1007–8.
48. **Herrick A, et al.** Nervous system involvement in association with vasculitis and anticardiolipin antibodies in a patient with systemic sclerosis. *Ann Rheum Dis.* 1994;**53**(5):349–50.
49. **Dyck PJ, Hunder GG.** A case-control and nerve biopsy study of CREST multiple mononeuropathy. *Neurology.* 1997;**49**(6):1641–5.
50. **Kibler R, Rose F.** Peripheral neuropathy in the 'collagen diseases': a case of scleroderma neuropathy. *Br Med J.* 1960;**1**(5188):1781–4.
51. **Dyck P, Conn D, Okazaki H.** Necrotizing angiopathic neuropathy. Three-dimensional morphology of fiber degeneration related to sites of occluded vessels. *Mayo Clinic Proc.* 1972;**47**(7):461–75.
52. **Amaral TN, et al.** Neurologic involvement in scleroderma: a systematic review. *Sem Arthritis Rheum.* 2013;**43**(3):335–47.
53. **Klimiuk P, et al.** Autonomic neuropathy in systemic sclerosis. *Ann Rheum Dis.* 1988;**47**(7):542–5.
54. **Poncelet A, Connolly M.** Peripheral neuropathy in scleroderma. *Muscle Nerve.* 2003;**28**(3):330–5.
55. **Kostis JB, et al.** Prognostic importance of cardiac arrhythmias in systemic sclerosis. *Am J Med.* 1988;**84**(6):1007–15.
56. **Lock G, et al.** Association of autonomic nervous dysfunction and esophageal dysmotility in systemic sclerosis. *J Rheumatol.* 1998;**25**(7):1330–5.

57. **Bajocchi G, et al.** Evidence of a selective nociceptive impairment in systemic sclerosis. *Clin Exp Rheumatol.* 2009;**27**(3 Suppl. 54):S9–S14.
58. **Lee P, Bruni J, Sukenik S.** Neurological manifestations in systemic sclerosis (scleroderma). *J Rheumatol.* 1984;**11**(4):480–3.
59. **Hietaharju A, et al.** Peripheral neuromuscular manifestations in systemic sclerosis (scleroderma). *Muscle Nerve.* 1993;**16**(11):1204–12.
60. **Di Trapani G, et al.** Peripheral neuropathy in course of progressive systemic sclerosis. Light and ultrastructural study. *Acta Neuropathologica.* 1986;**72**(2):103–10.
61. **Blocka K, et al.** The arthropathy of advanced progressive systemic sclerosis. A radiographic survey. *Arthritis Rheum.* 1981;**24**(7):874–84.
62. **Armstrong R, Gibson T.** Scleroderma and erosive polyarthritis: a disease entity? *Ann Rheum Dis.* 1982;**41**(2):141–6.
63. **Lóránd V, Czirják L, Minier T.** Musculoskeletal involvement in systemic sclerosis. *La Presse Médicale.* 2014;**43**(10):e315–e328.
64. **Randone SB, Guiducci S, Cerinic MM.** Musculoskeletal involvement in systemic sclerosis. *Best Pract Res Clin Rheumatol.* 2008;**22**(2):339–50.
65. **Baron M, Keystone E.** The articular manifestations of progressive systemic sclerosis (scleroderma). *Ann Rheum Dis.* 1982;**41**(2):147–52.
66. **Avouac J, et al.** Characteristics of joint involvement and relationships with systemic inflammation in systemic sclerosis: results from the EULAR Scleroderma Trial and Research Group (EUSTAR) database. *J Rheumatol.* 2010;**37**(7):1488–501.
67. **Schumacher J, Ralph H.** Joint and periarticular involvement in systemic sclerosis. *Clin Dermatol.* 1994;**12**(2):277–82.
68. **Misra R, et al.** Arthritis in scleroderma. *Br J Rheumatol.* 1995;**34**(9):831–7.
69. **Ferri C, et al.** Heart involvement and systemic sclerosis. *Lupus* 2005;**14**(9):702–7.
70. **Clements P, Furst DE.** Heart involvement in systemic sclerosis. *Clin Dermatol.* 1994;**12**:267–75.
71. **Allanore Y, Avouac J, Kahan A.** Systemic sclerosis: an update in 2008. *Joint Bone Spine: Revue du Rhumatisme.* 2008;**75**(6):650–5.
72. **Doria A, et al.** Risk factors for subclinical atherosclerosis in a prospective cohort of patients with systemic lupus erythematosus. *Ann Rheum Dis.* 2003;**62**(11):1071–7.
73. **June RR, Scalzi LV.** Peripheral vascular disease in systemic lupus patients. *JCR: J Clin Rheumatol.* 2013;**19**(7):367–72.
74. **Williams AE, et al.** Patients' experience of lupus related foot problems: a qualitative investigation. *Lupus.* 2017;**26**(11): https://doiorg/101177/0961203317696590.
75. **Alcacer-Pitarch B, et al.** Foot health needs in people with systemic sclerosis: an audit of foot health care provision. *Clin Rheumatol.* 2011;**30**(12):1611–15.
76. **Cherry L, et al.** The prevalence of self-reported lower limb and foot health problems experienced by participants with systemic lupus erythematosus: results of a UK national survey. *Lupus.* 2017;**26**(4):https://doiorg/101177/0961203316670730.
77. **Moran M.** Scleroderma and evidence based non-pharmaceutical treatment modalities for digital ulcers: a systematic review. *J Wound Care.* 2014;**23**(10):510–16.
78. **Schady W, et al.** Peripheral nerve dysfunction in scleroderma. *QJM.* 1991;**80**(292):661–75.
79. **Florica B, et al.** Peripheral neuropathy in patients with systemic lupus erythematosus. *Sem Arthritis Rheum.* 2011;**41**(2):203–11.
80. **Kowal-Bielecka O, et al.** EULAR recommendations for the treatment of systemic sclerosis: a report from the EULAR Scleroderma Trials and Research group (EUSTAR). *Ann Rheum Dis.* 2009;**68**:620–8.
81. **Pham HT, et al.** A prospective randomized controlled double-blind study of a moisturizer for xerosis of the feet in patients with diabetes. *Ostomy/Wound Man.* 2002;**48**(5):30.

82. **Loden M.** Urea-containing moisturizers influence barrier properties of normal skin. *Arch Derm Res.* 1996;**288**(2):103–7.
83. **Bakker K, et al.** Practical guidelines on the management and prevention of the diabetic foot 2011. *Diabetes/Metab Res Rev.* 2012;**28** (Suppl. 1):225–31.
84. **Ademola J, et al.** Clinical evaluation of 40% urea and 12% ammonium lactate in the treatment of xerosis. *Am J Clin Dermatol.* 2002;**3**(3):217–22.
85. **Pavicic T, Korting HC.** Xerosis and callus formation as a key to the diabetic foot syndrome: dermatologic view of the problem and its management. *J der Deutschen Dermatologischen Gesellschaft.* 2006;**4**(11):935–41.
86. **Young MJ, et al.** The effect of callus removal on dynamic plantar foot pressures in diabetic patients. *Diabetic Med.* 1992;**9**(1):55–7.
87. **Singh N, Armstrong DG, Lipsky BA.** Preventing foot ulcers in patients with diabetes. *JAMA.* 2005;**293**(2):217–28.
88. **Davys HJ, et al.** Debridement of plantar callosities in rheumatoid arthritis: a randomized controlled trial. *Rheumatology.* 2005;**44**(2):207–10.
89. **NHS England Clinical Commissioning Policy: Sildenafil and bosentan for the treatment of digital ulceration in systemic sclerosis 2015 NHS England A13/P/e**, from https://wwwengageenglandnhsuk/consultation/specialised-services-policies/user_uploads/bosntn-sildnfl-syst-sclerosis-polpdf
90. **Dole WP.** Intravenous iloprost treatment of Raynaud's phenomenon and ischemic ulcers secondary to systemic sclerosis. *J Rheumatol.* 1992;**19**(9):1407.
91. **Wigley FM, et al.** Intravenous iloprost infusion in patients with Raynaud phenomenon secondary to systemic sclerosis: a multicenter placebo-controlled double-blind study. *Ann Intern Med.* 1994;**120**(3):199–206.
92. **Matucci-Cerinic M, et al.** Bosentan treatment of digital ulcers related to systemic sclerosis: results from the RAPIDS-2 randomised double-blind placebo-controlled trial. *Ann Rheum Dis.* 2011;**70**(1):32–8.
93. **Abraham S, Steen V.** Optimal management of digital ulcers in systemic sclerosis. *Ther Clin Risk Man.* 2015;**11**:939.
94. **Wu SC, et al.** Foot ulcers in the diabetic patient prevention and treatment. *Vasc Health Risk Man.* 2007;**3**(1):65–76.
95. **Fiori G, et al.** Vitamin E gel reduces time of healing of digital ulcers in systemic sclerosis. *Clin Exp Rheumatol.* 2009;**27**(3 Suppl. 54):51–4.
96. **Derrett-Smith EC, et al.** Revisiting ANCA-associated vasculitis in systemic sclerosis: clinical serological and immunogenetic factors. *Rheumatology.* 2013;**52**(10):1824–31.
97. **Denton CP, et al.** BSR and BHPR guideline for the treatment of systemic sclerosis. *Rheumatology.* 2016;**55**(10):1906–10
98. **Bottomley W, Goodfield M, Sheehan-Dare R.** Digital calcification in systemic sclerosis: effective treatment with good tissue preservation using the carbon dioxide laser. *Br J Dermatol.* 1996;**135**(2):302–4.
99. **Alcacer-Pitarch B.** *Multifactorial Pathways Contributing to the Development and Impact of Foot Problems in Systemic Sclerosis (Scleroderma).* University of Leeds, 2014.
100. **Redmond A, et al.** Simple insoles for managing foot problems in people with SSc: the Pisces Randomized Controlled Trial. *Rheumatology.* 2013
101. **Attal N, et al.** EFNS guidelines on the pharmacological treatment of neuropathic pain: 2010 revision. *Eur J Neurol.* 2010;**17**(9):1113–e88.
102. **Nakamura T, et al.** *Mycobacterium kansasii* arthritis of the foot in a patient with systemic lupus erythematosus. *Int Med.* 2001;**40**(10):1045–9.
103. **Mendelson BC, et al.** Surgical treatment of calcinosis cutis in the upper extremity. *J Hand Surg.* 1977;**2**(4):318–24.

104. **Hughes M, et al.** Consensus best practice pathway of the UK Scleroderma Study Group: digital vasculopathy in systemic sclerosis. *Rheumatology.* 2015;**54**(11):2015–24.
105. **Botzoris V, Drosos AA.** Management of Raynaud's phenomenon and digital ulcers in systemic sclerosis. *Joint Bone Spine.* 2011;**78**(4):341–6.
106. **Lambova S, Hermann W, Müller-Ladner U.** Capillaroscopic pattern at the toes of systemic sclerosis patients: does it "tell" more than those of fingers? *JCR: J Clin Rheumatol.* 2011;**17**(6):311–14.
107. **Cutolo M, Grassi W, Matucci Cerinic M.** Raynaud's phenomenon and the role of capillaroscopy. *Arthritis Rheum.* 2003;**48**(11):3023–30.
108. **Sebastiani M, et al.** Predictive role of capillaroscopic skin ulcer risk index in systemic sclerosis: a multicentre validation study. *Ann Rheum Dis.* 2012;**71**(1):67–70.
109. **Smith V, et al.** Nailfold capillaroscopy for prediction of novel future severe organ involvement in systemic sclerosis. *J Rheumatol.* 2013;**40**(12):2023–8.
110. **Herrick AL, et al.** Nail-fold capillary abnormalities are associated with anti-centromere antibody and severity of digital ischaemia. *Rheumatology.* 2010;**49**(9):1776–82.
111. **Bredemeier M, et al.** Nailfold capillary microscopy can suggest pulmonary disease activity in systemic sclerosis. *J Rheumatol.* 2004;**31**(2):286–94.
112. **Maricq HR, Spencer-Green G, LeRoy EC.** Skin capillary abnormalities as indicators of organ involvement in scleroderma (systemic sclerosis) Raynaud's syndrome and dermatomyositis. *Am J Med.* 1976;**61**(6):862–70.
113. **Hoogen F, et al.** 2013 classification criteria for systemic sclerosis: an American College of Rheumatology/European League against Rheumatism collaborative initiative. *Arthritis Rheum.* 2013;**65**(11):2737–47.
114. **Santiago T, et al.** A preliminary study using virtual touch imaging and quantification for the assessment of skin stiffness in systemic sclerosis. *Clin Exp Rheumatol.* 2016;**34**(Suppl. 100):137–41.
115. **Babalola O, et al.** Optical coherence tomography (OCT) of collagen in normal skin and skin fibrosis. *Arch Derm Res.* 2014;**306**(1):1–9.
116. **Abignano G, et al.** Virtual skin biopsy by optical coherence tomography: the first quantitative imaging biomarker for scleroderma. *Ann Rheum Dis.* 2013;**72**(11):1845–51.
117. **Zayat AS, et al.** The role of ultrasound in assessing musculoskeletal symptoms of systemic lupus erythematosus: a systematic literature review. *Rheumatology (Oxford).* 2016;**55**(3):485–94.

Chapter 9

Soft-tissue disorders

Karl B. Landorf, Anne-Maree Keenan, and Rebecca Kearney

Introduction

Soft-tissue disorders are frequently encountered in rheumatology, including focal pathologies involving periarticular tissues, which are particularly common in the foot. Tissues involved include muscle, ligament, fascia, bursa, nerve, and tendon, and, while they have shared clinical presentation, accurate diagnosis is essential for planning treatment targeted towards the soft-tissue pathology. This chapter provides a brief overview of 10 of the most common soft-tissue disorders of the foot in rheumatology and Figures 9.1a–d show the locations to which they correspond on the foot and ankle.

Achilles tendinopathy

The macroscopic structure of tendons displays a hierarchical arrangement of parallel aligned crimped collagen fibres surrounded by a matrix ground substance (1). These characteristics work together to resist high tensile forces with minimal loss of energy and deformation, characterized by the stress–strain curve (2). In addition to the structural properties of tendons it is important to recognize that tendons are viscoelastic in nature. This results in decreased stress with time under constant deformation (stress relaxation), increased deformation with time under constant load (creep), and strain energy lost as heat during a stretch recoil cycle (mechanical hysteresis) (3). These combined characteristics are important considerations when identifying mechanisms of injury.

The Achilles tendon connects the triceps surae (gastrocnemius, soleus, and plantaris) distally to the middle one-third of the posterior surface of the calcaneus (4). This enables the forces produced by the triceps surae to be transmitted. However, if the tendon is subject to large forces, or repetitive submaximal forces over a prolonged duration the collagen cross-links begin to fail. A subsequent process of remodelling and repair then follows. When there is an imbalance between these processes, characteristics associated with tendinopathy occur (5). In addition to these mechanical factors it is important to acknowledge other risks for the development of Achilles tendinopathy. These have been attributed to a range of factors, including systemic diseases (such as diabetes), drugs (e.g., fluoroquinolones), smoking, obesity, biomechanical faults (such as excessive pronation of the foot), and age (6), for which the underlying pathology is thought to be distinct from mechanical processes in isolation.

Achilles tendinopathy most commonly occurs at the mid-substance or insertion. In addition to the above considerations, these two areas have two specific predisposing factors attributed to them. In the case of mid-substance pathology, this is an area of poor vascularity, as the tendon

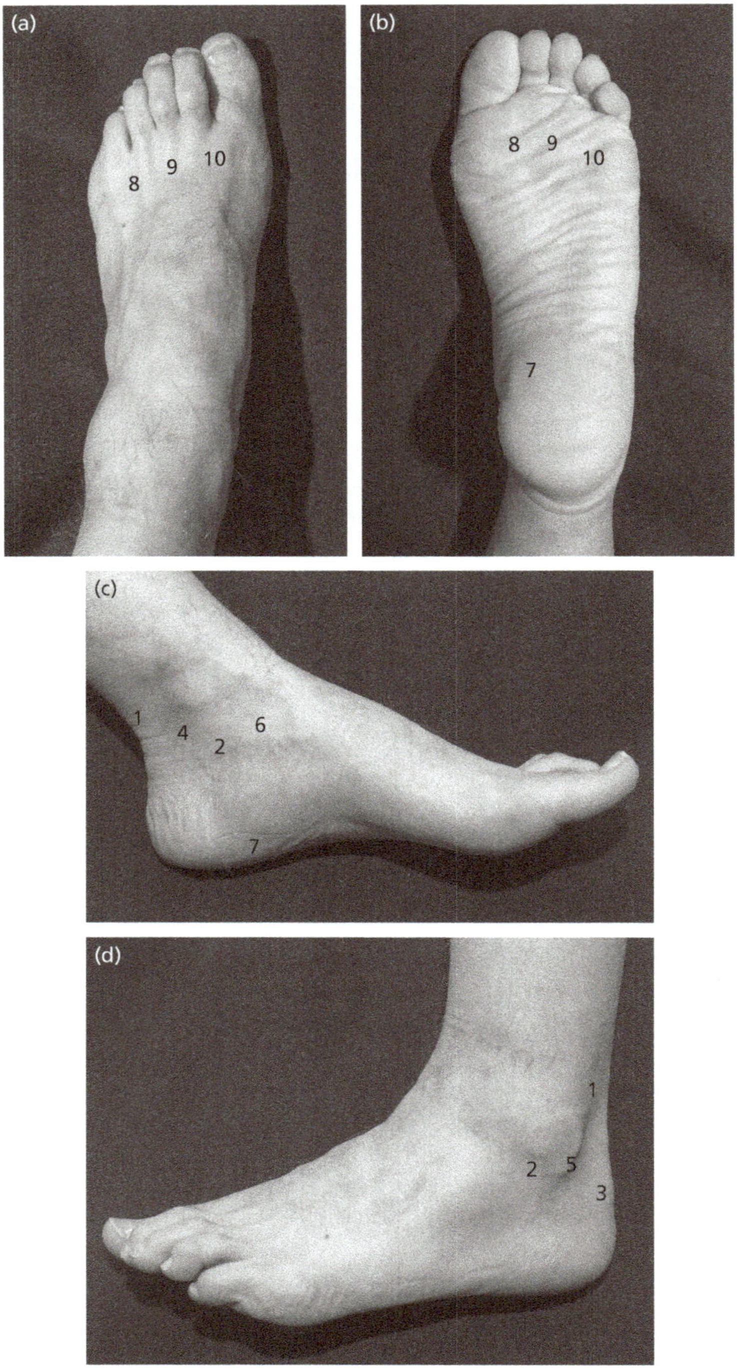

Figure 9.1 (a–d) Locations on the foot and ankle where 10 of the most common soft-tissue disorders in rheumatology occur.

NOTES. 1 = Achilles tendinopathy, 2 = Ankle sprains, 3 = Retrocalcaneal bursitis, 4 = Tarsal tunnel syndrome, 5 = Peroneal tendinopathy, 6 = Tibialis posterior tendinopathy, 7 = Plantar heel pain, 8 = Intermetatarsal bursitis, 9 = Intermetatarsal neuroma, 10 = Plantar plate pathology.

fibres spiral through 90° at this point. In the case of insertional pathology, this is an area subject to excessive shear and compressive forces (5).

In the general population, Achilles tendinopathy has a reported incidence of approximately 2.01 per 1000 people, affecting adults of around 40 years of age (7). On a cellular level there are a number of changes in the tendon that characterize Achilles tendinopathy, which include decreased matrix organization and cellularity and increased blood vessel infiltration and type III collagen expression (5). These features disrupt the important hierarchical structure that is inherent to the functioning of the tendon to resist high tensile forces, predisposing it to injury.

Patients with Achilles tendinopathy will commonly present with pain and stiffness over the Achilles area. This is often worse in the morning and is aggravated by weightbearing activities, with an area of thickening over the painful area (8). This triad of pain, thickening, and decreased activity is classical of a clinical presentation. Over time, there is no evidence to suggest that this is a self-limiting condition or is reversible in nature, which is in keeping with the first-line management strategies of activity modification and simple analgesia (9). Imaging is generally not required to diagnose Achilles tendinopathy; however, prior to any invasive procedure (such as injection or surgery) ultrasound or magnetic resonance imaging (MRI) is used to confirm the diagnosis.

Although common management strategies for foot and ankle pathologies are addressed in Chapters 14 and 15, there are some site-specific management strategies for mid-substance and insertional Achilles tendinopathy that are worthy of note. More specifically, it is important to recognize that, because the two sites of Achilles tendinopathy are thought to be caused by two different modes of action, the subsequent management strategies are also different for the two presentations (9).

A landmark study published in 1998 on an athletic sample described a specific exercise programme called an 'eccentric loading programme' (10). These exercises are performed two times per day, 7 days a week, for 12 weeks, and, at each session, the patient completes 180 repetitions. This has long been seen as the 'gold standard' treatment for patients with mid-substance Achilles tendinopathy (11, 12). However, more recent literature has discussed the problems with compliance with such a rigorous programme and whether the results are reproducible in a non-athletic population. This has led to a programme of research investigating alternative modalities that are currently under review in two ongoing Cochrane meta-analyses—one addressing the use of exercise, orthoses, and splinting, and the other addressing injection therapies (13, 14).

Two recent systematic reviews in this area, by Kearney and colleagues and updated by Wiegerinck and co-workers (9, 15), have pointed to the lack of evidence for this clinical area. However, both reviews highlighted the promising effects seen by extracorporeal shockwave therapy. This is a non-invasive treatment in which the equipment passes acoustic shockwaves through the skin to the affected area. This is thought to cause a short-term analgesic effect via stimulation of the peripheral nerves and a longer-term effect through a microtrauma-mediated healing response (16).

For both mid-substance and insertional Achilles tendinopathy presentations the evidence is not clear on how the pathologies should be managed. In the case of mid-substance Achilles tendinopathy, injection therapies have gained widespread popularity, in particular platelet-rich plasma injections. This rapid gain in popularity has led to national review of the treatment by National Institute for Health and Care Excellence (NICE) and a call for further research. In the case of insertional tendinopathy, again the widespread popularity of extracorporeal shockwave therapy has also led to a national review by NICE and a call for further research. They recognize that the treatment has no safety concerns, but robust evidence for its effectiveness is lacking.

Ankle sprains

Ankle sprains are a common soft-tissue injury in the general population (17). From the aspect of the foot in rheumatology, ankle sprains are important in three areas: first, there is an increased risk of ankle sprain associated with inherited conditions, including Marfan's syndrome, Ehlers–Danlos syndrome, and joint hypermobility syndrome (18), where tissue laxity predisposes the ankle to inversion injury; second, there is evidence to suggest a correlation with chronic ankle sprains and post-traumatic ankle osteoarthritis (19); and third, ankle sprains can be a consequence of the increased incidence of falls in rheumatoid arthritis (20).

As described in Chapter 2, the ankle joint is a complex structure. The medial aspect of the joint is stabilized by a strong, flat band of ligament known as the deltoid ligament: its structure means that it is not a common site for ankle sprain. The lateral side of the ankle is much more vulnerable, supported by three narrow bands of ligament: the anterior talofibular ligament, the posterior talofibular ligament, and the calcaneofibular ligament. While the anterior talofibular ligament is the most common site of injury, damage to the other ligaments and surrounding structures is often related to the nature of the injury, particularly of the tibia–fibula syndesmosis, spring ligament, sinus tarsi, peroneal, flexor and extensor retinaculum, and osteochondral and osseous tissue (21). Such structures should be considered in clinical examination of the area, and pathology confirmed with imaging (see Chapter 12).

Sprains are graded according to the extent of damage, from grade 1 (mild ligamentous damage which, on clinical examination, involves pain with no increased laxity), grade 2 (partial tear of the ligament, which is painful on extension of the ligament with slight increased laxity), to grade 3 (complete tear of the ligament, with no tension against extension of the ligament). Bruising and swelling are evident, often reflective of the nature of the injury. Imaging is generally not required to diagnose ankle sprains; however, X-ray examination can be used to identify a fracture in severe cases but should be considered in light of the Ottawa rules to avoid unnecessary X-rays: that is, X-rays are required only if there is pain in the lateral or medial malleolar zone along with bony tenderness and/or an inability to walk four weightbearing steps immediately after the injury (22). Ultrasound or MRI may be used in complex cases where other structures may have been injured or there is unexplained delayed healing.

For all ankle sprains, treatment has traditionally focused around the treatment approach known as RICE (rest, ice, compression, and elevation) (23), with oral anti-inflammatory medication to reduce inflammation and pain. For grade 1 and 2 ankle sprains, early mobilization and weightbearing with an external support, including bracing or taping (Figure 9.2), has been shown to have better functional outcomes (23) and is generally preferred by patients compared to plaster cast immobilization (23, 24). For grade 3 ankle sprains, immobilization with a plaster cast is recommended (25) and, while surgery is advocated, there is limited research to indicate its superiority: clearly more research is required. The choice is generally made in consideration to other patient comorbidity and preferences.

Retrocalcaneal bursitis

Retrocalcaneal bursitis, also referred to as Haglund's disease, refers to a condition characterized by pain and swelling at the posterolateral aspect of the heel in the region of the insertion of the Achilles tendon. The condition is often associated with an enlarged posterior superior calcaneal shelf adjacent to the Achilles tendon insertion. Retrocalcaneal bursitis is common when a tight heel counter of a shoe directs sufficient pressure on the region for the retrocalcaneal bursae to become inflamed (in addition, a subcutaneous bursa can also develop

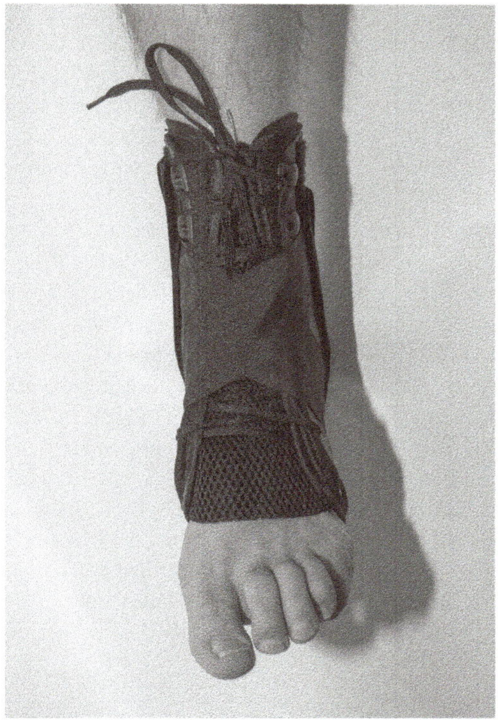

Figure 9.2 Example of external support for grade 1 and 2 ankle sprains.

and become inflamed at the site of pressure). Indeed, fashion footwear and shoes worn by running athletes, if tight or poorly fitting, can contribute to the condition. However, this region of the heel is also commonly affected by pathology in the spondyloarthropathies (26), so care is needed when diagnosing the condition, particularly if the symptoms are bilateral and associated with systemic changes.

The key structure to become inflamed in this condition is the retrocalcaneal tendon bursa, situated between the smooth upper part of the posterior calcaneus and the deep surface of the distal Achilles tendon (27). The retrocalcaneal bursa is intimately connected with Kager's fat pad and the Achilles tendon enthesis. The distal aspect of Kager's fat pad plays a role in minimizing pressure changes in the bursa by assisting retraction of the bursal wedge during dorsiflexion (28). Pathology of the Achilles tendon enthesis in insertional Achilles tendon problems (see section on 'Achilles tendinopathy', above) is often difficult to isolate from retrocalcaneal bursitis owing to its proximity and interrelated configuration (29). The term 'enthesis organ' has been designated to such complex tissue and the Achilles tendon enthesis is prone to pathological changes in spondyloarthropathy (26). Furthermore, retrocalcaneal bursitis may be associated with an underlying exostosis of the posterolateral calcaneus (30). Alignment and shape of the calcaneus has also been implicated in the condition, with the angle of the posterior superior calcaneus, the inclination of the calcaneus, and whether the calcaneus is abnormally inverted all being suggested as contributing factors (31). Accordingly, because of the interrelated and complex anatomy of this region, the condition may be more of a syndrome (Haglund's syndrome) rather than a distinct entity, where only the bursa is affected.

As retrocalcaneal bursitis progresses, the bursa enlarges and the excessive bursal fluid will easily be palpated. If the underlying periosteum is irritated sufficiently over time, an exostosis may form. However, it should be noted that retrocalcaneal exostoses associated with insertional calcific Achilles tendinopathy may form posterior to the tendon between the posterior tendon and the subcutaneous skin tissue (30). If allowed to progress, the bursa and any associated exostosis will enlarge to an extent that makes it difficult for a person with the condition to wear shoes that are closed in around the heel.

Medical imaging is not really necessary for this condition; however, conventional radiography will identify any associated posterior calcaneal spurring (Figure 9.3a) and ultrasound may be used to image the bursa and the distal Achilles tendon for pathology. In the early stages of the retrocalcaneal bursitis, treatment involves minimizing pressure on the heel that is irritating the bursae. Choosing footwear that minimizes pressure from the heel counter is the key to treatment. Periods of open shoes, such as sandals, may be necessary to alleviate all pressure, or, if this is not an option, appropriate padding can be used (Figure 9.3b). Heel lifts, either within a shoe or added externally, may be beneficial as they will plantar flex the ankle and, by doing so, reduce the prominence of the posterior superior calcaneus. In addition, anti-inflammatory measures may be helpful, including ice application and oral or topical anti-inflammatory medication. Corticosteroid injection directly into the bursae (see Chapter 14) has been advocated; however, ultrasound guidance is recommended to minimize any adverse effects of the corticosteroid on the Achilles tendon (32). In extreme cases, surgery may be warranted to resect part of the underlying calcaneus (33), thus minimizing the potential for ongoing shoe pressure. In these

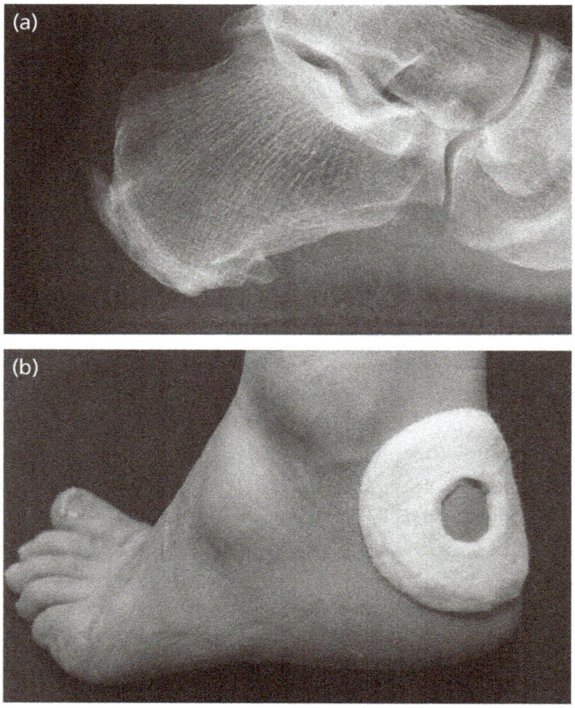

Figure 9.3 (a) Associated posterior calcaneal spurring. (b) Padding to alleviate pressure in retrocalcaneal bursitis.

cases, care is needed, though, as the insertion of the Achilles tendon and the enthesis organ need to be considered.

Retrocalcaneal bursitis can be a challenging condition. There has been little research conducted and the interrelationship of the retrocalcaneal bursa to its surrounding structures has only relatively recently been discovered, which is important in rheumatological conditions of the foot. Prevalence of retrocalcaneal bursitis has not been established, so large cross-sectional studies using representative samples would be of use. In addition, high-quality randomized trials are required to provide evidence for current treatment options and to compare new interventions against established interventions as they become available.

Tarsal tunnel syndrome

Tarsal tunnel syndrome is a relatively infrequent condition in which the tibial nerve is entrapped within the fibro-osseous tarsal tunnel as it passes around the distal tibia (medial malleolus). The term tarsal tunnel syndrome also refers to entrapment of the more major distal branches of the tibial nerve as it passes around the ankle: the medial and lateral plantar nerves, and the medial calcaneal nerve (34). Entrapment of these nerves leads to entrapment neuropathy, which presents as diffuse pain in the medial heel and plantar foot. Patients may have difficulty describing the pain, but burning, shooting, tingling, numbing, or electric sensations are common, and these may radiate distally into the plantar foot (34). Dysaesthesia, or an abnormal and unpleasant sensation under the foot and/or heel, may also cause sleep disturbance (35).

A positive Tinel's sign may be present (36), in which symptoms radiate distally when the posterior tibial nerve is externally percussed or even under palpation of the tarsal tunnel region. However, this test has been found to have only poor to moderate sensitivity in carpal tunnel syndrome, so care is needed when interpreting its findings (37). The dorsiflexion-eversion provocation test (Figure 9.4a), which aims to place tension on the posterior tibial nerve, can be used to assist in diagnosis of entrapment of the nerve (38); however, this test mechanically affects multiple structures (39), so its specificity, which to date has not been assessed, may not be good. With this test, where the metatarsophalangeal (MTP) joints are passively extended and then the ankle dorsiflexed and everted, the posterior tibial nerve is stretched, which frequently reproduces or aggravates the symptoms. If symptoms are bilateral, patients should be further investigated for systemic disease or back-related issues (35).

The tarsal tunnel spans from the distal, lower leg to the level of the plantar aspect of the navicular. There are two components to it—the upper tarsal tunnel and lower tarsal tunnel. The upper tarsal tunnel corresponds to the posterior aspect of the distal tibia, the retromedial aspect of the medial malleolus, the posterior border of the talus, and the medial talar surface (27). Overlying these structures, and what converts it into a tunnel, is the deep aponeurosis of the leg (27). The lower tarsal tunnel is formed by the medial surface of the calcaneus, which is flanked anterosuperiorly by the posteromedial aspect of the talus and the sustentaculum tali, and posteroinferiorly by the medial calcaneal tuberosity (27). Overlying these structures, and what converts it into the lower tunnel, is the flexor retinaculum above and the posterior segment of the abductor hallucis muscle below (27).

Important structures that pass through the tarsal tunnel include the tibialis posterior, flexor digitorum longus and flexor hallucis longus tendons, and the posterior tibial neurovascular bundle. Because of the physical constraints of the tarsal tunnel, space-occupying lesions or fibrosis within the tunnel will affect the function of these structures. Common space-occupying lesions include ganglionic cysts from the sinus tarsi (Figures 9.4b and 9.4c), lipomas, tenosynovitis of the tendons that pass around the posteromedial aspect of the ankle, varicosities, bony enlargements

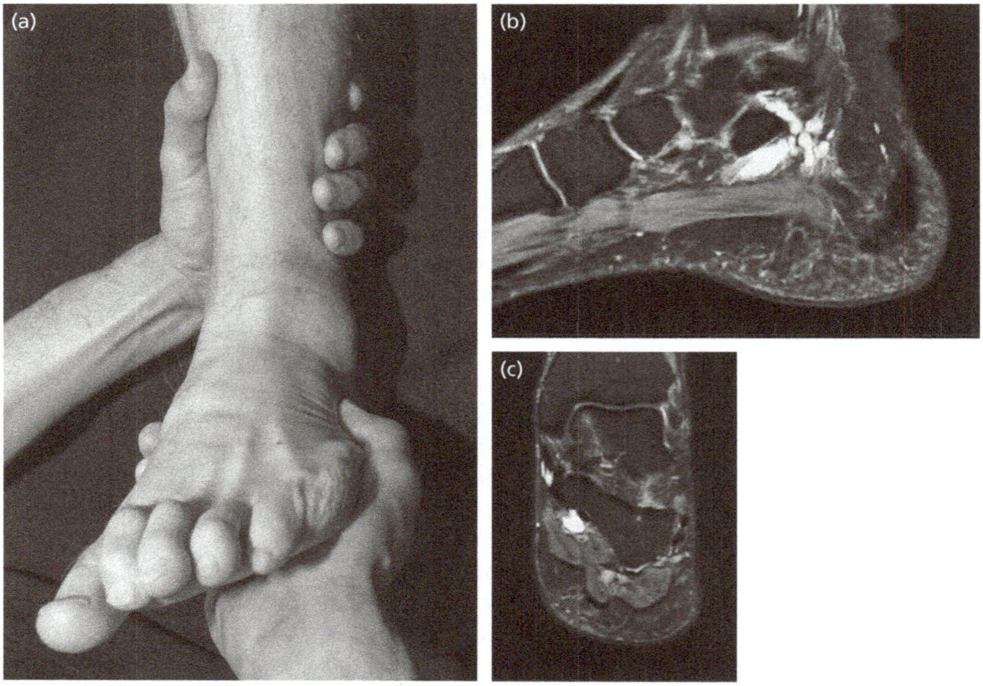

Figure 9.4 (a) The dorsiflexion-eversion provocation test. (b and c) A ganglionic cyst arising from the sinus tarsi.

or fragments from an ankle fracture, or accessory muscles (36). Excessive hindfoot pronation, which places tension on the posterior tibial nerve, and generalized oedema have also been suggested as a cause or aggravating factor (40). Direct trauma that causes a haematoma or deep scarring within the tarsal tunnel can also cause the condition (40).

The primary diagnosis of tarsal tunnel syndrome is clinical, although medical imaging can assist, particularly in the case of identifying the location, extent, and nature of the space-occupying lesions. Ultrasound and MRI are useful for soft-tissue lesions that may be related to the condition (41). While not necessary, electrodiagnostic tests, including nerve conduction studies and quantitative sensory testing, are also used (42).

It is generally accepted that the longer tarsal tunnel syndrome is present, the worse the prognosis is (36), so early intervention is recommended (34). If space-occupying lesions are present these frequently worsen over time, thus compressing the posterior tibial nerve and its branches more. With worsening symptoms, dysaesthesia and sleep disturbance may become problematic. Treatment of tarsal tunnel syndrome ranges from conservative to surgical, with surgery being a last resort (34). Non-surgical options include activity modifications, minimizing compressive clothing or footwear, physical therapy, nerve mobilization techniques, oral anti-inflammatory medication, night splinting, removable walking boot (e.g., Aircast boot or Cam Walker), and corticosteroid injections (see Chapter 14) (42). If foot orthoses are prescribed for excessive hindfoot pronation, a 'nerve relief' channel has been suggested by one author to minimize pressure on the posterior tibial nerve from external forces (36). Medications aimed at relieving the neurological symptoms, such as gabapentin, are recommended where symptoms have a substantial impact on health status, including disrupting sleep (36). Surgical intervention is primarily aimed at decompressing the tarsal tunnel (e.g., removal of a space-occupying lesion) and freeing the posterior tibial nerve of entrapment or fibrosis (35, 36). However, postoperative recovery can be slow, and patients need to be carefully educated and managed (40).

Tarsal tunnel syndrome has received little in the way of high-quality investigation. Many studies are expert opinion, relatively simple case series of surgical interventions, or non-systematic literature reviews. Accordingly, more investigation is needed on this relatively complex condition, which should include epidemiological studies to establish prevalence, high-quality evaluations of diagnostic tests, and well-controlled randomized trials to evaluate interventions for the condition.

Peroneal tendinopathy

Pain around the lateral ankle behind the distal fibula (lateral malleolus) is most commonly because of peroneal tendinopathy, a condition where the peroneal tendons and their tendon sheath become pathological. The condition is most common following an ankle sprain but can also develop in laterally unstable footwear and excessive hindfoot varus (i.e., cavovarus, pes cavus), which may cause the peroneal muscles to contract abnormally. Swelling and crepitus may be present if there is tenosynovitis. Pain can be elicited when inverting the foot, as well as on active muscle testing of the peroneals (i.e., eversion of the foot) and with isometric muscle testing of the peroneal muscles against resistance by the examiner; that is, resisted eversion Figure 9.5a) (43). Palpation along the course of the tendons during muscle testing can further isolate the location of tendon pathology.

The key structures involved in peroneal tendinopathy are the peroneus brevis and peroneus longus tendons. The peroneal muscles evert and plantar flex the foot, and peroneus longus also acts to stabilize and plantar flex the first ray. The peroneus brevis and peroneus longus muscles originate from the lateral side of the fibula and their tendons course distally until they wrap around the distal fibula (27). The peroneus brevis tendon inserts onto the base of the fifth metatarsal and the peroneus longus tendon, after wrapping around the cuboid, courses distally and medially to its distal insertions on the base of the first metatarsal and the medial cuneiform (27). In addition, the peroneal tendons are supported by the superior and inferior peroneal retinacula at the lateral ankle, and the peroneus longus also enters the plantar tunnel as it turns around the cuboid (27). If a lateral ankle sprain has occurred, the peroneal retinacula, most likely the superior retinaculum, can be torn or ruptured, and there is a possibility of an avulsion fracture of the retinacula from the underlying bone (44). In addition, an os peroneum (Figure 9.5b) may be present in the peroneus longus tendon as it wraps around the cuboid. This accessory bone can also be injured or become arthritic, and, as such, cause symptoms.

If the condition is allowed to progress without treatment, including reducing the aggravating factors, further tenosynovitis and degeneration of the tendons may occur. If a traumatic incident is the inciting factor, such as a lateral ankle sprain, and the retinaculum is ruptured, the tendons may end up subluxing or even dislocating out of the peroneal groove. When this occurs, the person may experience a painful popping or snapping sensation (45).

Care is needed with imaging, particularly with MRI, as the positive predictive value is quite low (46) and a substantial percentage of asymptomatic individuals have peroneal tendon pathology on MRI (47). Treatment initially involves resting the tendons by decreasing aggravating activities, and the use of ice and oral anti-inflammatory medication to control inflammation (44). Once settled, physical therapies, including mobilization of the hindfoot and stretching/strengthening the peroneal muscles, have been suggested (44). In addition, factors such as inappropriate footwear and abnormal biomechanics need to be addressed. For example, laterally supportive shoes should be recommended to address lateral shoe instability, and foot orthoses or lateral wedges may be

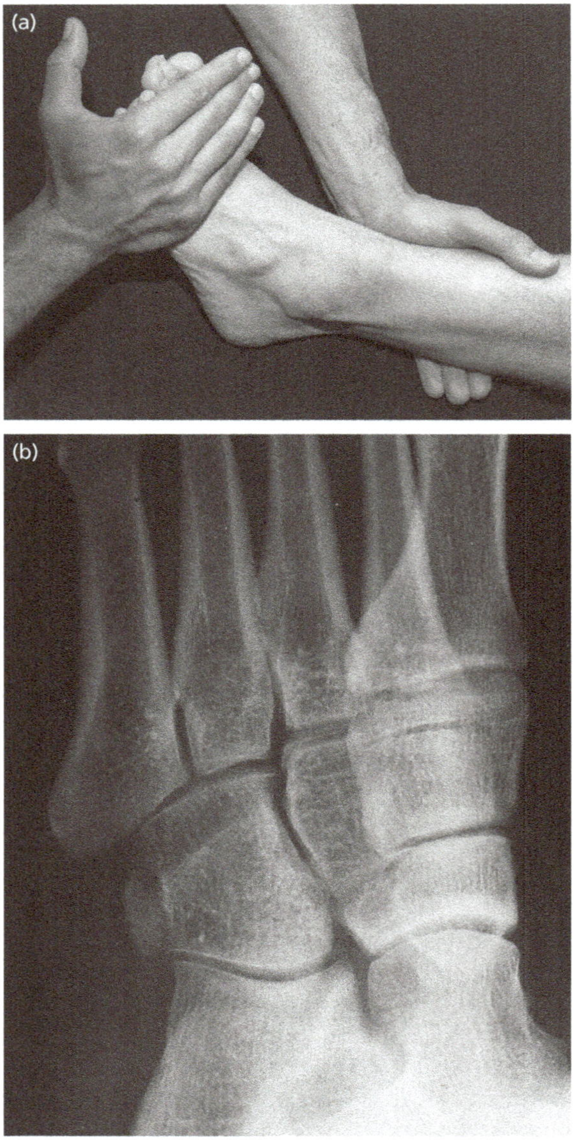

Figure 9.5 (a) Isometric muscle testing of the peroneal muscles against resistance by the examiner. (b) An os peroneum located lateral and plantar to the cuboid.

required if there is hindfoot varus leading to lateral instability. If ongoing tenosynovitis, tendon degeneration, or tendon tears are present, surgery may be required (45). Underlying anatomical anomalies, such as an enlarged peroneal tubercle, may also need to be addressed, as will tears or rupture of retinacula (48).

While peroneal tendinopathy has increasingly been recognized over the past few decades, there has been surprisingly little robust investigation of this condition. Prevalence has not been established, so large cross-sectional studies using representative samples would be of use. In addition, as with most tendinopathies, further understanding of the mechanisms involved in the pathology would be of benefit for prevention and treatment. Finally, there is no high-quality evidence for interventions for this condition, so well-controlled randomized trials are required.

Tibialis posterior tendinopathy

Tibialis posterior tendinopathy presents as pain and swelling located medially and posteriorly to the medial malleolus (distal tibia) and the medial hindfoot. It can develop without obvious underlying pathology; however, it occurs relatively frequently in people with rheumatoid arthritis (49). Pain can be elicited when palpating the tibialis posterior tendon as it courses around the medial malleolus and more distally onto its insertion onto the navicular tuberosity. Active movement (i.e., supination of the foot) and isometric muscle testing against resistance by the examiner of the tibialis posterior; that is, resisted inversion and plantar flexion (Figure 9.6a) should reproduce symptoms (43). Pain or tenderness will be present upon palpation of the tendon while doing these tests. Swelling around the medial ankle and hindfoot indicates tenosynovitis.

The key structures involved in tibialis posterior tendinopathy are the tibialis posterior tendon and its tendon sheath. The tibialis posterior musculotendinous complex inverts and plantar flexes the foot and is a key dynamic stabilizer of the medial longitudinal arch of the foot (50). The tibialis posterior muscle originates from the posterior tibia, fibula, and the adjacent interosseous membrane. Its tendon courses distally until it wraps around the distal tibia (medial malleolus) where it is deep to the flexor retinaculum but superficial to the deltoid ligament (27). From here, it continues distally to insert onto the following bones: primary insertion onto the navicular, with insertions onto all tarsus bones except the talus, and the bases of the middle three cuneiforms (27). Its synovial sheath is 7–9 cm in length, starting approximately 6 cm proximal to the medial malleolus and terminating close to the navicular tuberosity (27). Cadaveric studies have demonstrated that the tendon has a zone of hypovascularity distal to the medial malleolus, which has been associated with the area in which degeneration and rupture of the tibialis posterior can occur (51), although many other aetiologies, in addition to poor blood supply, have been proposed (52). An accessory bone, the os tibiale externum, can also be present at the insertion of tibialis posterior onto the navicular. This accessory bone can be problematic and contribute to the symptoms of distal tibialis posterior tendinopathy. Three types of os tibiale externum have been described, and the type II accessory, which forms a fibrocartilaginous joint with the navicular (Figure 9.6b), can be particularly troublesome if injured (53).

If the condition is treated early and the individual is otherwise healthy, tibialis posterior tendinopathy generally settles relatively quickly. However, if the inciting aetiological factors are allowed to continue or the individual is predisposed to the condition, the tendon can progress to a state of disrepair and degeneration. If degeneration occurs, and particularly if the tendon weakens and elongates, the 'too many toes sign' may be present when viewing the patient from behind, as the forefoot abducts on the rearfoot (Figure 9.6c). In addition, the patient may have difficulty performing a one-legged heel raise on the affected side. A lack of inversion of the heel during this test when the patient has the heel off the ground (Figure 9.6d) indicates a substantially damaged and elongated tendon, leading to a loss of muscle power and stabilization of the foot. In addition, other support structures, such as the spring ligament, become pathological, further compounding the condition. If the condition progresses to this level it is referred to as tibialis posterior tendon dysfunction or adult acquired flatfoot. People with rheumatoid arthritis that experience this condition have been found to demonstrate altered muscle function in conjunction with suboptimal mechanical function (49).

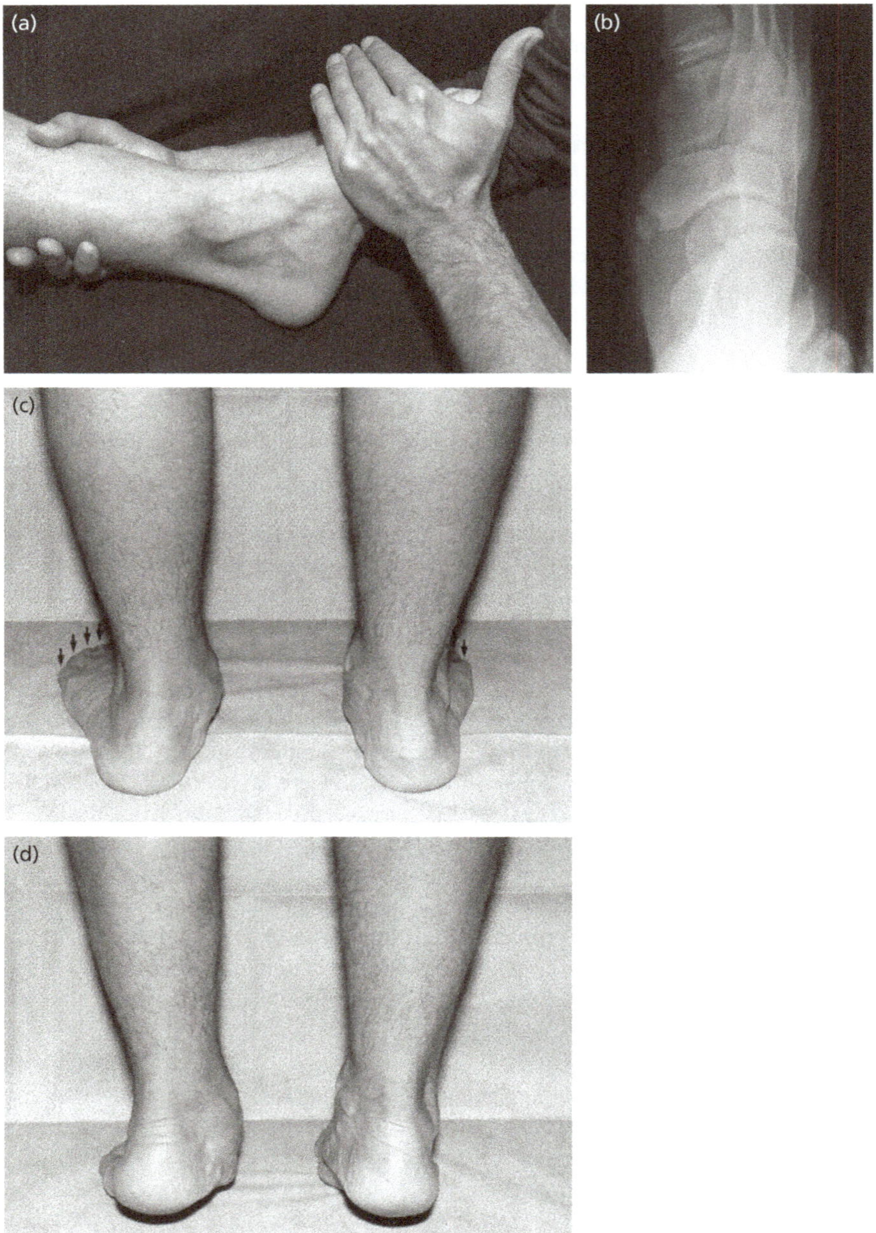

Figure 9.6 (a) Isometric muscle testing of tibialis posterior against resistance by the examiner. (b) A type II os tibiale externum located proximally and medially to the navicular tuberosity. (c) The 'too many toes sign', indicating tendon degeneration in tibialis posterior tendinopathy. (d) Lack of inversion of the left heel during a one-legged heel raise (both heels shown for comparison).

A three-stage categorization of tibialis posterior tendon dysfunction is commonly used, with stage 3 being the most severe (54), although more complex staging systems have been developed as understanding of the condition improves (55, 56). One study of a random sample of 1000 women over 40 years of age in England found the prevalence of stage 1 and 2 tibialis posterior tendon dysfunction to be 3.3% (57). Left untreated, tibialis posterior tendon dysfunction can result in a severe, painful flatfoot with relatively marked arthritic change in the hindfoot and ankle (54). Accordingly, targeted therapy to reduce inflammation and limit degeneration is necessary to off-load the affected tendon (49).

While medical imaging is not essential, X-ray can be used to evaluate arthritic change associated with the condition, and ultrasound and MRI can assist with staging the deformity or for surgical planning. If caught early, then tibialis posterior tendinopathy can be treated like most tendinopathies, including decreasing aggravating activities, and the use of ice and oral non-steroidal anti-inflammatory medications to control inflammation (44). Once settled, physical therapies, including antipronatory taping (e.g., low-Dye/augmented low-Dye taping) and stretching and strengthening the tibialis posterior, have been suggested (44, 58, 59). In addition, factors such as inappropriate footwear and biomechanics need to be addressed. For example, medially supportive shoes should be recommended to minimize excessive hindfoot pronation and medial longitudinal arch collapse, and foot orthoses may be required to limit foot pronation, particularly if the condition is resistant to more conservative treatment (59). Customized foot orthoses have been shown to alter foot motion and muscle activation in people with rheumatoid arthritis with tibialis posterior tendon dysfunction (60). For severe cases, some practitioners recommend high-top walking boots with substantial hindfoot and ankle support. If foot orthoses are prescribed, then specific antipronatory measures are recommended, including a deep heel cup, heel stabilizer (rearfoot post), medial heel skive, and even ankle stirrup support (58). If ongoing tenosynovitis, tendon degeneration, or tendon tears are present, surgery is usually required to limit the acquired flatfoot deformity that can occur if the tendon begins to elongate (56).

Although tibialis posterior tendinopathy has received some research attention, mainly because of the relatively severe consequences if not treated, there is still a need to further research the epidemiology, risk factors, and management of the condition. Further high-quality randomized trials are required to evaluate the effectiveness of new interventions against established interventions. Long-term follow-up studies are also needed to investigate whether there is re-occurrence following treatment, particularly for conservative treatments in less severe cases.

Plantar heel pain

Plantar heel pain (also known as plantar fasciitis or plantar fasciosis) is one of the most common musculoskeletal complaints of the foot and ankle (61–64). It can lead to significant levels of disability and poor health-related quality of life (65, 66), and causes substantial economic burden to the population (67).

Plantar heel pain presents as pain under the plantar heel, usually the anteromedial plantar heel, although the central plantar heel and the borders of the heel can also be affected. The pain generally worsens during the day with activity and is alleviated with rest. First-step pain (pain when first arising from bed in the morning or after an extended period of sitting) is a characteristic symptom; however, this is not present in all individuals with the condition. Pain may also be experienced after rest, such as after going to bed, but this does not occur in the majority of cases.

There are generally few outward signs of plantar heel pain, although some individuals may have some swelling of the anteromedial plantar heel. There are two primary subgroups of patients presenting with plantar heel pain. These are: (i) middle- to older-aged adults, typically who are overweight;

or (ii) running athletes with high-training loads (68). However, there are also patients that do not fit into these categories, and even younger individuals can experience plantar heel pain (62).

The primary structure that is involved in this condition is the plantar fascia (plantar aponeurosis); however, plantar calcaneal spurs, the calcaneus, and the first branch of the lateral plantar nerve have also been associated with the condition (69, 70). Although the traditional theory for the cause of plantar heel pain is excessive tension in the plantar fascia, which causes microtears at its origin at the plantar calcaneus, other investigators have proposed a vertical compression hypothesis, where there is a bone stress reaction and growth of plantar calcaneal spurs as an adaptive response to changes in loading of the plantar heel (71).

There are many causes of plantar heel pain, although the most frequent aetiology is that of mechanical overload (72). Key risk factors include being overweight (high body mass index), distance running, and increased number of hours standing on hard floors (68, 73, 74). There is also some evidence to demonstrate an association between certain biomechanical factors, such as cavus foot type (74, 75), and rate of loading has been found to be greater in individuals with the condition (76). Plantar heel pain is also common in spondyloarthropathies (72). Bilateral heel pain that does not respond to usual care may be the result of systemic inflammatory disease, particularly if symptoms are more widespread.

Because of the weightbearing nature of the heel and the difficulty in off-loading the area, plantar heel pain frequently worsens over time, particularly if the aggravating factors are not minimized. It is also not uncommon for one heel to be affected, and then, over time, for the contralateral heel to be affected also. However, most research indicates that individuals with the condition eventually improve, although this may take up to several years (77). The plantar fascia itself can become degenerated and thickened; however, in surgical cases there are no signs of inflammation so, more recently, the term plantar fasciitis has lost favour (78).

Medical imaging is not usually needed to diagnose plantar heel pain but may be helpful in cases that are unresponsive to treatment or where the symptoms suggest that other structures, such as the plantar fat pad or calcaneus, may be involved (79). X-rays can be used to determine the presence of a calcaneal spur, and particularly for the possibility of a fractured spur. Ultrasound and MRI are the modalities of choice to evaluate other tissues. People with plantar heel pain generally have a thickened plantar fascia (>4.0 mm) that shows signs of heterogeneity, degeneration, and/or tears (Figure 9.7a). Bone marrow oedema and plantar fat pad oedema have been reported on MRI, with bone marrow oedema (Figure 9.7b) being linked with atypical symptoms of night pain (69).

Many treatments have been proposed for plantar heel pain; however, a three-tiered approach has been recommended in one clinical practice guideline (80). This approach essentially runs the spectrum of conservative to more invasive treatment, and two systematic reviews provide evidence for most recommended treatments (81, 82). The first tier involves minimizing aggravating activity, wearing of appropriate footwear, supportive foot taping (e.g., low-Dye taping) (Figure 9.7c), prefabricated contoured foot orthoses, and stretching the plantar fascia and calf muscles. Anti-inflammatory oral drugs may also be prescribed. The second tier includes customized foot orthoses (if prefabricated foot orthoses are not appropriate), dry needling (83), and corticosteroid injections. The third tier involves night stretch splints (although compliance can be a problem and the evidence for this intervention is weak), extracorporeal shock wave therapy, and, as a last resort, surgery (again, there is weak evidence).

Because plantar heel pain is common, it has received a relatively large amount of research attention. Nevertheless, high-quality prevalence studies are still required and further risk factor studies would be useful. There have been many randomized trials evaluating the effectiveness of interventions for plantar heel pain, but many are of low quality and are at risk of bias, thus calling into question their believability (82). Therefore, further high-quality randomized trials would be worthwhile.

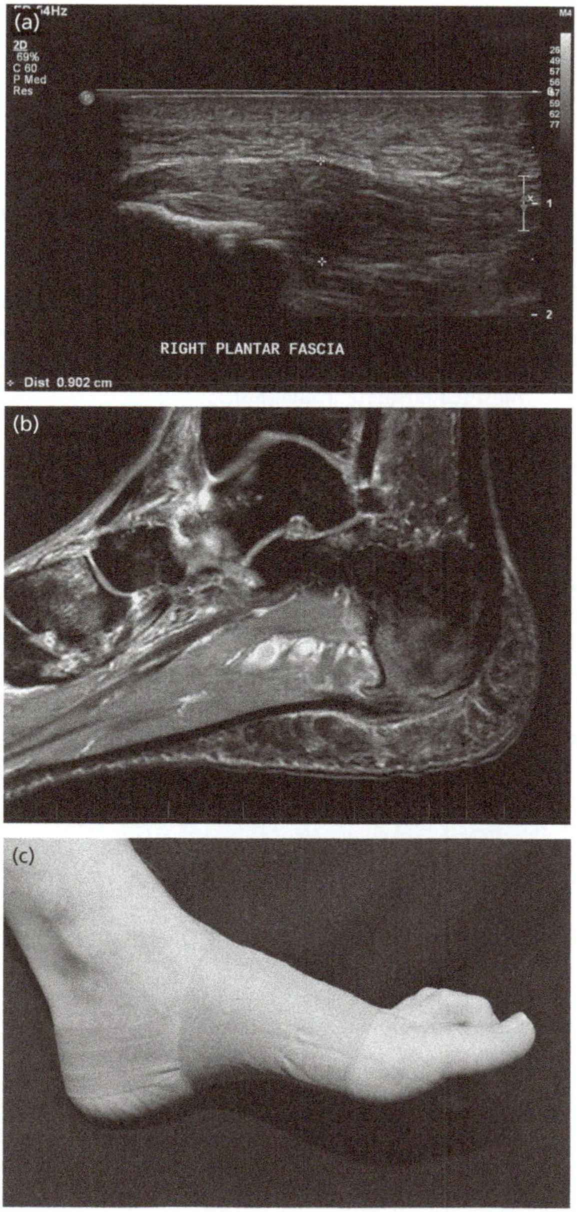

Figure 9.7 (a) An ultrasound scan showing plantar fasciopathy. (b) A magnetic resonance image showing bone marrow oedema in the calcaneus. (c) Supportive foot taping for plantar heel pain.

Intermetatarsal bursitis

Bursae are small pockets containing synovial fluid that act as a cushion in areas of friction. There are two types of bursae that exist within the body.

(i) *Anatomical* bursae, or those that are common to most people, which are found in areas of expected friction. This type of bursa is generally asymptomatic.

(ii) *Adventitious* bursae, or those that develop in response to local extreme stress, such as over bony prominences. This type of bursa is a physiological response to overloading, generally friction and pressure, but becomes inflamed if the overloading continues.

Bursitis is an inflammation of the bursae, which can be caused by mechanical overload or secondary to systemic synovitis, as seen with rheumatoid arthritis (see Chapter 6).

Intermetatarsal bursitis is an inflammation of the anatomical bursae between the MTP joints that lie superior to the transverse metatarsal ligament: they act to reduce friction and stress between the metatarsal heads. Given the forces generated at the MTP joint area with walking, together with the close proximity of bone, ligament, interosseous muscles, and tendon (84), and compounded by the mechanical effects of poor footwear, it is not surprising that the intermetatarsal bursae are common sites for overloading. While bursitis may affect any of the intermetatarsal bursae, the most common presentation is between the second and third (85) and third and fourth metatarsal heads, particularly with intermetatarsal neuroma (86).

Inflammation of adventitious bursae is particularly common in rheumatoid arthritis and is often seen in areas of bone prominences, including around the interphalangeal joints with digital deformities and under the metatarsal heads when the plantar fat pad is denuded or displaced, and where local pressures are elevated with greater joint degeneration (87). In osteoarthritis, bursitis is also commonly seen around bony prominences and is the most commonly reported feature of hallux abducto valgus, or bunions (88).

Bursitis presents with the classic signs of inflammation (painful on direct pressure, red, hot, and swollen), which is particularly evident in adventitious bursae over bony prominences. Symptoms of intermetatarsal bursitis are reasonably characteristic: pain on weightbearing, often worsened by narrow footwear, and is easily replicated by palpating the bursae and squeezing the metatarsal area. In chronic cases, the thickening of the bursal lining may be palpable: swelling in the dorsal

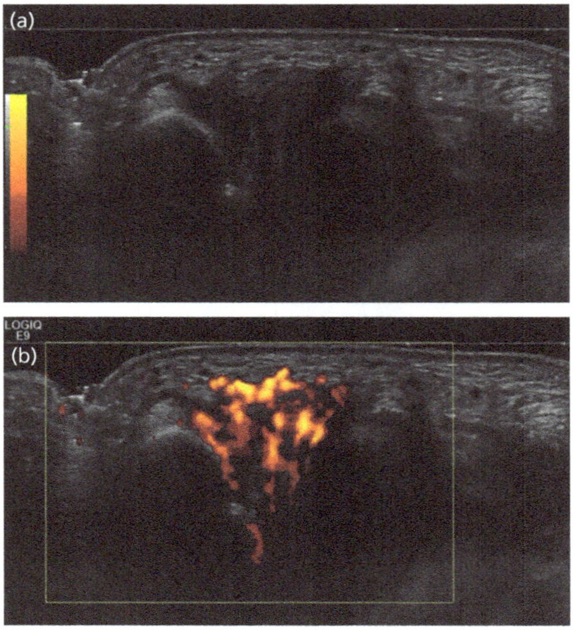

Figure 9.8 (a) B mode ultrasound image of the intermetatarsal bursitis. (b) Intermetatarsal bursitis with grade 3 power Doppler signal.

region may also be present. While the clinical presentation is relatively easy to detect, distension of the inflamed bursae can be detected on both ultrasound (Figure 9.8a, b) (89) and MRI (90) (see Chapter 12). In addition, ultrasound or MRI may be used in complex cases to assist in differential diagnosis of intermetatarsal bursitis from intermetatarsal neuroma and plantar plate pathology.

Inflamed bursae often benefit from aspiration and injection with a corticosteroid (see Chapter 14) (85). Aspiration prior to injection is also helpful to indicate the presence of infection, in which case a corticosteroid should not be given. Oral non-steroidal anti-inflammatory medication is recommended to reduce symptoms in the short term (91). Ultimately, however, long-term management of the condition means that pressure should be deflected from the inflamed bursae where possible, through either accommodative footwear, padding, orthotic therapy, or, in recalcitrant cases, surgery. High-quality randomized trials are needed to evaluate these interventions properly.

Intermetatarsal neuroma

Intermetatarsal neuroma, also known as Morton's neuroma, is an impingement syndrome of the plantar nerve, most commonly seen in the third metatarsal space, between the third and fourth metatarsal heads (86). It was first thought to be an impingement of the nerve caused by friction between the metatarsal heads: this has long been questioned owing to the local anatomy of the intermetatarsal space and is more likely to be caused by an impingement associated with thickened and dysregulated local soft tissue, including of the intermetatarsal ligament and inflamed bursae (85). In rheumatoid arthritis, nodules may also be present, further impinging the nerve. The neuroma refers to fibrosis of the perineural tissue, but cadaveric and imaging studies have demonstrated that this thickening has been found in people with and without symptoms (92), and may indicate a tissue response to trauma, which causes the impingement.

Symptoms are consistent with other nerve impingement syndromes and include pain on weightbearing, throbbing, burning, numbness, and shooting pains distally to the toes (93). As with intermetatarsal bursitis, the pain is often exacerbated by narrow and/or high-heeled footwear. People often describe the discomfort as like walking on a pebble, with symptoms initially mild, but gradually worsening. The clinical appearance of the area is generally unremarkable: pain is replicated by squeezing the ball of the foot combined with direct pressure on the metatarsal space. This clinical test may result in an audible pop, known as a 'Mulder's click' (94).

While ultrasound is useful to detect the perineural thickening, medical imaging is most useful to assist in common differential diagnoses, including stress fractures, capsulitis, and plantar plate pathology. Indeed, clinical assessment has been found to be more sensitive and specific than MRI or ultrasound assessment (95). The neuroma can be successfully managed in the short term by injection therapy of corticosteroid (96), with or without ultrasound guidance. As with bursitis, however, long-term management of the condition ultimately requires pressure to be deflected from the area where possible, through either accommodative footwear, padding (Figure 9.9), orthotic therapy, or, in recalcitrant cases, surgery. Again, high-quality randomized trials are needed to evaluate these interventions properly.

Plantar plate pathology

An increasingly recognized condition that causes forefoot pain is that of plantar plate pathology, which manifests as pain beneath the metatarsal heads. The onset of pain is generally gradual and oedema around the affected MTP joint may be present (97). The condition may also have a more acute onset if there is a hyperextension of the MTP joint, which results in damage to the plantar plate (98). In addition, plantar plate pathology is common in the painful forefoot of patients with rheumatoid arthritis, where it is associated with features of disease and deformity in the lesser

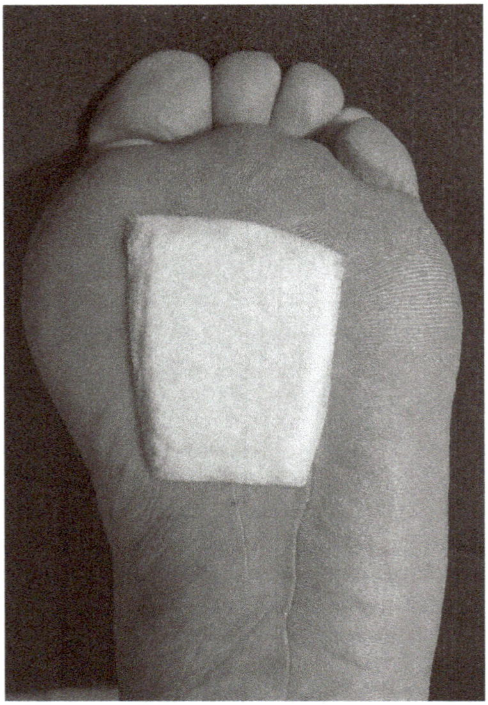

Figure 9.9 Padding to deflect pressure in intermetatarsal neuroma.

MTP joints (99). The second MTP joint appears to be the most frequently reported joint to be affected, but other MTP joints can be involved (100). In contrast, for patients with rheumatoid arthritis, it has been found to be more common in the fourth and fifth MTP joints (101). On examination, pain is elicited when palpating the plantar MTP joint region and more distally onto the proximal phalanx, which worsens when the proximal phalanx is passively dorsiflexed. A positive drawer sign (Figure 9.10a) may be present, where the proximal phalanx can be dorsally translated by an examiner while stabilizing the metatarsal (98, 102).

The plantar plate is the main restraining mechanism of the MTP joint, preventing the proximal phalanx from subluxing or dislocating dorsally on the corresponding metatarsal head (98). It is a complex fibrocartilaginous structure that sits underneath the MTP joint measuring 2–5 mm thick, 16–23 mm long, and 8–13 mm wide. The plantar plate is attached to the proximal phalanx and suspended from the sides of the metatarsal head through the collateral and the suspensory glenoid ligaments (27). It is also connected on each side by the deep transverse intermetatarsal ligament and provides insertion on its plantar aspect to the flexor tendon sheath, the plantar aponeurosis, and the transverse head of adductor hallucis. Importantly, its relationship with surrounding structures makes the plantar plate essential for stability of the MTP joint, and, when injured, stability is lost, which contributes to the symptoms of plantar plate pathology (97).

Dorsal subluxation or dislocation of the proximal phalanx on the corresponding metatarsal head occurs as the MTP joint becomes more unstable, and the toe may cross over adjacent toes in more extreme cases (98). As the condition advances, there may be frank dislocation of the MTP joint and a relatively unrestricted drawer test will be present. This progression is associated with

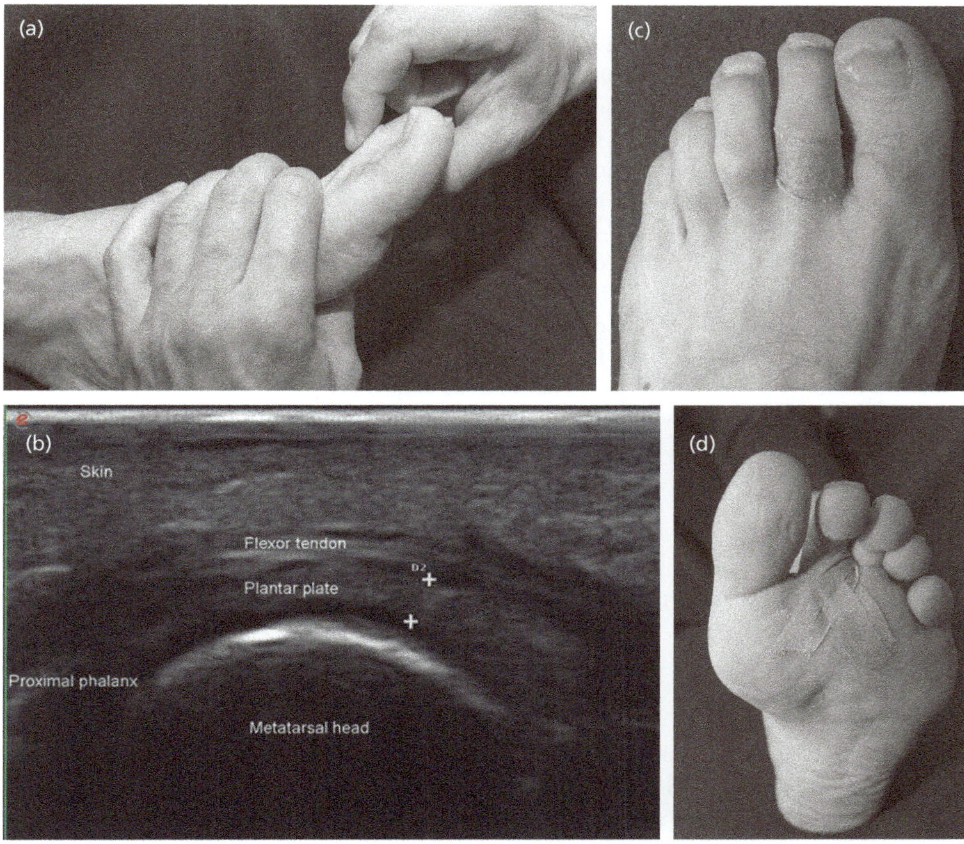

Figure 9.10 (a) Examination for a positive drawer sign related to plantar plate pathology. (b) Ultrasound longitudinal view of the plantar plate of the second metatarsophalangeal (MTP) joint. The longitudinal image is acquired from the plantar aspect of the second MTP joint, the homogeneous structure of the plantar plate (between + and +) is visualized between the flexor tendon and the thin hypoechoic line of cartilage against the hyperechoic skeletal cortex of the metatarsal head. (c and d) Tape applied in a sling configuration for plantar plate pathology.

increased transverse tearing of the plantar plate and attenuation or rupture of other connected structures, such as the collateral ligaments (100).

Ultrasound (Figure 9.10b) (or MRI) may be used in complex cases to assist in differential diagnosis of plantar plate pathology from MTP joint synovitis, intermetatarsal bursitis, and intermetatarsal neuroma. However, while both imaging modalities are sensitive for detecting plantar plate pathology, one study found that these modalities demonstrate poor specificity (103). A relatively small, but more recent, study of 15 participants with rheumatoid arthritis found that magnetic resonance arthrography can demonstrate lesser MTP joint capsule and plantar plate pathology, which are associated with disease duration, biomechanical changes in the forefoot, and radiographic damage (99). This study highlighted the improved visualization and delineation of tears in the plantar plate with magnetic resonance arthrography, but also demonstrated moderate sensitivity for unenhanced magnetic resonance.

If plantar plate pathology is caught early, then conservative treatment may be successful. The mainstay of conservative treatment is supportive taping of the corresponding toe. Tape is applied in a sling configuration (Figures 9.10c, d) to attempt to prevent the toes from dorsiflexing, which places strain on the plantar plate. Shoe modifications (stiff-soled or rocker bottom shoes), metatarsal pads (metatarsal domes), and foot orthoses (with metatarsal pads) may also be of benefit, as they will also minimize dorsiflexion of the toes (98). If conservative care fails, then surgery is required, where the plantar plate is repaired with or without a metatarsal osteotomy and flexor tendon transfer (104).

While the general understanding of plantar plate pathology has improved substantially in the past 30 years, there is still a need to further research the epidemiology and treatment options for this condition. Prevalence has not been established, so large cross-sectional studies using representative samples would be of use. In addition, high-quality randomized trials are required to provide evidence for the current treatment options and to compare new interventions against established interventions as they become available. Long-term follow-up studies are also needed to evaluate whether there is re-occurrence following treatment.

References

1. **Evans NA, Stanish WD.** The basic science of tendon injuries. *Curr Orthop.* 2000;**14**(6):403–12.
2. **Wang JH, Iosifidis MI, Fu FH.** Biomechanical basis for tendinopathy. *Clin Orthop Rel Res.* 2006;**464**:320–32.
3. **Maganaris CN, Narici MV, Maffulli N.** Biomechanics of the Achilles tendon. *Disabil Rehabil.* 2008;**30**(20–22):1542–7.
4. **Standring S.** *Gray's Anatomy*, 39th edn. London: Elsevier: Churchill Livingstone; 2005.
5. **Riley G.** Tendinopathy—from basic science to treatment. *Nat Clin Pract Rheumatol.* 2008;**4**(2):82–9.
6. **van Sterkenburg MN, van Dijk CN.** Mid-portion Achilles tendinopathy: why painful? An evidence-based philosophy. *Knee Surg Sports Traumatol Arthrosc.* 2011;**19**(8):1367–75.
7. **de Jonge S, van den Berg C, de Vos RJ, et al.** Incidence of midportion Achilles tendinopathy in the general population. *Br J Sports Med.* 2011;**45**(13):1026–8.
8. **Maffulli N, Longo UG, Denaro V.** Novel approaches for the management of tendinopathy. *J Bone Joint Surg-Am.* 2010;**92**(15):2604–13.
9. **Kearney R, Costa ML.** Insertional achilles tendinopathy management: a systematic review. *Foot Ankle Int.* 2010;**31**(8):689–94.
10. **Alfredson H, Pietila T, Jonsson P, Lorentzon R.** Heavy-load eccentric calf muscle training for the treatment of chronic Achilles tendinosis. *Am J Sports Med.* 1998;**26**(3):360–6.
11. **Magnussen RA, Dunn WR, Thomson AB.** Nonoperative treatment of midportion Achilles tendinopathy: a systematic review. *Clin J Sport Med.* 2009;**19**(1):54–64.
12. **Andres BM, Murrell GA.** Treatment of tendinopathy: what works, what does not, and what is on the horizon. *Clin Orthop Rel Res.* 2008;**466**(7):1539–54.
13. **Kearney R, Parsons N, Metcalfe D, Costa ML.** Injection therapies for Achilles tendinopathy. Cochrane Database Syst Rev. 2015;**26**(5):CD010960.
14. **Wilson FBC, Bennett K, Mockler D.** Exercise, orthoses and splinting for treating Achilles tendinopathy. *Cochrane Database Syst Rev.* 2017;**9**:CD010874.
15. **Wiegerinck JI, Kerkhoffs GM, van Sterkenburg MN, Sierevelt IN, van Dijk CN.** Treatment for insertional Achilles tendinopathy: a systematic review. *Knee Surg Sports Traumatol Arthrosc.* 2013;**21**(6):1345–55.
16. **Costa ML, Shepstone L, Donell ST, Thomas TL.** Shock wave therapy for chronic Achilles tendon pain: a randomized placebo-controlled trial. *Clin Orthop Rel Res.* 2005;**440**:199–204.

17. **Hiller CE, Nightingale EJ, Raymond J, et al.** Prevalence and impact of chronic musculoskeletal ankle disorders in the community. *Arch Phys Med Rehab.* 2012;**93**(10):1801–7.
18. **Grahame R, Kazkaz H.** The rheumatological heritable disorders of connective tissue. *Medicine.* 2014;**42**(5):275–8.
19. **Delco ML, Kennedy JG, Bonassar LJ, Fortier LA.** Post-traumatic osteoarthritis of the ankle: a distinct clinical entity requiring new research approaches. *J Orthop Res.* 2016;**35**(3):440–53.
20. **Stanmore EK, Oldham J, Skelton DA, et al.** Fall incidence and outcomes of falls in a prospective study of adults with rheumatoid arthritis. *Arthritis Care Res.* 2013;**65**(5):737–44.
21. **Roemer FW, Jomaah N, Niu J, et al.** Ligamentous injuries and the risk of associated tissue damage in acute ankle sprains in athletes: a cross-sectional MRI study. *Am J Sports Med.* 2014;**42**(7):1549–57.
22. **Beckenkamp PR, Lin CC, Macaskill P, Michaleff ZA, Maher CG, Moseley AM.** Diagnostic accuracy of the Ottawa Ankle and Midfoot Rules: a systematic review with meta-analysis. *Br J Sports Med.* 2017;**51**(6):504–10.
23. **Naeem M, Rahimnajjad MK, Rahimnajjad NA, Idrees Z, Shah GA, Abbas G.** Assessment of functional treatment versus plaster of Paris in the treatment of grade 1 and 2 lateral ankle sprains. *J Orthop Traumatol.* 2015;**16**(1):41–6.
24. **Kemler E, van de Port I, Backx F, van Dijk CN.** A systematic review on the treatment of acute ankle sprain: brace versus other functional treatment types. *Sports Med.* 2011;**41**(3):185–97.
25. **Petersen W, Rembitzki IV, Koppenburg AG, et al.** Treatment of acute ankle ligament injuries: a systematic review. *Arch Orthop Trauma Surg.* 2013;**133**(8):1129–41.
26. **Benjamin M, McGonagle D.** The anatomical basis for disease localisation in seronegative spondyloarthropathy at entheses and related sites. *J Anat.* 2001;**199**(5):503–26.
27. **Sarrafian SK.** *Sarrafian's Anatomy of the Foot and Ankle*, 3rd edn. Philadelphia: Lippincott Williams & Wilkins; 2011.
28. **Theobald P, Bydder G, Dent C, Nokes L, Pugh N, Benjamin M.** The functional anatomy of Kager's fat pad in relation to retrocalcaneal problems and other hindfoot disorders. *J Anat.* 2006;**208**(1):91–7.
29. **Benjamin M, Moriggl B, Brenner E, Emery P, McGonagle D, Redman S.** The 'enthesis organ' concept: why enthesopathies may not present as focal insertional disorders. *Arthritis Rheum.* 2004;**50**(10):3306–13.
30. **Chao W, Deland JT, Bates JE, Kenneally SM.** Achilles tendon insertion: an in vitro anatomic study. *Foot Ankle Int.* 1997;**18**(2):81–4.
31. **Ross JA.** Sports medicine and injuries. In: Lorimer D, French G, Burrow JG, Wall B. (Eds). *Neale's Disorders of the Foot*, 7th edn. Edinburgh: Churchill Livngstone; 2006, pp. 327–416.
32. **Chu NK, Lew HL, Chen CP.** Ultrasound-guided injection treatment of retrocalcaneal bursitis. *Am J Phys Med Rehabil.* 2012;**91**(7):635–7.
33. **Wiegerinck JI, Kok AC, van Dijk CN.** Surgical treatment of chronic retrocalcaneal bursitis. *Arthroscopy.* 2012;**28**(2):283–93.
34. **Pomeroy G, Wilton J, Anthony S.** Entrapment neuropathy about the foot and ankle: an update. *J Am Acad Orthop Surg.* 2015;**23**(1):58–66.
35. **Lareau CR, Sawyer GA, Wang JH, DiGiovanni CW.** Plantar and medial heel pain: diagnosis and management. *J Am Acad Orthop Surg.* 2014;**22**(6):372–80.
36. **Gould JS.** Tarsal tunnel syndrome. *Foot Ankle Clin.* 2011;**16**(2):275–86.
37. **Wiesman IM, Novak CB, Mackinnon SE, Winograd JM.** Sensitivity and specificity of clinical testing for carpal tunnel syndrome. *Can J Plast Surg.* 2003;**11**(2):70–2.
38. **Kinoshita M, Okuda R, Morikawa J, Jotoku T, Abe M.** The dorsiflexion-eversion test for diagnosis of tarsal tunnel syndrome. *J Bone Joint Surg—Am.* 2001;**83**(12):1835–9.
39. **Alshami AM, Babri AS, Souvlis T, Coppieters MW.** Biomechanical evaluation of two clinical tests for plantar heel pain: the dorsiflexion-eversion test for tarsal tunnel syndrome and the windlass test for plantar fasciitis. *Foot Ankle Int.* 2007;**28**(4):499–505.

40. **Ahmad M, Tsang K, Mackenney PJ, Adedapo AO.** Tarsal tunnel syndrome: a literature review. *Foot Ankle Surg.* 2012;**18**(3):149–52.
41. **Lopez-Ben R.** Imaging of nerve entrapment in the foot and ankle. *Foot Ankle Cllin.* 2011;**16**(2):213–24.
42. **Alshami AM, Souvlis T, Coppieters MW.** A review of plantar heel pain of neural origin: differential diagnosis and management. *Manual Ther.* 2008;**13**(2):103–11.
43. **Kendall FP, McCreary EK, Provance PG, Rodgers MM, Romani WA.** *Muscles, Testing and Function*, 5th edn. Baltimore: Lippincott Williams & Wilkins; 2005.
44. **Brukner P, Clarsen B, Cook J, et al.** *Brukner & Khan's Clinical Sports Medicine: Injuries*, 5th edn. North Ryde, Australia: McGraw-Hill; 2017.
45. **Heckman DS, Gluck GS, Parekh SG.** Tendon disorders of the foot and ankle, part 1: peroneal tendon disorders. *Am J Sports Med.* 2009;**37**(3):614–25.
46. **Giza E, Mak W, Wong SE, Roper G, Campanelli V, Hunter JC.** A clinical and radiological study of peroneal tendon pathology. *Foot Ankle Specialist.* 2013;**6**(6):417–21.
47. **O'Neil JT, Pedowitz DI, Kerbel YE, Codding JL, Zoga AC, Raikin SM.** Peroneal tendon abnormalities on routine magnetic resonance imaging of the foot and ankle. *Foot Ankle Int.* 2016;**37**(7):743–7.
48. **Roster B, Michelier P, Giza E.** Peroneal tendon disorders. *Clin Sports Med.* 2015;**34**(4):625–41.
49. **Barn R, Turner DE, Rafferty D, Sturrock RD, Woodburn J.** Tibialis posterior tenosynovitis and associated pes plano valgus in rheumatoid arthritis: electromyography, multisegment foot kinematics, and ultrasound features. *Arthritis Care Res.* 2013;**65**(4):495–502.
50. **Semple R, Murley GS, Woodburn J, Turner DE.** Tibialis posterior in health and disease: a review of structure and function with specific reference to electromyographic studies. *J Foot Ankle Res.* 2009;**2**:24.
51. **Frey C, Shereff M, Greenidge N.** Vascularity of the posterior tibial tendon. *J Bone Joint Surg—Am.* 1990;**72**(6):884–8.
52. **Bowring B, Chockalingam N.** Conservative treatment of tibialis posterior tendon dysfunction—a review. *Foot (Edinburgh, Scotland).* 2010;**20**(1):18–26.
53. **Sella EJ, Lawson JP.** Biomechanics of the accessory navicular synchondrosis. *Foot Ankle.* 1987;**8**(3):156–63.
54. **Johnson KA, Strom DE.** Tibialis posterior tendon dysfunction. *Clin Orthop Rel Res.* 1989;**239**:196–206.
55. **Abousayed MM, Tartaglione JP, Rosenbaum AJ, Dipreta JA.** Classifications in brief: Johnson and Strom classification of adult-acquired flatfoot deformity. *Clin Orthop Rel Res.* 2016;**474**(2):588–93.
56. **Nair P, Deland J, Ellis SJ.** Current concepts in adult acquired flatfoot deformity. *Curr Orthop Pract.* 2015;**26**(2):160–8.
57. **Kohls-Gatzoulis J, Woods B, Angel JC, Singh D.** The prevalence of symptomatic posterior tibialis tendon dysfunction in women over the age of 40 in England. *Foot Ankle Surg.* 2009;**15**(2):75–81.
58. **Houck J, Neville C, Tome J, Flemister A.** Randomized controlled trial comparing orthosis augmented by either stretching or stretching and strengthening for stage II tibialis posterior tendon dysfunction. *Foot Ankle Int.* 2015;**36**(9):1006–16.
59. **Kulig K, Reischl SF, Pomrantz AB, et al.** Nonsurgical management of posterior tibial tendon dysfunction with orthoses and resistive exercise: a randomized controlled trial. *Phys Ther.* 2009;**89**(1):26–37.
60. **Barn R, Brandon M, Rafferty D, et al.** Kinematic, kinetic and electromyographic response to customized foot orthoses in patients with tibialis posterior tenosynovitis, pes plano valgus and rheumatoid arthritis. *Rheumatology (Oxford).* 2014;**53**(1):123–30.
61. **Dunn JE, Link CL, Felson DT, Crincoli MG, Keysor JJ, McKinlay JB.** Prevalence of foot and ankle conditions in a multiethnic community sample of older adults. *Am J Epidemiol.* 2004;**159**(5):491–8.
62. **Hill CL, Gill TK, Menz HB, Taylor AW.** Prevalence and correlates of foot pain in a population-based study: the North West Adelaide health study. *J Foot Ankle Res.* 2008;**1**(2):1–7.
63. **Menz HB, Jordan KP, Roddy E, Croft PR.** Characteristics of primary care consultations for musculoskeletal foot and ankle problems in the UK. *Rheumatology (Oxford).* 2010;**49**(7):1391–8.

64. **Riddle DL, Schappert SM.** Volume of ambulatory care visits and patterns of care for patients diagnosed with plantar fasciitis: a national study of doctors. *Foot Ankle Int.* 2004;**25**(5):303–10.
65. **Riddle DL, Schappert SM.** Impact of demographic and impairment-related variables on disability associated with plantar fasciitis. *Foot Ankle Int.* 2004;**25**(5):311–17.
66. **Irving DB, Cook JL, Young MA, Menz HB.** Impact of chronic plantar heel pain on health-related quality of life. *J Am Pod Med Assoc.* 2008;**98**(4):283–9.
67. **Tong KB, Furia J.** Economic burden of plantar fasciitis treatment in the United States. *Am J Orthop.* 2010;**39**(5):227–31.
68. **van Leeuwen KDB, Rogers J, Winzenberg T, van Middelkoop M.** Higher body mass index is associated with plantar fasciopathy/'plantar fasciitis': systematic review and meta-analysis of various clinical and imaging risk factors. *Br J Sports Med.* 2016;**50**(16):972–81.
69. **Chimutengwende-Gordon M, O'Donnell P, Singh D.** Magnetic resonance imaging in plantar heel pain. *Foot Ankle Int.* 2010;**31**(10):865–70.
70. **Baxter DE, Thigpen CM.** Heel pain—operative results. *Foot Ankle.* 1984;**5**(1):16–25.
71. **Kumai T, Benjamin M.** Heel spur formation and the subcalcaneal enthesis of the plantar fascia. *J Rheumatol.* 2002;**29**:1957–64.
72. **Rome K.** Etiologic and extrinsic risk factors associated with plantar heel pain during physical activity: a review. *The Lower Extremity.* 1998;**5**(1):3–10.
73. **Waclawski ER, Beach J, Milne A, Yacyshyn E, Dryden DM.** Systematic review: plantar fasciitis and prolonged weight bearing. *Occup Med (Oxford, England).* 2015;**65**(2):97–106.
74. **Di Caprio F, Buda R, Mosca M, Calabro A, Giannini S.** Foot and lower limb diseases in runners: assessment of risk factors. *J Sports Sci Med.* 2010;**9**(4):587–96.
75. **Irving D, Cook J, Young M, Menz H.** Obesity and pronated foot type may increase the risk of chronic plantar heel pain: a matched case-control study. *BMC Musculoskel Dis.* 2007;**8**(1):41.
76. **Pohl MB, Hamill J, Davis IS.** Biomechanical and anatomic factors associated with a history of plantar fasciitis in female runners. *Clin J Sport Med.* 2009;**19**(5):372–6.
77. **Wolgin M, Cook C, Graham C, Mauldin D.** Conservative treatment of plantar heel pain: long-term follow-up. *Foot Ankle.* 1994;**15**(3):97–102.
78. **Lemont H, Ammirati KM, Usen N.** Plantar fasciitis: a degenerative process (fasciosis) without inflammation. *J Am Pod Med Assoc.* 2003;**93**(3):234–7.
79. **McMillan AM, Landorf KB, Barrett J, Menz HB, Bird A.** Diagnostic imaging for chronic plantar heel pain: a systematic review and meta-analysis. *J Foot Ankle Res.* 2009;**2**(1):32.
80. **Thomas JL, Christensen JC, Kravitz SR, et al.** The diagnosis and treatment of heel pain: a clinical practice guideline-revision 2010. *J Foot Ankle Surg.* 2010;**49**(3, Suppl. 1):S1–S19.
81. **Martin RL, Davenport TE, Reischl SF, et al.** Heel pain—plantar fasciitis: revision 2014. *J Orthop Sports Phys Ther.* 2014;**44**(11):A1–33.
82. **Landorf KB.** Plantar heel pain and plantar fasciitis. *BMJ Clinical Evidence.* 2015;pii:1111.
83. **Cotchett M, Landorf KB, Munteanu SE.** Effectiveness of trigger point dry needling for plantar heel pain: a randomized controlled trial. *Phys Ther.* 2014;**94**:1083–94.
84. **Theumann NH, Pfirrmann CW, Chung CB, et al.** Intermetatarsal spaces: analysis with MR bursography, anatomic correlation, and histopathology in cadavers. *Radiology.* 2001;**221**(2):478–84.
85. **Hassouna H, Singh D.** Morton's metatarsalgia: pathogenesis, aetiology and current management. *Acta Orthop Belg.* 2005;**71**(6):646–55.
86. **Espinosa N, Schmitt JW, Saupe N, et al.** Morton neuroma: MR imaging after resection—postoperative MR and histologic findings in asymptomatic and symptomatic intermetatarsal spaces. *Radiology.* 2010;**255**(3):850–6.
87. **Bowen C, Culliford D, Dewbury K, et al.** The clinical importance of ultrasound detectable forefoot bursae in rheumatoid arthritis. *Rheumatology.* 2010;**49**(1):191–2.

88. **Hurn SE, Vicenzino BT, Smith MD.** Non-surgical treatment of hallux valgus: a current practice survey of Australian podiatrists. *J Foot Ankle Res.* 2016;**9**:16.
89. **Bowen CJ, Hooper L, Culliford D.** Assessment of the natural history of forefoot bursae using ultrasonography in patients with rheumatoid arthritis: a twelve month investigation. *Arthritis Care Res.* 2010;**62**(12):1756–62.
90. **Cherry L, King L, Thomas M, et al.** The reliability of a novel magnetic resonance imaging-based tool for the evaluation of forefoot bursae in patients with rheumatoid arthritis: the FFB score. *Rheumatology (Oxford).* 2014;**53**(11):2014–17.
91. **Choices N.** Bursitis Treament 2016 [cited 2016 31st October]. Available from: http://www.nhs.uk/Conditions/Bursitis/Pages/Treatment.aspx.
92. **Bencardino J, Rosenberg Z, Beltran J, Lui X, Marty-Delfaut E.** Morton's neuroma: is it always symptomatic. *Am J Radiol.* 2000;**175**(3):649–53.
93. **Rajput K, Reddy S, Shankar H.** Painful neuromas. *Clin J Pain.* 2012;**28**(7):639–45.
94. **Mulder JD.** The causative mechanism in Morton's neuroma. *J Bone Joint Surg—Br.* 1951;**33-B**(162):94–5.
95. **Sharp RJ, Wade CM, Hennessy MS, Saxby TS.** The role of MRI and ultrasound imaging in Morton's neuroma and the effect of size of lesion on symptoms. *J Bone Joint Surg—Br.* 2003;**85**(7):999–1005.
96. **Mahadevan D, Attwal M, Bhatt R, Bhatia M.** Corticosteroid injection for Morton's neuroma with or without ultrasound guidance: a randomised controlled trial. *J Bone Joint Surg—Br.* 2016;**98–B**(4):498–503.
97. **Maas NMG, van der Grinten M, Bramer WM, Kleinrensink G-J.** Metatarsophalangeal joint stability: a systematic review on the plantar plate of the lesser toes. *J Foot Ankle Res.* 2016;**9**(1):32.
98. **Suero EM, Meyers KN, Bohne WH.** Stability of the metatarsophalangeal joint of the lesser toes: a cadaveric study. *J Orthop Res.* 2012;**30**(12):1995–8.
99. **Siddle HJ, Hodgson RJ, O'Connor P, et al.** Magnetic resonance arthrography of lesser metatarsophalangeal joints in patients with rheumatoid arthritis: relationship to clinical, biomechanical, and radiographic variables. *J Rheumatol.* 2012;**39**(9):1786–91.
100. **Coughlin MJ, Schutt SA, Hirose CB, et al.** Metatarsophalangeal joint pathology in crossover second toe deformity: a cadaveric study. *Foot Ankle Int.* 2012;**33**(2):133–40.
101. **Siddle HJ, Hodgson RJ, Redmond AC, et al.** MRI identifies plantar plate pathology in the forefoot of patients with rheumatoid arthritis. *Clin Rheumatol.* 2012;**31**(4):621–9.
102. **Klein EE, Weil L, Jr., Weil LS, Sr., Coughlin MJ, Knight J.** Clinical examination of plantar plate abnormality: a diagnostic perspective. *Foot Ankle Int.* 2013;**34**(6):800–4.
103. **Gregg J, Silberstein M, Schneider T, Marks P.** Sonographic and MRI evaluation of the plantar plate: a prospective study. *Eur Radiol.* 2006;**16**(12):2661–9.
104. **Flint WW, Macias DM, Jastifer JR, Doty JF, Hirose CB, Coughlin MJ.** Plantar plate repair for lesser metatarsophalangeal joint instability. *Foot Ankle Int.* 2017;**38**(3):234–42.

Chapter 10

Juvenile idiopathic arthritis

Gordon Hendry

Introduction

The impact of a chronic, painful, and destructive arthritis occurring during childhood would historically have resulted in severe joint damage, deformities, disability, and a poor quality of life. Thankfully the management of juvenile idiopathic arthritis (JIA) has evolved in recent decades and now has similar management goals to that of adult rheumatoid arthritis (RA), which are firmly based around a zero tolerance approach to the primary disease process: synovitis. However, in spite of improvements in the medical management of JIA, many young children will continue to experience active inflammatory disease into adulthood; many will be diagnosed too late and the damage will have been done before they reach paediatric rheumatology services; and symptoms such as joint pain and stiffness often persist even for those who are considered to be well managed. In addition, a somewhat obvious complicating factor is that the disease targets the joints and periarticular soft tissues of the growing and developing child or adolescent. As a result, there are some additional challenges for clinicians involved in the management of children with JIA, including communication challenges during the consultation with the very young patient, the hormonal adolescent, and parents/guardians; necessity for knowledge and understanding of key developmental milestones; awkwardness of physical examination of small foot joints and soft tissues; compliance issues surrounding prescription of exercise programmes, footwear advice, and wearing of foot orthoses; contraindication of joint injections in the young child without sedation or general anaesthetic; and cost issues with regard to outgrowing recommended shoes and prescribed foot orthoses. There are also disease-specific complications concerning the growing child/adolescent that require consideration, such as growth disruption due to inflammation in the region of epiphyseal growth plates and poor physical condition owing to physical inactivity, resulting in cumulative health risks associated with poor bone health and fractures and cardiovascular disease.

Children with JIA are largely managed in paediatric rheumatology outpatient settings by a team that includes a paediatric rheumatologist, paediatric rheumatology nurse specialist, a paediatric physiotherapist, and a paediatric occupational therapist. The overall aim of the multidisciplinary team is to improve functional, educational, social, and employment outcomes. Podiatrists and orthotists are considered to be part of the extended multidisciplinary team and are often not integrated within the immediate paediatric rheumatology care team. Current evidence suggests that podiatry input, which is based predominantly around the use of foot orthoses for pain reduction, can be beneficial. However, evidence in support of other podiatric interventions or, indeed, multi-faceted podiatry interventions remains scarce, and, as such, many recommendations for management are based on expert opinion. This chapter will provide summary background information about JIA and its subtypes and general medical management strategies prior to the main focus on disease presentations affecting the foot and ankle and related podiatric assessment and management strategies.

Juvenile idiopathic arthritis nomenclature and classification

JIA is an umbrella term for a group of paediatric rheumatic disorders that are associated by the primary disease pathology, which is unexplained, and persistent synovitis, which occurs prior to the sixteenth birthday and persists for at least 6 weeks (1). The current and most widely accepted disease classification criteria is the Edmonton 2001 revision of the International League of Associations for Rheumatism (ILAR) criteria for JIA (Table 10.1).

Persistent and extended oligoarthritis

Persistent oligoarthritis is the commonest presentation of JIA and affects around 40–60% of those with JIA (1, 2). It is typified by asymmetrical large joint involvement and has a tendency for the knee, ankle, and subtalar joints (3–7). Persistent oligoarthritis affects four joints or less throughout the disease course and is generally relatively benign and well managed medically in contrast to other subtypes. In contrast, extended oligoarthritis initially affects four joints or less within the first 6 months, and then a total of more than four joints after the first 6 months of the disease. Extended oligoarthritis is a more destructive form of JIA and is associated with radiographic progression (erosive disease) and poorer functional outcomes (8, 9).

Rheumatoid factor-negative and -positive polyarticular juvenile idiopathic arthritis

Rheumatoid factor-negative (RhF–) polyarticular JIA affects around 20–25% of those with JIA and has a polyarticular disease pattern (five joints or more), affecting large and small joints with variable degrees of symmetry. It is a destructive form of JIA, which has a propensity for synovitis of lower limb joints. Children with this form of the disease often fail to achieve remission or low disease activity states (8–10) and experience poor long-term outcomes characterized by erosive

Table 10.1 Summary of the International League of Associations for Rheumatism classification criteria for juvenile idiopathic arthritis

	International League of Associations for Rheumatism criteria
Name	Juvenile idiopathic arthritis
Age at onset	<16 years
Diagnosis duration	≥ 6 weeks
Subtypes	Persistent oligoarthritis Extended oligoarthritis Polyarthritis (RF–) Polyarthritis (RF+) Enthesitis-related arthritis Psoriatic arthritis Systemic arthritis Other/undifferentiated arthritis

RF, rheumatoid factor; –, negative; +, positive.

joint destruction and more severe disability. Rheumatoid factor-positive (RhF+) polyarticular JIA is confirmed where two or more tests for RhF at least 3 months apart during the first 6 months of the disease are positive (1). It is similar in presentation to RhF– JIA but often has a bilateral and symmetrical pattern of joint involvement. Erosive changes have been described as most common in this subtype, suggestive that it can be an extremely destructive form of JIA (11).

Juvenile enthesitis-related arthritis

Juvenile enthesitis-related arthritis (jERA) is formally defined as the presence of arthritis and enthesitis, or arthritis or enthesitis with at least two of the following: sacroiliac joint tenderness or lumbosacral pain, HLA-B27 antigen positivity, onset in a male over 6 years of age, acute anterior uveitis, or a history of ankylosing spondylitis, enthesitis-related arthritis, sacroiliitis with inflammatory bowel disease, reactive arthritis, or acute anterior uveitis in a first-degree relative (1). Synovitis can affect large and small joints and occasionally presents as an oligoarticular pattern. Enthesitis (see Section on 'Enthesitis') commonly affects the entheses of the Achilles tendon and the proximal and distal aspects of the plantar fascia, but may also be more widespread throughout the ligamentous attachments of the foot, resulting in widespread tenderness (12). Tarsitis, defined as inflammation of the midfoot resulting in severe dorsal swelling and tenderness in the region of the Lisfranc joint, is a hallmark feature of jERA and can be debilitating (12).

Juvenile psoriatic arthritis

Juvenile psoriatic arthritis (JPsA) is defined as arthritis and psoriasis, or arthritis and at least two of the following: dactylitis, nail pitting/onycholysis, and/or psoriasis in a first-degree relative (1). It often results in large- and small-joint disease, which is asymmetrical and often follows an oligoarticular pattern. The ankle and small joints of the forefoot are often affected, and, where there is additional tendon sheath and entheseal inflammation, the toes can exhibit a sausage-like appearance known as dactylitis, which can be extremely painful (Figure 10.1) (13). Typical psoriatic skin and nail lesions are more subtle and are less common in the juvenile version relative to adult PsA. However, JPsA is associated with unfavourable physical functional outcomes (14).

Systemic juvenile idiopathic arthritis

Systemic onset JIA (SoJIA) is defined as arthritis in one or more joints with quotidian fever (fever spikes occurring at least daily and returning to normal) for at least 3 days within a 2-week period and accompanied by at least one of the following: evanescent erythematous rash, generalized lymph node enlargement, hepatomegaly and/or splenomegaly, and serositis (1). It typically presents as a florid polyarthritis which is bilateral and symmetrical synovitis affecting large and small joints (15). Foot disease is common at the hindfoot as well as the forefoot (16, 17) and the child can often be very unwell as a result of the systemic pathology. Several commentaries have called for a re-classification of JIA that does not include SoJIA as recent research has demonstrated clear aetiopathogenetic differences between SoJIA and other forms of JIA, and its medical management is substantially different (18, 19).

Undifferentiated juvenile idiopathic arthritis

Undifferentiated JIA is defined as JIA that fulfils criteria in either no category or in two or more categories (1). The main factors that contribute to the classification of undifferentiated JIA are the presence of a first-degree relative with psoriasis (in children fulfilling criteria categories other than JPsA), presence of rheumatoid factor positivity (in children fulfilling criteria in categories

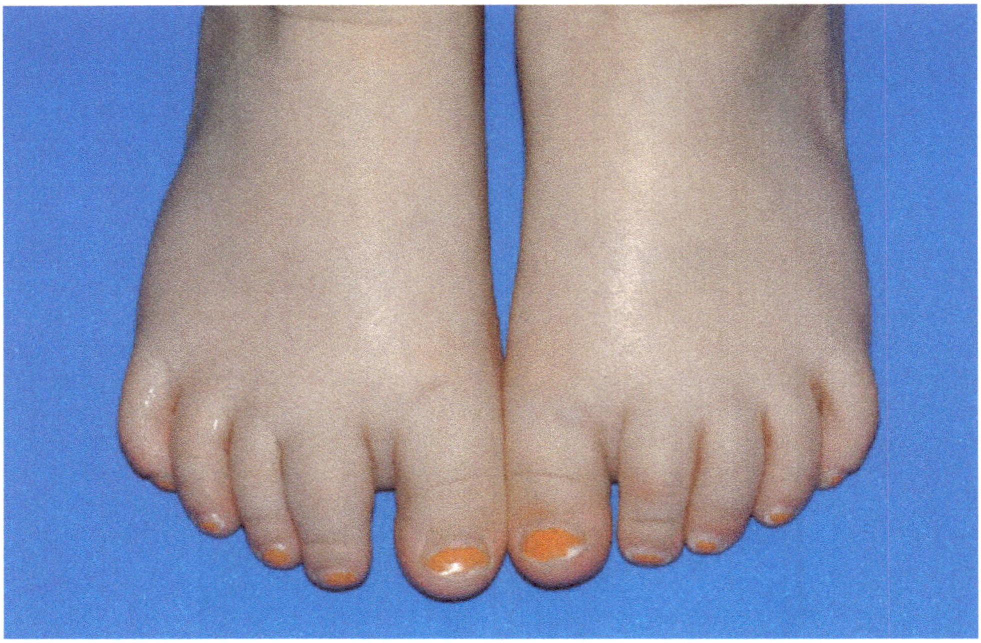

Figure 10.1 Dactylitis with characteristic sausage-like swelling of the right second toe in a young girl with juvenile psoriatic arthritis.

other than RhF+ JIA), and the presence of HLA-B27 positivity and/or presence of enthesitis (in children fulfilling criteria in categories other than jERA) (20).

Prevalence

JIA, when considered as a whole group, is largely considered to be the commonest rheumatic disorder of childhood and awareness of the condition is on the rise. Its worldwide prevalence is variable but is estimated as 0.7–4 per 1000 children, with an annual incidence of 0.008 to 0.226 per 1000 children (21). A recent systematic review of 43 articles suggests a European pooled annual incidence and overall prevalence rates of 7.8 and 32.6 per 100,000 children, respectively (22). The UK-wide prevalence of JIA is estimated at approximately 0.65 to 2 per 1000 children, with an annual incidence rate of 10 per 100,000 children (21, 23). Whilst the disease is uncommon relative to adult RA, it is certainly not rare and its prevalence rates in the UK are comparable to that of juvenile-onset type 1 diabetes (24).

Diagnosis

The diagnosis of JIA is recognized as challenging and relies upon the clinical skills of consultant paediatric rheumatologists for taking a relevant history and undertaking physical examinations. Whilst there is no specific laboratory test to establish a diagnosis of JIA, they are helpful in excluding other disorders (for example, synovial fluid analysis to rule out septic arthritis) or confirming and/or excluding ILAR subtypes (HLA-B27 for jERA, RhF for RhF+ polyarthritis). Imaging techniques such as musculoskeletal ultrasound (MSUS) and magnetic resonance imaging (MRI) can be useful to identify signs of synovitis such as effusions, synovial hypertrophy, erosions, and hypervascularity (power Doppler signal), but radiographs are not considered to be useful for diagnoses of JIA except for ruling out other conditions (25).

Delayed access to paediatric rheumatology care has been identified as an important and potentially avoidable predictor of poor disease outcomes in JIA owing to progressive damage caused by prolonged and untreated inflammatory disease activity (26, 27). As a result, there is a clear rationale for early referral to paediatric rheumatology services to facilitate timely diagnosis of JIA and targeting of inflammatory disease at an early stage with aggressive systemic pharmacological regimens (28). Recent research has demonstrated that persistent delayed access to paediatric rheumatology care remains problematic (26) and has been attributed to reports of a lack of confidence and training in paediatric musculoskeletal examination skills amongst many doctors in primary care (28). Whilst it is relatively unlikely that a paediatric patient with undiagnosed JIA will present in podiatry settings, podiatrists should be aware that unexplained large-joint swelling (especially knee or ankle), limp, and a recent history of reduced physical activity in the paediatric patient should be considered a 'red flag', which should trigger immediate urgent referral to paediatric rheumatology services. Detailed examinations using paediatric musculoskeletal screening systems, such as the paediatric Gait, Arms, Legs, Spine (pGALS) and paediatric Regional Examination of the Musculoskeletal System (pREMS) tools (29, 30), can help to confirm diagnostic suspicions and facilitate referral to the necessary specialists. Details on how to conduct and score pGALS and pREMS are available as online resources from Arthritis Research UK (now known as Versus Arthritis) (31, 32).

General medical management

Similar to the treatment goals in adult RA and the concepts of the window of opportunity (early treatment to improve long-term outcomes), the primary aim of medical management of JIA is to suppress inflammation prior to the development of irreparable joint damage and functional limitation (2). Whilst treat-to-target and tight control strategies are less well established in JIA, there are criteria for disease activity states based on three-variable JIA disease activity scores known as the clinical Juvenile Arthritis Disease Activity Score (cJADAS) (33). The cJADAS is derived from core outcome variables, including physician's global rating of overall disease activity, parent/child ratings of wellbeing (both on 100-mm visual analogue scales), and a count of active joints based on either 71, 27, or 10 joints. The cJADAS is calculated as the sum of the scores of its three components, which yields a global score of 0–91, 0–47, and 0–30 for the cJADAS71, cJADAS27, and cJADAS10, respectively (33). Cut-offs for the cJADAS permit allocation of children with JIA to inactive, low-, moderate-, and high-disease activity and thus provide a means of targeting lower disease activity categories.

Recent recommendations for medical management of JIA endorsed by the American College of Rheumatology provide guidance on therapeutic agents according to disease subtype and safety monitoring (34). Typically for oligoarthritis, medical management includes intra-articular glucocorticoid injections with triamcinolone hexacetonide, adjunct non-steroidal anti-inflammatory drugs (NSAIDs), and escalations to methotrexate and then a tumour necrosis factor alpha (TNF-α) inhibitor such as etanercept (34). Polyarthritis is managed in a similar fashion but often requires escalation to abatacept if disease activity is high after receipt of TNF-α inhibitor (34). For SoJIA, management includes NSAIDs with systemic glucocorticoids and possible escalation to anakinra, with additional TNF-α inhibitor and abatacept for persistently active synovitis (34). Early and aggressive medical management of JIA with disease-modifying antirheumatic drugs (DMARDs) and biologic class drugs appears to have resulted in improvements in short- and long-term outcomes; however, a significant proportion of children continue to experience at least mild disability after 1 year of medical management (35). Moreover, many adolescents with JIA will continue to experience active disease into adulthood, resulting in poor long-term outcomes (2, 36, 37).

Juvenile idiopathic arthritis: synovitis and the foot

Inflammatory foot disease has been cited as a common manifestation of JIA (17). Recent longitudinal research suggests that ankle joint synovitis affects approximately 60% of patients at disease onset, and, following the introduction of systemic antirheumatic and biologic therapies, this reduces to approximately 50% after 1 year, 40% at year 2, and 30% at year 3 and thereafter (3). In terms of cumulative frequency, the best available evidence suggests that ankle joint synovitis will affect approximately 80% of all patients with JIA within 5 years of diagnosis, making it the second most frequently affected joint after the knee (3). Recent research has demonstrated that the presence of ankle arthritis at diagnosis is strongly predictive of poor disease outcomes (38), and this suggests that existing rehabilitation strategies that appear beneficial for hip and knee problems may not be sufficient for ankle problems.

Relatively little is known regarding the frequency of synovitis affecting other foot joints, and this has been attributed at least partly to the challenging nature of clinical assessments of the foot or a lack of recognition (39–42). In particular, the subtalar joint is believed to be frequently affected with synovitis and often presents with concomitant ankle joint disease. However, clinical assessment is considered to be challenging in the region of the subtalar joint owing to the multiplicity of joint recesses, surrounding tendons, small articular compartments, and abundant fat (39). Relative to adult RA, forefoot synovitis appears to be far less common, with previous reports suggesting that forefoot synovitis may affect up to 16% of patients with JIA (17). Persistent active synovitis is associated with progressive joint destruction, which is characterized by factors detectable using radiographs, including reduced cartilage thickness, joint space narrowing, juxta-articular osteoporosis, bone growth abnormality, bony erosions, and severe deformation/loss of congruity of articular surfaces (11). Radiographic joint destruction can occur early in the disease course if left untreated or treated suboptimally, and it is strongly predictive of severe physical disability, which can persist into adulthood (36, 43, 44).

Juvenile idiopathic arthritis in the ankle and lower limb

Periarticular disease

The prevalence of lower limb periarticular manifestations of disease activity in JIA has not been studied in great detail and is most likely underreported. Documented periarticular inflammatory lesions in JIA include tenosynovitis of the periarticular tendon sheaths of the ankle joint complex (40, 45–48), bursitis affecting the retrocalcaneal bursa (40, 49), and enthesitis affecting various tendinous and ligamentous attachments (12).

Tenosynovitis

Tenosynovitis is an inflammation of the synovial lining of the sheath that surrounds a tendon. Tenosynovitis is clinically detectable by palpation of a 'boggy' swelling along the course of the tendon in question, which is often tender. Few studies have sought to describe the presence of lower limb tenosynovitis in JIA (40, 46, 48). Tynjala et al. (48), in a retrospective study of 19 patients with JIA who had 22 clinically swollen ankles, reported that tenosynovitis was present in 17/22 ankles/feet using MRI. Similarly, Rooney et al. (46), in a cross-sectional observational study

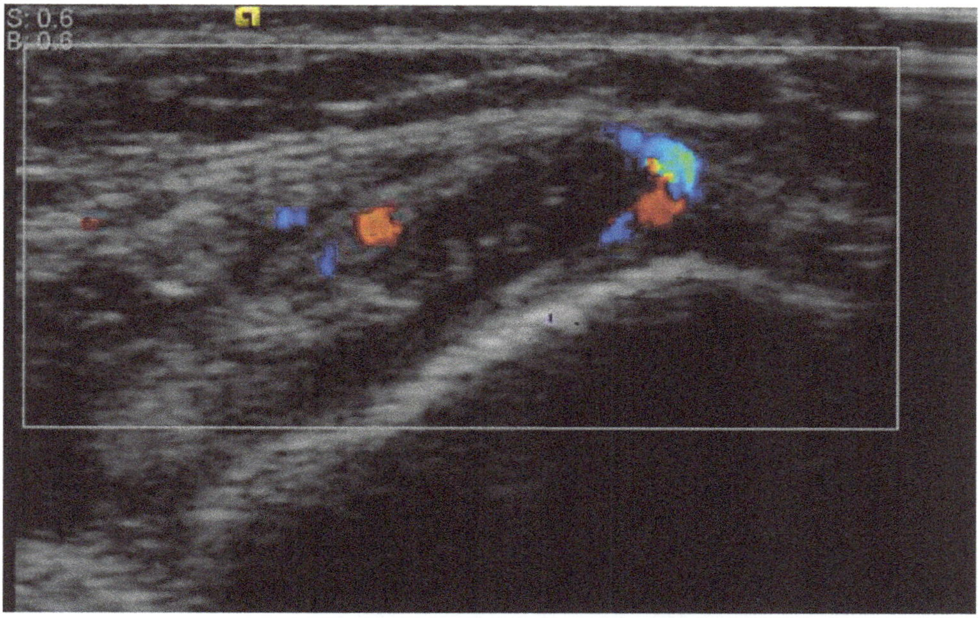

Figure 10.2 Cross-sectional ultrasound scan with power Doppler signal of the tibialis posterior tendon in a boy with oligoarticular juvenile idiopathic arthritis indicative of active tenosynovitis.

using MSUS (visible using B-mode and power Doppler [Figures 10.2 and 10.3]), found a high frequency of tenosynovitis affecting 35 of 49 clinically swollen ankles, 19 of which were affected by tenosynovitis in the absence of active ankle joint synovitis. Tenosynovitis of the tibialis posterior tendon was found most frequently in this study (46), and anecdotally this presentation appears to be associated with walking-related disability and progressive pes plano valgus foot deformity in a similar fashion to adult RA (50). Tenosynovitis of the extrinsic muscle tendons surrounding the ankle appear to be more frequently involved where there is concomitant ankle and subtalar joint synovitis.

Enthesitis

Enthesitis is a feature of JIA that is considered a subtype-specific manifestation, occurring exclusively in jERA (1). However, it is widely recognized that this classification is contentious (51) given that JPsA is considered to be a separate category of JIA whilst enthesitis is widely recognized as a common manifestation in adult PsA (52). As such, many children with enthesitis tend to be allocated an undifferentiated JIA classification. Peripheral enthesitis typically affects the Achilles tendon insertion, the patellar tendon insertion, and, in rarer cases, the plantar fascia origin (53). The commonest symptom is often superficial tenderness, which can be elicited upon palpation, and the pain can often be severe enough to be disabling (54).

Bursitis

Goldenstein-Schainberg et al. (49) suggested that inflammation of the retrocalcaneal bursa (RCB), which lies between the Achilles tendon and the calcaneus proximal to the tendon insertion, is frequently both underreported and underrecognized in JIA. Clinical assessment of

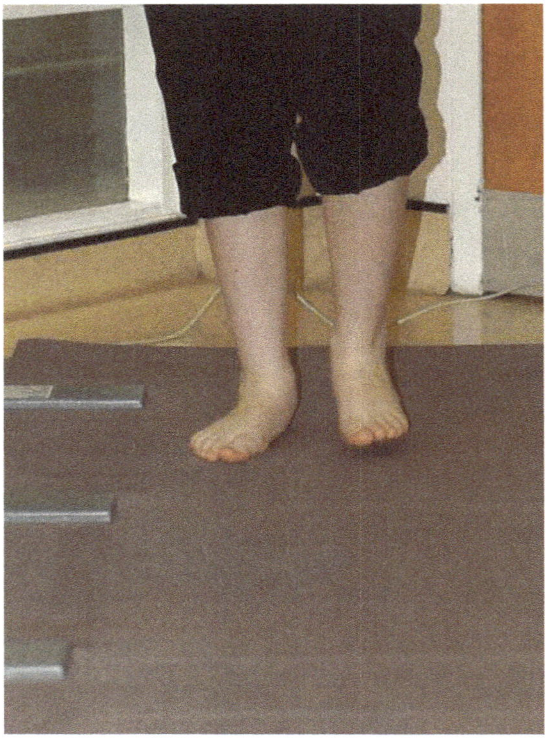

Figure 10.3 Abnormal hindfoot posture during single limb (right) stance in a boy with oligoarticular juvenile idiopathic arthritis and tibialis posterior tenosynovitis.

the RCB is not routinely conducted and it can often be overlooked where there is swelling in the region of the ankle joint complex. In addition, it is often difficult to distinguish between RCB bursitis and enthesitis at the Achilles tendon insertion. A study comparing clinical versus ultrasound-based examinations of foot disease activity in JIA found that tenderness and swelling detected via mediolateral palpation and ultrasound-detected effusions were present in a small number of participants (40). Relative to adult RA, where forefoot bursitis has been identified as an important prognostic indicator for foot-related disability (55), very little is known concerning the significance of bursitis affecting the foot in JIA and its impact on foot function. However, where RCB bursitis is present, it can cause pain and discomfort during terminal stance and can be disabling.

Foot impairments and disability

Cross-sectional studies suggest that foot and ankle problems and disability are common in JIA and often persist despite the recent improvements in medical management (56, 57). The presence of active synovitis affecting the foot and ankle appears to be associated with higher levels of foot pain, reduced abilities to perform activities of daily living, and reduced standing and walking abilities (56, 57). In terms of foot function, observational studies employing instrumented gait analyses have demonstrated that children with JIA may experience abnormal lower limb and foot joint ranges-of-motion, reduced ankle joint power, and altered plantar

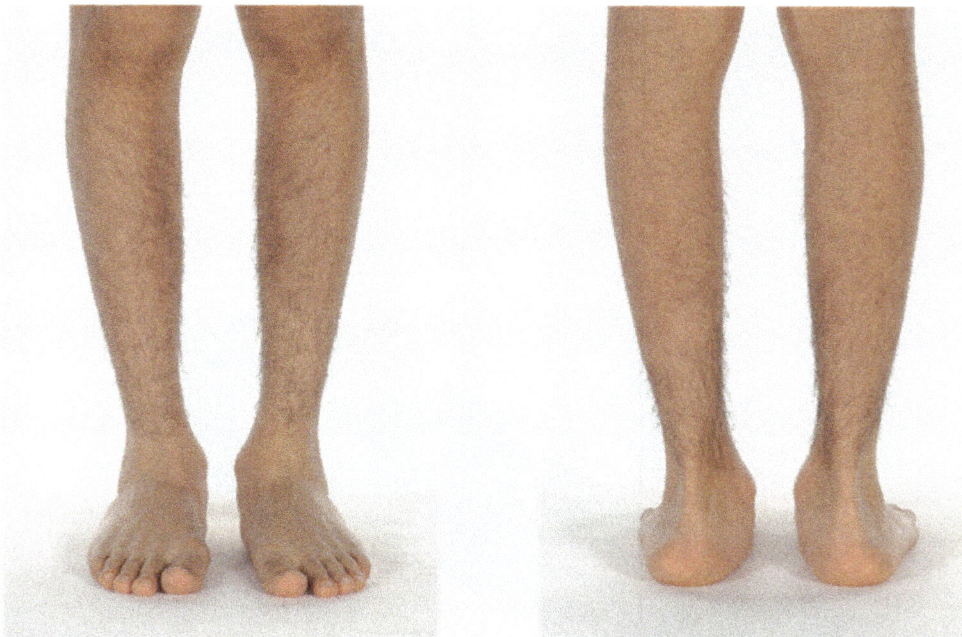

Figure 10.4 Severe pes plano valgus foot posture in an adolescent with rheumatic factor-positive juvenile idiopathic arthritis.

foot loading characteristics (58–60). Merker et al. (61) recently demonstrated that children with JIA and pes plano valgus foot posture (Figures 10.4 and 10.5) exhibit excessive hindfoot eversion and reduced medial longitudinal arch height during walking relative to age-matched healthy controls, and suggested such misalignments could potentially overburden muscles and cause further impairments. However, there is little evidence to suggest that current therapeutic strategies for pes plano valgus can correct the deformity or halt its progression. While these studies have been useful in identifying potential associations between impairments, suboptimal mechanics, and disability, robust statistical evaluations of these associations have not been possible as testing has been conducted on small heterogeneous samples. Identification of the key factors associated with foot-related disability in clinically meaningful homogenous groups of children with JIA would serve to assist rehabilitation specialists who routinely evaluate the burden of foot and ankle disease in response to either medical or conservative foot interventions.

Global functional capacity as well as localized anatomical functions may be affected as a result of foot involvement, and several studies have demonstrated that children with JIA tend to walk more slowly than healthy age-matched controls (58, 62, 63). This can be particularly problematic as walking is recognized as the commonest type of physical activity in children and adolescents (64). Impaired mobility as a result of disease-related lower limb problems translates as being unable to keep up with peers, and research suggests that there may be associations with subsequent feelings of depression and isolation (65). Unsurprisingly, many children with JIA are often significantly less physically active than healthy children and lower physical activity is inversely associated with higher pain intensity (66–68). The importance of physical activity during childhood

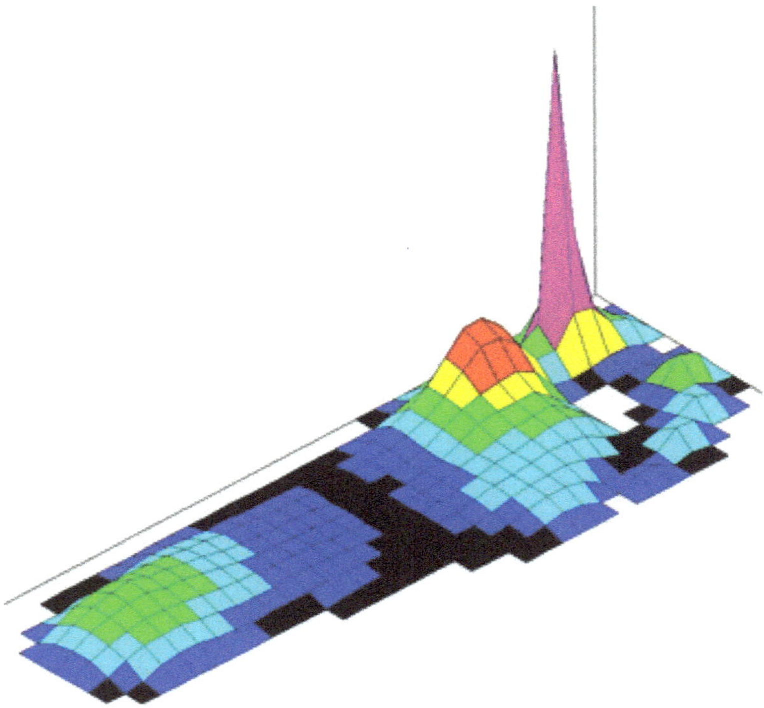

Figure 10.5 Corresponding plantar pressure profile for the right foot of the adolescent in Figure 10.4, indicating abnormal and excessive midfoot contact area.

is well established and documented benefits include better cardiovascular health, healthy body weight, improved bone health, improved self-confidence, and better social skills (64).

It is likely that low physical activity levels in JIA are driven by avoidance of the activities that are perceived to cause pain and discomfort. Subsequently, children with JIA may have localized reduced muscle strength adjacent to joints with active synovitis (69–71) and, possibly, impaired balance and proprioception (72). Singh-Grewal et al. (73) proposed a model of deconditioning whereby avoidance of physical activity amongst children with JIA results in further deconditioning and limited participation, culminating in prolonged and worsening disability. In addition, preliminary findings suggest that the adoption of avoidant coping strategies amongst children with JIA is predictive of poorer functional outcomes (74, 75). As such, it is possible that avoidant coping strategies may contribute to a downward spiral of deconditioning in children with JIA. The avoidance model of activity limitations is well established in paediatric chronic pain patients (75) and adults with localized chronic pain such as that experienced in knee osteoarthritis (76). According to this model, a patient initially experiences the unpleasant sensation of pain during activity, which leads to subsequent avoidance of that activity, which, in the longer term, results in physical deconditioning and activity limitations (75, 76). While the avoidance model is conceptually appealing in JIA, this has yet to be empirically tested. Nevertheless, there appears to be an unmet need for evidence-based therapies to maintain and/or improve foot function, restore and preserve normal gait, and promote physical activity.

Foot deformities and footwear

In the rearfoot, synovitis of the ankle and subtalar joints have been associated with a reduction in joint range of motion and the development of valgus, or occasionally varus, deformities (17, 57, 77, 78). Forefoot synovitis has been associated with the development of deformities such as hallux abducto valgus and a variety of lesser toe deformities, including claw toes (Figure 10.6) (17, 57, 77, 78). Small-sample observational studies suggest that persistent synovitis may disrupt foot growth and maturation, causing pain, stiffness, and the development of foot deformities at a relatively early age (17, 78). Growth disruption can be characterized by initial overgrowth, followed by premature fusion of the epiphyseal growth plates, leading to a net loss of local growth potential (11, 79). This can result in the development of unusual asymmetrical deformities, particularly in the region of the distal tibial and fibular epiphyses where there is adjacent ankle synovitis (80).

In comparison to adult RA, the consequences of JIA-related foot deformities are neither well described nor understood. It is likely that foot pain has more of an influence on functional ability in JIA and that foot deformities may be less of an influence on disability, but more troublesome in terms of obtaining comfortable footwear (81, 82). Indeed, footwear difficulties in JIA have been identified recently as an important issue to parents of children with JIA, and adults and adolescents who have the disease (65, 83, 84). Participants have reported having experienced difficulties in finding appropriate footwear owing to a number of factors, including the presence of pain/deformity, concerns over poor-fitting shoes and styles, suitability of styles for specific occasions, including physical activity/sports and employment (adult JIA patients), and the negative influence of fashion trends (65). There may be a bidirectional link between foot problems and poor footwear characteristics in JIA where: 1) the presence of joint swelling, joint tenderness, and/or foot deformities may restrict footwear choices; and 2) persistence with wearing inappropriate footwear in the presence of joint swelling, joint tenderness, and/or foot deformities may contribute to increased foot pain levels and the maladaptation of foot function and gait. Poor footwear habits may be an important contributory but potentially modifiable factor for higher levels of foot-related disability in JIA, which could be targeted through improved footwear education

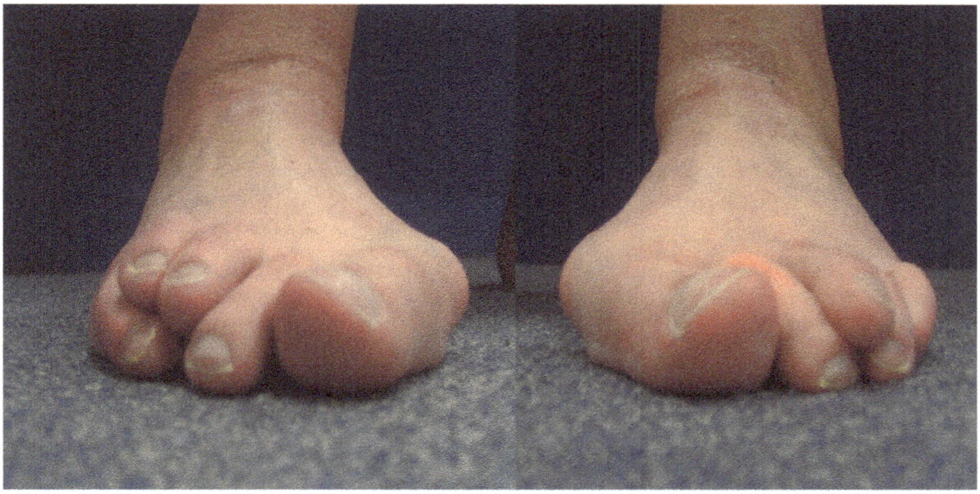

Figure 10.6 Severe asymmetrical foot deformities, including hallux valgus, and a variety of lesser toe deformities in an adult woman with a long history of juvenile idiopathic arthritis.

and behaviour-change strategies. At present, there is a major need to explore in greater detail the perceptions, experiences, and preferences of parents and children/adolescents with JIA regarding obtaining suitable and desirable footwear.

Specific management and assessment

Management

The management of foot problems in JIA is complex and challenging, involving a multidisciplinary team of health professionals to deliver coordinated medical and rehabilitative treatments (65, 84, 85). Podiatrists have been identified as essential members of the core paediatric rheumatology multidisciplinary team, and UK standards of care for JIA indicate that access to podiatry is a requirement for every child or young person with JIA (86). Podiatry care is centred on customized foot orthoses, footwear education and advice, footwear modification, and muscle-endurance and strengthening exercises (84). General advice and education surrounding foot health and physical activity may also be beneficial and can help to reinforce the advice provided by other members of the multidisciplinary team. Detailed clinical practice guidelines for foot care in JIA are lacking, but preliminary guidelines produced by the Ottawa Panel recommend that both customized and prefabricated foot orthoses are a good treatment option for managing foot pain and function in JIA (86).

Assessment

History-taking and physical examinations of the paediatric patient can be challenging relative to the adult patient. The first key consideration is that clinicians may have to rely on the parent or guardian for information where the patient is very young (87). For a new paediatric patient, a detailed history, including details of the chief complaint, full medical history, review of systems (neurological, musculoskeletal, dermatological, and vascular), thorough detailed physical examinations and observations of gait, is recommended (87). A detailed account of examinations of the paediatric patient can be found elsewhere (87).

Where a diagnosis of JIA is suspected but has not yet been confirmed by a paediatric rheumatologist, there are some key considerations that merit attention. Should a tender and swollen joint be identified (often at the knee or ankle), the clinician should seek to establish the date of onset, duration, and degree of persistence. If the joint pain is mainly related to physical activity, it is more likely to be of mechanical origin. Secondly, if the child appears to be ill and/or has a fever, the clinician should suspect infection or malignancy initially and consider appropriate onward referral. Next, the clinician should seek to rule out trauma as a cause of injury. Neurological symptoms such as general muscle weakness and loss of sensation should be ruled out at this stage, as should inherited causes of musculoskeletal dysfunction such as hypermobility syndromes. pGALS and pREMS screening tools can be useful to confirm suspicions where the patient history and presentation suggests a musculoskeletal disorder.

When a diagnosis of JIA has been obtained, an essential component of the management of foot problems in JIA is a detailed patient assessment, which takes into account examinations of primary disease pathology (inflammatory disease activity) or its surrogates (pain/swelling), foot structure, and foot and global gait function. Clinical examination of the foot and ankle should involve palpation of foot joints and relevant soft tissues to detect the presence of tenderness or swelling as clinical surrogates of synovitis, tenosynovitis, enthesitis, and bursitis. Tenderness and swelling is normally detected at the joint margin with pressure exerted by the examiner's thumb and index finger that is sufficient to cause 'whitening' of the examiner's nail bed (88), with the examiner looking for signs that the pressure stimulus has caused the patient to experience localized tenderness or pain. However, it is often challenging to obtain verbal cues from the paediatric patient and the examiner has to be vigilant for non-verbal cues such as wince or withdrawal of the lower limb. If localized 'new' disease activity is detected or suspected, the patient's paediatric rheumatologist should be informed promptly to allow him or her to escalate systemic DMARD and/or biologic therapies and/or administer intra-articular corticosteroids (under sedation or general anaesthetic) as appropriate. The location of suspected disease activity within the foot will help to guide non-medical therapeutic intervention with foot orthoses, exercises, and footwear advice. Where there is synovitis and associated symptoms at the ankle joint complex and/or midfoot in normal to pronated foot postures, the treatment goal should be to maintain medial longitudinal arch height and limit excessive hindfoot eversion. Where foot posture is more supinated, the treatment goal should be to increase contact area under the midfoot. Where forefoot disease is present, the goal should be to limit peak pressures in the forefoot through cushioning and deflection.

The examination of static and dynamic foot posture should be a core component of the assessment of the patient with JIA to allow evaluation of progression of deformities over time. Semi-quantitative tools such as the Structural Index (originally developed for adult RA) and the Foot Posture Index (FPI-6) can be useful for scoring specific foot deformities and general foot posture (89, 90). In particular, the FPI-6 has been found to be reliable for assessment of the paediatric foot (91, 92) and normal comparative values are available (93). The FPI-6 has good face validity for use in JIA given the propensity for synovitis resulting in deformity or postural changes of the hindfoot.

Evaluation of physical function should include at least one performance-based measure of global physical function such as walking speed (using a stopwatch and a set distance such as 10 metres) and self-report utilizing patient-reported outcome measures. There is only one measure of foot-related impairments and disability that has been developed and validated for use in JIA; the Juvenile Arthritis Foot Disability Index (JAFI) (94). The JAFI is a 27-item questionnaire organized by three dimensions related to impairment (nine items), activity limitation (fourteen items), and participation restriction (four items). Each item is scored on a five-point Likert scale, which describes the frequency of foot-related problems (0 = never, 1 = less than once a week, 2 = once a week, 3 = two or three times a week, 4 = always), and a median score derived from individual items is calculated for each dimension. The JAFI has been shown to be valid and reliable for assessing foot-related disability in JIA and has been found to be responsive to change (94, 95). Therefore administration of the JAFI as an appendage to routine medical note-taking could permit objective monitoring of patients over time as well as response to foot-specific interventions. Parents or guardians should complete patient-reported outcomes as a proxy for the young child of 8–10 years of age or younger.

Musculoskeletal ultrasound

MSUS has emerged as an increasingly popular tool for the examination of inflammatory joint diseases owing to its well-documented benefits relative to other imaging strategies (96, 97). For JIA, several additional benefits of MSUS have been identified: 1) sedation is not required for younger children as compared to MRI; 2) it is non-invasive and non-ionizing; and 3) its real-time imaging capabilities appear to be parent- and child-friendly (Figure 10.7) and help to facilitate understanding of the inflammatory disease process. MSUS can be utilized to guide joint and tendon sheath injections and subsequently visualize the correct placement of steroid crystals (98, 99).

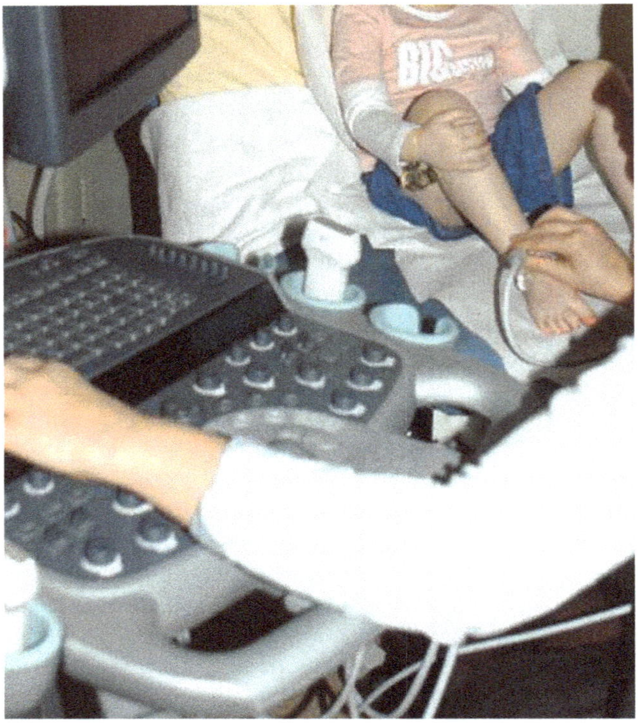

Figure 10.7 Child-friendly ultrasound scan of the ankle joint being performed in a young girl with juvenile psoriatic arthritis.

The ability to visualize correct placement of long-acting steroids is particularly useful for awkward and/or small joints of the feet such as the subtalar and midtarsal joints. A recent systematic review has demonstrated that ultrasound has superior sensitivity over clinical examination for detecting synovitis in JIA (99). It can be used to detect subclinical disease that would not otherwise have been identified using clinical examination techniques. However, there are also challenges when using ultrasound in JIA that require consideration. These include the unique features of the growing skeleton, such as age-related variation of cartilage thickness, incomplete ossification, and metaphyseal blood vessels, which can be confused with disease activity when power Doppler signal is employed (98).

Foot orthoses

Foot orthoses are recommended for the management of foot pain in JIA, and evidence from three randomized controlled trials and a systematic review suggests that they are beneficial in reducing pain, activity limitations, and disability (84, 86, 100, 101). There is evidence of effectiveness for both semi-rigid customized foot orthoses (made from polyolefin) (101) and prefabricated foot orthoses (Slimflex-Plus, Algeos UK) (100). However, there is a paucity of evidence available to guide specific foot orthosis prescriptions for children with JIA owing to a lack of information concerning the specific mechanisms of action of foot orthoses in this population. The best available evidence, which is drawn from a review of mechanistic studies, suggests that benefits are achieved through provision of greater hindfoot motion control via posting and attenuated loading through increased midfoot contact area (102). Prescribers of foot orthoses for JIA patients should consider a set of design rules (such as outlined for adult RA in the section on 'Foot orthoses' in Chapter 14) such as the level of dynamic peak rearfoot eversion to guide rearfoot posting, minimum navicular height during the stance phase of gait to guide foot orthosis medial arch height, and presence of forefoot disease and/or deformity to guide presence/absence of cushioned forefoot extensions. Should a patient present with tenosynovitis affecting the tibialis posterior tendon, podiatrists should consider whether or not customized foot orthoses will provide sufficient rearfoot motion control. In some cases a hinged ankle–foot orthosis with medial and lateral support such as a Richie Brace may be more appropriate for short-term use whilst the inflammatory lesion is addressed by the paediatric rheumatologist with ultrasound-guided steroid injections. In some cases, a total contact cast for up to 2 weeks post-injection would be appropriate to maximize the action of the locally administered steroid and limit potential for subsequent rupture owing to raised intra-sheath pressures.

There are some important considerations with the provision of foot orthoses for children with JIA. Firstly, clinicians should recognize that they are providing a device that may be outgrown within a relatively short period of time and therefore cost for replacement foot orthosis prescriptions can be a factor. In addition, children have a habit of losing or damaging their existing pair of foot orthoses. Secondly, very little is known about adherence to foot orthoses in the paediatric patient. Qualitative research suggests that some paediatric rheumatologists and parents of children with JIA are sceptical about the effectiveness of foot orthoses and that non-compliance is a major problem (103). Young children can often be persuaded to wear customized foot orthoses by allowing them to choose from a variety of colourful top covers. However, older children often do not want to be perceived as different, and therefore they will be reluctant to transfer foot orthoses from one pair of shoes to another in sight of other children in certain environments or circumstances (such as for physical education classes). Perceptions of comfort may also be an issue and many children will comment that their foot orthoses feel strange inside their shoes. Unfortunately, adherence to wearing foot orthoses as recommended remains a significant clinical challenge.

Exercises and physical activity

Podiatrists and physiotherapists should seek to work closely to avoid conflicting advice concerning exercise and physical activity recommendations for the patient with JIA. There is increasing evidence to suggest that specific foot muscle strengthening exercises can help to maintain or improve foot muscle strength in adults (104–106). Lower limb strength, proprioception, and balance exercises are underpinned by well-established evidence for adults with RA (106–112). A small randomized controlled trial recently compared an exercise programme incorporating 100 repetitions of a two-footed jump with rope (skipping) and demonstrated improvements in leg muscle strength (70). However, at present there have been no trials of specific foot muscle strengthening exercises in JIA. Simple foot muscle strengthening and endurance exercises may be beneficial, and a simple regime can be recommended incorporating calf and toe raises (with body weight resistance or no resistance as appropriate), and ankle inversion and eversion against resistance using therapeutic elastic bands or ankle weights. To produce improvements in muscle strength and endurance, physiological principles of overload (muscles need to perform more work than usual, resulting in fatigue), specificity (muscles must be trained using tasks that replicate the functional movement required, including acceleration and deceleration), and reversibility (benefits from undertaking functional tasks are reversible if not undertaken regularly) should be adhered to as part of a routine (113). General physical activity should also be recommended where possible. Every effort should be made to ensure that targeted exercise programme and physical activity recommendations are made fun and/or interesting to maximize the child's adherence. Importantly, no detrimental effects of exercise therapy for children with JIA have been found (114).

Footwear advice

Several important footwear characteristics have been identified from studies of adults and children generally, which should be considered when recommending footwear to parents of children with JIA or adolescents/adults with JIA. Current recommendations emphasize that: 1) a shoe heel height of less than 4 cm may reduce the risk of high forefoot pressures and pain, foot deformities, skin lesions, ankle sprain risk, and impaired balance (115–119); 2) strapping or another fixation method (i.e., laces) over the instep may be protective against foot pain, discomfort, or localized muscle fatigue (120, 121); 3) non-slip sloes may reduce the risk of injury due to falls/slipping (122, 123); 4) heel counter-rigidity may provide additional desirable rearfoot motion control (124); 5) the sole flexion point should correspond to the location of flexion of the first metatarsophalangeal (MTP) joint to prevent abnormal MTP function and associated pain and discomfort (120, 121, 125, 126); and 6) longitudinal sole rigidity provides torsional stability to reduce pain, discomfort, or localized fatigue owing to insufficient motion control (127, 128). In addition, three main factors concerning fit should be considered to prevent foot pain, discomfort, skin lesions, and the development of forefoot deformities (115, 121, 127, 128). Shoe length should be between 1 cm and 2 cm longer than the length of the foot itself; shoe width should be wide enough at the uppers in the region of the metatarsal heads to accommodate the forefoot without exerting lateral pressure; and shoe toe box height should be sufficient to allow space for movement of the toes (115, 121, 127, 128).

Conclusion

JIA is a complex group of paediatric rheumatic disorders that all affect the foot and ankle. Awareness of the disease appears to be increasing and medical management strategies are improving, but more high-quality research evidence is required to investigate the role of non-medical rehabilitation strategies for the foot and lower limb. This chapter has highlighted some of the key considerations for managing the child with suspected or diagnosed JIA as part of the wider multidisciplinary team. The overall aim of management of foot and ankle problems should be to reduce pain levels and maximize physical function through provision of foot orthoses where appropriate and promotion of good foot health, exercise, and physical activity.

References

1. **Petty RE, Southwood TR, Manners P, et al.** International league of associations for rheumatology classification of juvenile idiopathic arthritis: second revision, Edmonton, 2001. *J Rheumatol.* 2004;**31**:390–2.
2. **Hashkes, P.J., Laxer, R.M.** Medical treatment of juvenile idiopathic arthritis. *JAMA*. 2005;**294**:1671–84.
3. **Hemke R, Nusman CM, van der Heijde DMFM, et al.** Frequency of joint involvement in juvenile idiopathic arthritis during a 5-year follow-up of newly diagnosed patients: implications for MR imaging as outcome measure. *Rheumatol Int*. 2015;**35**(2):351–7.
4. **Al-Matar MJ, Petty RE, Tucker LB, Malleson PN, Schroeder ML, Cabral DA.** The early pattern of joint involvement predicts disease progression in children with oligoarticular (pauciarticular) juvenile rheumatoid arthritis. *Arthritis Rheum*. 2002;**46**:2709–15.
5. **Cahill AM, Cho SS, Baskin KM, et al.** Benefit of fluoroscopically guided intraarticular, long-acting corticosteroid injection for subtalar arthritis in juvenile idiopathic arthritis. *Pediat Radiol.* 2007;**37**:544–8.

6. **Beukelman T, Arabshahi C AM, Kaye RD, Cron RQ.** Benefit of intraarticular corticosteroid injection under fluoroscopic guidance for subtalar arthritis in juvenile idiopathic arthritis. *J Rheumatol.* 2006;**33**:2330–2336.
7. **Remedios D, Martin K, Kaplan G, Mitchell R, Woo P, Rooney M.** Juvenile chronic arthritis: diagnosis and management of tibio-talar and sub-talar disease. *Br J Rheumatol.* 1997;**36**:1214–17.
8. **Flato B, Lien G, Smerdel A, Vinje O, Dale K, Johnston V.** Prognostic factors in juvenile rheumatoid arthritis. *J Rheumatol.* 2003;**30**:386–93.
9. **Flato B, Aasland A, Vinje O, Forre O.** Outcome and predictive factors in juvenile rheumatoid arthritis. *J Rheumatol.* 1998;**25**:366–75.
10. **Wallace CA, Bandeira M, Ravelli A, Giannini EH.** Patterns of clinical remission in select categories of juvenile idiopathic arthritis. *Arthritis Rheum.* 2005;**52**:3554–62.
11. **Selvaag AM, Flato B, Dale K, et al.** Radiographic and clinical outcome in early juvenile rheumatoid arthritis and juvenile spondylarthropathy: a 3-year prospective study. *J Rheumatol.* 2006;**33**:1382–91.
12. **Burgos-Vargas R, Pacheco-Tena C, Vazquez-Mellado J.** A short-term follow-up of enthesitis and arthritis in the active phase of juvenile onset spondyloarthropathies. *Clin Exp Rheumatol.* 2002;**20**:727–31.
13. **Huemer C, Malleson PN, Cabral DA, et al.** Patterns of joint involvement at onset differentiate oligoarticular juvenile psoriatic arthritis from pauciarticular juvenile rheumatoid arthritis. *J Rheumatol.* 2003;**29**:1531–5.
14. **Flato B, Lien G, Smerdel-Ramoya A,Vinje O.** Juvenile psoriatic arthritis: longterm outcome and differentiation from other subtypes of juvenile idiopathic arthritis. *J Rheumatol.* 2009;**36**:642–50.
15. **Ravelli A, Martini A.** Juvenile idiopathic arthritis. *The Lancet.* 2007;**369**:767–78.
16. **Pay S, Turkcapar N, Kalyoncu M, et al., and the Ankara Rheumatology Study Group**. A multicenter study of patients with adult-onset Still's disease compared with systemic juvenile idiopathic arthritis. *Clin Rheumatol.* 2006;**25**:639–44.
17. **Spraul G, Koenning G.** A descriptive study of foot problems in children with juvenile rheumatoid arthritis (JRA). *Arthritis Care Res* 1994;**7**:144–50.
18. **Martini A.** Systemic juvenile idiopathic arthritis. *Autoimmun Rev* 2012;**12**:56–9.
19. **Martini A.** It is time to rethink juvenile idiopathic arthritis classification and nomenclature. *Ann Rheum Dis.* 2012;**71**:1437–9.
20. **Chan MO, Petty RE, Oen K, et al.**, The ReACCh Out Investigators. A67: Factors that contribute to classification of children as having undifferentiated juvenile idiopathic arthritis. *Arthritis Rheumatol.* 2014;**66**:S98.
21. **Manners PJ, Bower C.** Worldwide prevalence of juvenile arthritis—why does it vary so much? *J Rheumatol.* 2002;**29**:1520–30.
22. **Thierry S, Fautrel B, Lemelle I, Guillemin F.** Prevalence and incidence of juvenile idiopathic arthritis: a systematic review. *Joint Bone Spine.* 2014;**81**:112–17.
23. **Adib N, Hyrich K, Thornton J, et al.** Association between duration of symptoms and severity of disease at first presentation to paediatric rheumatology: results from the Childhood Arthritis Prospective Study. *Rheumatology.* 2008;**47**:991–5.
24. **Gale EAM.** The rise of childhood type 1 diabetes in the 20th century. *Diabetes.* 2002;**51**:3353–61.
25. **Szer I.** Clinical skills in the evaluation of arthritis. In: IS Szer, Y Kimura, PN Malleson, TR Southwood (eds). *Arthritis in Children and Adolescents*, 1st edn; 2006. Oxford: Oxford University Press, pp. 3–18.
26. **McErlane F, Foster HE, Carrasco R, et al.** Trends in paediatric rheumatology, referral times and disease activity indices over a ten-year period among children and young people with juvenile idiopathic arthritis: results from the childhood arthritis prospective study. *Rheumatology.* 2016;**55**(7):1225–34.
27. **Foster H, Rapley T, May C.** Juvenile idiopathic arthritis: improved outcome requires improved access to care. *Rheumatology.* 2010;**49**:401–3.

28. **Foster HE, Eltringham MS, Kay LJ, Friswell M, Abinun M, Myers A.** Delay in access to appropriate care for children presenting with musculoskeletal symptoms and ultimately diagnosed with juvenile idiopathic arthritis. *Arthritis Rheum.* 2007;**57**:921–7.
29. **Foster HE, Kay LJ, Friswell M, Coady D, Myers A.** Musculoskeletal screening examination (pGALS) for school age children based on the adult GALS screen. *Arthritis Rheum.* 2006;**55**:709–16.
30. **Foster H, Kay L, May C, Rapley T.** Pediatric regional examination of the musculoskeletal system: a practice and consensus based approach. *Arthritis Care Res.* 2011;**63**:1503–10.
31. **Arthritis Research UK.** Paediatric Gait Arms Legs Spine videos: http://www.arthritisresearchuk.org/health-professionals-and-students/video-resources/pgals.aspx.
32. **Arthritis Research UK. Regional examination of the Musculoskeletal System (REMS):** http://www.arthritisresearchuk.org/health-professionals-and-students/video-resources/rems.aspx
33. **Consolaro A, Negro G, Gallo MC, et al.** Defining crtieria for disease activity states in non-systemic juvenile idiopathic arthritis based on a three-variable juvenile disease activity score. *Arthritis Care Res.* 2014;**66**:1703–9.
34. **Beukelman T, Patkar NM, Saag KG, et al.** 2011 American College of Rheumatology recommendations for the treatment of juvenile idiopathic arthritis: initiation and safety monitoring of therapeutic agents for the treatment of arthritis and systemic features. *Arthritis Care Res.* 2011;**63**:465–82.
35. **Hyrich KL, Lal SD, Foster HE, et al.** Disease activity and disability in children with juvenile idiopathic arthritis one year following presentation to paediatric Rheumatology. Results from the Childhood Arthritis Prospective Study. *Rheumatology.* 2010;**49**:116–22.
36. **Flato B, Lien G, Smerdel-Ramoya A, Vinje O.** Juvenile psoriatic arthritis: longterm outcome and differentiation from other subtypes of juvenile idiopathic arthritis. *J Rheumatol.* 2009;**36**:642–50.
37. **Packham JC, Hall MA.** Long-term follow-up of 246 adults with juvenile idiopathic arthritis: functional outcome. *Rheumatology.* 2002;**41**:1428–35.
38. **Esbjornsson AC, Aalto K, Brostom EW, et al.**, on behalf of the Nordic Study Group of Paediatric Rheumatology (NoSPeR). *Clin Exp Rheumatol.* 2015;**33**:751–7.
39. **Lanni S, Bovis F, Ravelli A, et al.** Delineating the application of ultrasound in detecting synovial abnormalities of subtalar joint in juvenile idiopathic arthritis. *Arthritis Care Res.* 2016;doi:10.1002/acr.22846.
40. **Hendry GJ, Gardner-Medwin J, Steultjens MPM, Woodburn J, Sturrock RD, Turner DE.** Frequent discordance between clinical and musculoskeletal ultrasound examinations of foot disease in juvenile idiopathic arthritis. *Arthritis Care Res* 2012;**64**:441–7.
41. **Magni-Manzoni S, Epis O, Ravelli A, et al.** Comparison of clinical versus ultrasound determined synovitis in juvenile idiopathic arthritis. *Arthritis Rheum.* 2009;**61**:1497–504.
42. **Guzman J, Burgos-Vargas R, Duarte-Salazar C, Gomez-Mora R.** Reliability of the articular examination in children with juvenile rheumatoid arthritis: interobserver agreement and sources of disagreement. *J Rheumatol.*1995;**22**:2331–6.
43. **Magni-Manzoni S, Rossi F, Pistorio A, et al.** Prognostic factors for radiographic progression, radiographic damage, and disability in juvenile idiopathic arthritis. *Arthritis Rheum.* 2003;**48**:3509–17.
44. **Foster HE, Marshall N, Myers A, Dunkley P, Griffiths ID.** Outcome in adults with juvenile idiopathic arthritis. *Arthritis Rheum.* 2003;**48**:767–75.
45. **Pascoli L, Wright S, McAllister C, Rooney M.** Prospective evaluation of clinical and ultrasound findings in ankle disease in juvenile idiopathic arthritis: importance of ankle ultrasound. *J Rheumatol.* 2010;**37**:1–6.
46. **Rooney M, McAllister C, Burns JFT.** Ankle disease in juvenile idiopathic arthritis: ultrasound findings in clinically swollen ankles. *J Rheumatol.* 2009;**36**:1725–9.
47. **Karmazyn B, Bowyer SL, Schmidt KM, et al.** US findings of metacarpophalangeal joints in children with idiopathic juvenile arthritis. *Pediat Radiol.* 2007;**37**:475–82.

48. **Tynjala P, Honkanen V, Lahdenne P.** Intra-articular steroids in radiologically confirmed tarsal and hip synovitis of juvenile idiopathic arthritis. *Clin Exp Rheumatol.* 2004;**22**:643–8.
49. **Goldenstein-Schainberg C, Homsi C, Pereira RMR, Cossermelli W.** Retrocalcaneal bursitis in juvenile chronic arthritis. *Ann Rheum Dis.* 1992;**51**:1162–3.
50. **Barn R, Turner DE, Rafferty D, Sturrock RD, Woodburn J.** Tibialis posterior tenosynovitis and associated pes plano valgus in rheumatoid arthritis: electromyography, multisegment foot kinematics, and ultrasound features. *Arthritis Care Res* 2013;**65**:495–502.
51. **Colbert RA.** Classification of juvenile spondyloarthritis: enthesitis related arthritis and beyond. *Nature Rev Rheumatol.* 2010;**6**:477–85.
52. **Hyslop E, McInnes IB, Woodburn J, Turner DE.** Foot problems in psoriatic arthritis: high burden and low care provision. *Ann Rheum Dis.* 2010;**69**:928.
53. **Jousse-Joulin S, Breton S, Cangemi C, et al.** Ultrasonography for detecting enthesitis in juvenile idiopathic arthritis. *Arthritis Care Res.* 2011;**63**:849–55.
54. **Burgos-Vargas R.** Juvenile onset spondyloarthropathies: therapeutic aspects. *Arch Dis Child.* 2003;**88**:312–18.
55. **Hooper L, Bowen CJ, Gates L, et al.** Prognostic indicators of foot-related disability in patients with rheumatoid arthritis: results of a prospective three-year study. *Arthritis Care Res.* 2012;**64**:1116–24.
56. **Dekker M, Hoeksma AF, Dekker JHM, et al.** Strong relationships between disease activity, foot-related impairments, activity limitations and participation restrictions in children with juvenile idiopathic arthritis. *Clin Exp Rheumatol.* 2010;**28**:905–11.
57. **Hendry G, Turner D, Gardner-Medwin J, Watt G, Woodburn J.** A survey of foot problems in juvenile idiopathic arthritis. *Musculoskeletal Care.* 2008;**6**(4):221–32.
58. **Hartmann M, Kreuzpointer F, Haefner R, Michels H, Schwirtz A, Haas JP.** Effects of juvenile idiopathic arthritis of the lower extremities: call for consequences in physical activities recommendations. *Int J Ped.* 2010;**2010**:835984.
59. **Broström E, Haglund-Åkerlind Y, Hagelberg S, Cresswell AG.** Gait in children with juvenile chronic arthritis. *Scand J Rheumatol.* 2002;**31**(6):317–23.
60. **Fairburn PS, Panagamuwa B, Falkonakis A, et al.** The use of multidisciplinary assessment and scientific measurement in advanced juvenile idiopathic arthritis can categorise gait deviations to guide treatment. *Arch Dis Child.* 2002;**87**:160–5.
61. **Merker J, Hartmann M, Kreuzpointner F, Schwirtz A, Haas JP.** Pathophysiology of juvenile idiopathic arthritis induced pes planovalgus in static and walking condition—a functional view using 3d gait analysis. *Ped Rheumatology.* 2015;**13**:21.
62. **Hendry GJ, Rafferty D, Barn R, Gardner-Medwin J, Turner DE, Woodburn J.** Foot function is well preserved in children and adolescents with juvenile idiopathic arthritis who are optimally managed. *Gait Posture.* 2013;**38**(1):30–6.
63. **Lechner DE, McCarthy CF, Holden MK.** Gait deviations in patients with juvenile rheumatoid arthritis. *Phys Ther.* 1987;**67**:1335–41.
64. **Department of Health.** *Start Active, Stay Active: A Report on Physical Activity for Health from the Four Home Countries' Chief Medical Officers.* London: Crown Copyright; 2011.
65. **Hendry GJ, Turner DE, Gardner-Medwin J, Lorgelly PK, Woodburn J.** An exploration of parents' preferences for foot care in juvenile idiopathic arthritis: a possible role for the discrete choice experiment. *J Foot Ankle Res.* 2014;**7**:10.
66. **Hulsegge G, Henschke N, McKay D, et al.** Fundamental movement skills, physical fitness and physical activity among Australian children with juvenile idiopathic arthritis. *J Ped Child Health.* 2015;**51**:425–32.
67. **Limenis E, Grosbein HA, Feldman BM.** The relationship between physical activity levels and pain in children with juvenile idiopathic arthritis. *J Rheumatol.* 2014;**41**:345–51.

68. **Lelieveld OT, Armbrust W, van Leeuwen MA, et al.** Physical activity in adolescents with juvenile idiopathic arthritis. *Arthritis Rheum*. 2008;**59**:1379–84.
69. **Sandstedt E, Fasth A, Eek MN, Beckung E.** Muscle strength, physical fitness and well-being in children and adolescents and the effect of an exercise programme: a randomized controlled trial. *Ped Rheumatology*. 2013;**11**:7.
70. **van Oort C, Tupper SM, Rosenberg AM, Farthing JP, Baxter-Jones AD.** Safety and feasibility of a home-based six week resistance training program in juvenile idiopathic arthritis. *Ped Rheumatology*. 2013;**11**:46.
71. **McKay D, Ostring G, Broderick C, Chaitow J, Singh-Grewal D.** A feasibility study of the effect of intra-articular corticosteroid injection on isokinetic muscle strength in children with juvenile idiopathic arthritis. *Ped Ex Sci*. 2013;**25**:221–37.
72. **Baydogan SN, Tarakci E, Kasapcopur O.** Effect of strengthening versus balance-proprioceptive exercises on lower extremity function in patients with juvenile idiopathic arthritis. *Am J Phys Med Rehabil*. 2015;**00**:1–12.
73. **Singh-Grewal D, Schneiderman-Walker J, Wright V, et al.** The effects of vigorous exercise training on physical function in children with arthritis: a randomized controlled, single-blinded trial. *Arthritis Care Res*. 2007;**57**:1202–10.
74. **Feinstein AB, Forman EM, Masuda A, et al.** Pain intensity, psychological inflexibility, and acceptance of pain as predictors of functioning in adolescents with juvenile idiopathic arthritis: a preliminary investigation. *J Clin Psychol Med Settings*. 2001;**18**:291–8.
75. **Simons LE, Kaczynski KJ.** The fear avoidance model of chronic pain: examination for pediatric application. *J Pain*. 2012;**13**(9):827–35.
76. **Holla JFM, van der Leeden M, Knol DL, et al.** Avoidance of activities in early symptomatic knee osteoarthritis: results from the CHECK cohort. *Ann Behav Med*. 2012;**44**:33–42.
77. **Ferrari J.** A review of the foot deformities seen in juvenile chronic arthritis. *The Foot*. 1998;**8**:193–6.
78. **Mavidrou A, Klenerman L, Swann M, Hall MA, Ansell BM.** Conservative management of the hindfoot in juvenile chronic arthritis. *The Foot*. 1991;**1**:143.
79. **MacRae VE, Farquharson C, Ahmed SF.**The pathophysiology of the growth plate in juvenile idiopathic arthritis. *Rheumatology*. 2006;**45**:19.
80. **Murray K, Ferrari J.** Rheumatic conditions of childhood. In: P. Thomson (ed.). *Introduction to Podopaediatrics*, 2nd edn. Edinburgh: Churchill Livingstone; 2001, pp. 105–19.
81. **Turner DE, Helliwell PS, Siegel KL, Woodburn J.** Biomechanics of the foot in rheumatoid arthritis: identifying abnormal function and the factors associated with localised disease 'impact'. *Clin Biomech (Bristol, Avon)*. 2008;**23**:93–100.
82. **Turner DE, Woodburn J.** Characterising the clinical and biomechanical features of severely deformed feet in rheumatoid arthritis. *Gait Posture*. 2008;**28**:574–80.
83. **Hendry GJ, Brenton-Rule A, Barr G, Rome K.** Footwear experiences of people with chronic musculoskeletal diseases. *Arthritis Care Res*. 2015;**67**:1164–72.
84. **Hendry GJ, Watt GF, Brandon M, et al.** The effectiveness of a multidisciplinary foot care program for children and adolescents with juvenile idiopathic arthritis: an exploratory trial. *J Rehabil Med*. 2013;**45**:467–76.
85. **Davies K, Cleary G, Foster H, Hutchinson E, Baildam E**, on behalf of the British Society of Paediatric and Adolescent Rheumatology. BSPAR Standards of Care for children and young people with juvenile idiopathic arthritis. *Rheumatology*. 2010;**49**:1406–8.
86. **Brosseau L, Toupin-April K, Wells G, et al.** Ottawa panel evidence-based clinical practice guidelines for foot care in the management of juvenile idiopathic arthritis. *Arch Phys Med Rehabil*. 2016;doi:10.1016/j.apmr.2015.11.011.
87. **Thomson P.** History-taking and the physical examination. In: R. Thomson & R. Volpe (eds). *Introduction to Podopaediatrics*, 2nd edn. Edinburgh: Churchill Livingstone Elsevier; 2001, pp. 31–46.

88. **Helliwell P, Woodburn J, Redmond A, Turner D, Davys H.** Clinical assessment. In: Helliwell P, **et al.** (eds). *The Foot and Ankle in Rheumatoid Arthritis*, 1st edn. London: Churchill Livingstone Elsevier; 2007, pp. 75–98.
89. **Redmond AC, Crosbie J, Ouvrier RA.** Development and validation of a novel rating system for scoring standard foot posture: the foot posture index. *Clin Biomech.* 2006;**21**:89–98.
90. **Platto J, O'Connell PG, Hicks JE, Gerber LH.** The relationship of pain and deformity of the rheumatoid foot to gait and an index of functional ambulation. *J Rheum.* 1991;**18**:38–43.
91. **Evans AM, Rome K, Peet L.** The foot posture index, ankle lunge test, Beighton scale and the lower limb assessment score in health children: a reliability study. *J Foot Ankle Res.* 2012;**5**:1.
92. **Morrison SC, Ferrari J.** Inter-rater reliability of the Foot Posture Index (FPI-6) in the assessment of the paediatric foot. *J Foot Ankle Res.* 2009;**2**:26.
93. **Redmond AC, Crane YZ, Menz HB.** Normative values for the foot posture index. *J Foot Ankle Res.* 2008;**1**:6.
94. **Andre M, Hagelberg S, Stenstrom, CH.** The juvenile arthritis foot disability index: development and evaluation of measurement properties. *J Rheum.* 2004;**31**(12):2488–93.
95. **Esbjornsson AC, Iversen MD, Brostrom EW, Hagelberg S, Andre M.** Responsiveness of the juvenile arthritis foot disability index. *Ped Rheumatology.* 2013;**11**:P37.
96. **Szkudlarek M, Klarlund M, Narvestad E, et al.** Ultrasonography of the metacarpophalangeal and proximal interphalangeal joints in rheumatoid arthritis: a comparison with magnetic resonance imaging, conventional radiography and clinical examination. *Arthritis Res Ther.* 2006;**8**:R52.
97. **Wakefield RJ, Balint PV, Szkudlarek M, et al.** Musculoskeletal ultrasound including definitions for ultrasonographic pathology. *J Rheumatol.* 2005;**32**:2485–7.
98. **Magni-Manzoni S.** Ultrasound in juvenile idiopathic arthritis. *Ped Rheumatology.* 2016;**14**:33.
99. **Collado P, Jousse-Joulin S, Alcalde M, Naredo E, D'Agostino MA.** Is ultrasound a validated tool for the diagnosis and management of synovitis in juvenile idiopathic arthritis: a systematic literature review. *Arthritis Care Res* 2012;**64**:1011–19.
100. **Coda A, Fowlie PW, Davidson JE, Walsh J, Carline T, Santos D.** Foot orthoses in children with juvenile idiopathic arthritis: a randomised controlled trial. *Arch Dis Child.* 2014;doi:10.1136/archdischild-2013-305166.
101. **Powell M, Seid M, Szer IS.** Efficacy of custom foot orthotics in improving pain and functional status in children with juvenile idiopathic arthritis: a randomized trial. *J Rheumatol.* 2005;**32**:943–50.
102. **Mills K, Blanch P, Chapman AR, McPoil TG, Vicenzio B.** Foot orthoses and gait: a systematic review and meta-analysis of literature pertaining to potential mechanisms. *Br J Sports Med.* 2010;**44**:1035–46.
103. **Hendry GJ, Turner DE, Lorgelly PK, Woodburn J.** Room for improvement: patient, parent and practitioners' perceptions of foot problems and foot care in juvenile idiopathic arthritis. *Arch Phys Med Rehabil.* 2012;**93**:2062–7.
104. **Alvarez RG, Marini A, Schmitt C, Saltzman CL.** Stage I and II posterior tibial tendon dysfunction treated by a structured nonoperative management protocol: an orthosis and exercise program. *Foot Ankle Int.* 2006;**27**(1):2–8.
105. **Kulig K, Lederhaus ES, Reischl S, Arya S, Bashford G.** Effect of eccentric exercise program for early tibialis posterior tendinopathy. *Foot Ankle Int.* 2009;**30**(9):877–85.
106. **Spink MJ, Menz HB, Fotoohabadi MR, et al.** Effectiveness of a multifaceted podiatry intervention to prevent falls in community dwelling older people with disabling foot pain: randomised controlled trial. *BMJ.* 2011;**342**:d3411.
107. **da Silva KNG, de Paiva Teixeira LEP, Imoto AM, Atallah AN, Peccin MS, Trevisani VFM.** Effectiveness of sensorimotor training in patients with rheumatoid arthritis: a randomized controlled trial. *Rheumatol Int.* 2012,**33**:2269–75.

108. **Williams SB, Brand CA, Hill KD, Hunt SB, Moran H.** Feasibility and outcomes of a home based exercise program on improving balance and gait stability in women with lower-limb osteoarthritis or rheumatoid arthritis: a pilot study. *Arch Phys Med Rehabil*. 2010,**91**:106–14.
109. **Baillet A, Vaillant M, Guinot M, Juvin R, Gaudin P.** Efficacy of resistance exercises in rheumatoid arthritis: meta-analysis of randomized controlled trials. *Rheumatology*. 2012,**51**:519–27.
110. **Lemmey AB, Marcora SM, Chester K, Wilson S, Casanova F, Maddison PJ.** Effects of high intensity resistance training in patients with rheumatoid arthritis: a randomized controlled trial. *Arthritis Rheum*. 2009;**61**:1726–34.
111. **Bearne LM, Scott DL, Hurley MV.** Exercise can reverse quadriceps sensorimotor dysfunction that is associated with rheumatoid arthritis without exacerbating disease activity. *Rheumatology*. 2002;**41**:157–66.
112. **Hakkinen A, Sokka T, Kotaniemi A, Hannonen P.** A randomized two-year study of the effects of dynamic strength training on muscle strength, disease activity, functional capacity, and bone mineral density in early rheumatoid arthritis. *Arthritis Rheum*. 2001;**44**:515–22.
113. **McArdle WD, Katch FI, Katch VL.** *Exercise Physiology: Energy, Nutrition and Human Performance*, 3rd edn. United States of America: Lea & Febiger; 1991.
114. **Takken T, van Brussel M, Englebert RHH, van der Net J, Kuis W, Helders PJM.** Exercise therapy in juvenile idiopathic arthritis: a Cochrane Review. *Eur J Phys Rehabil Med*. 2008;**44**:287–97.
115. **Menz HB, Morris ME.** Footwear characteristics and foot problems in older people. *Gerontology*. 2005;**51**:346–51.
116. **Klein C, Groll-Knapp E, Kundi M, Kinz W.** Increased hallux angle in children and its association with insufficient length of footwear: a community based cross-sectional study. *BMC Musculoskel Dis*. 2009;**10**:159.
117. **Foster A, Blanchette MG, Chou YC, Powers CM.** The influence of heel height on frontal plane ankle biomechanics: implications for lateral ankle sprains. *Foot Ankle Int*. 2012;**33**:64–9.
118. **Lord S, Bashford G.** Shoe characteristics and balance in older women. *J Am Geriatr Soc*. 1996;**44**:429–33.
119. **Menant J, Perry S, Steele J, Menz H, Munro B, Lord S.** Effects of shoe characteristics on dynamic stability when walking on even and uneven surfaces in young and older people. *Arch Phys Med Rehabil*. 2008;**89**:1970–6.
120. **van der Zwaard BC, van der Horst HE, Knol DL, Elders PJM.** Treatment of forefoot problems in older people: a randomized clinical trial comparing podiatric treatment with standardized shoe advice. *Ann Fam Med*. 2014;**12**:432–40.
121. **Barton CJ, Bonnano D, Menz HB.** Development and evaluation of a tool for the assessment of footwear characteristics. *J Foot Ankle Res*. 2009;**2**:10.
122. **Menz H, Lord S, McIntosh A.** Slip resistance of casual footwear: implications for falls in older adults. *Gerontology*. 2001;**47**:145–9.
123. **Baker M, Bell R.** The role of footwear in childhood injuries. *Pediatr Emerg Care*. 1991;**7**:353–5.
124. **Frey C.** Foot health and shoewear for women. *Clin Orthop Relat Res*. 2000;**372**:32–44.
125. **Byrne M, Curran M.** The development and use of a footwear assessment score in comparing the fit of children's shoes. *The Foot*. 1998;**8**:215–18.
126. **Hall C, Nester C.** Sagittal plane compensations for artificially induced limitation of the first metatarsophalangeal joint: a preliminary study. *J Am Podiatr Med Assoc*. 2004;**94**:269–74.
127. **Burns S, Leese G, McMurdo M.** Older people and ill fitting shoes. *Postgrad Med J*. 2002;**78**:344.
128. **Frey C, Thompson F, Smith J, Sanders M, Horstman H.** American orthopaedic foot and ankle society women's shoe survey. *Foot Ankle*. 1993;**14**:78–81.

Chapter 11

Clinical assessment

Lindsey Cherry, Lucy Gates, and Catherine Bowen

Clinical history

A structured approach to history-taking

When assessing patients it is important to follow a structured approach that is inclusive of a complete clinical history. It is proposed that key elements of a patient history should include the following:

- Presenting complaint: to include main symptoms, symptom pattern, nature of onset (e.g., sudden or gradual), symptom duration, and known aggravating or alleviating factors.
- General health status: to include known health conditions. Consider a systems approach to aid full assessment, e.g., cardiovascular, respiratory, musculoskeletal, neurological, dermatological, immunological, endocrine, and renal.
- Current medication: to include patient-acquired over-the-counter remedies, prescribed, and hospital-administered drugs.
- Surgical history: to include all previous surgical or planned interventions and outcomes.
- Social history: to include activities of daily living or sports.
- Psychosocial history: to include previous or current episodes of mental ill-health.
- Occupation: to include evaluation of activities/level of sedentary behaviours and environmental factors (e.g., frequent working in cold spaces).
- Footwear: to include daily social, working, or sporting shoes in addition to indoor footwear.

A complete patient-reported history should be sufficient to identify the nature of the patient's presenting complaint, the impact of the complaint, and to provide some early indication regarding potential causative factors. Physical assessments can be used subsequently to develop a working diagnosis and form a treatment plan.

Psychosocial approach

Assessment of a patient's daily life and the broader impact that illness can have is an important part of history-taking. A fuller understanding of the external stresses or supports that are impacting a person living with a long-term condition has been previously demonstrated to be fundamental to developing good patient–practitioner partnerships (1). An assessment that includes a biopsychosocial approach is recommended, as this facilitates awareness of the complex relationships that exist between a person's physical, cognitive, and emotional state (2). There is a range of tools available to support psychosocial assessment; however, the timely referral of patients to health psychology services is increasingly recognized and included within clinical guidance, and is particularly well evidenced for patients with fibromyalgia (3).

Footwear history

As part of routine clinical care, health professionals need to assess footwear and, where necessary, modify footwear habits either as a primary intervention for foot symptoms or as a preventative measure in the development of lower limb pathology (4, 5). Guidance related to footwear advice for people who have rheumatoid arthritis exists (6) and the Osteoarthritis Research Society International (OARSI) recommendations state that 'every patient with hip or knee osteoarthritis should receive advice concerning appropriate footwear' (5). There are few specific recommendations in relation to other rheumatological conditions.

The supporting evidence for guidance on footwear advice for patients living with rheumatological conditions is at the level of 'expert opinion' and 'good clinical practice' and women's views on modifying their footwear habits often differ to those of the health professionals (7–9). Conflicts between the perceptions of the practitioner and the patient in terms of footwear acceptability and therapeutic effectiveness have been demonstrated (10, 11). Self-identity and body image issues have been identified as socially important in relation to footwear styles, particularly amongst women, who can feel less feminine, and this may restrict social engagements (12, 13). Consequently, adherence to footwear advice can be low, especially when there is a lack of choice (7).

When assessing footwear it is therefore critical for health professionals to understand the importance of the patient's beliefs and activities, and for this to form part of footwear assessment (11, 14, 15). A systematic approach to ascertaining footwear suitability should be considered in conjunction with any foot orthoses that are worn within the shoes.

Examination of the patient's footwear and its suitability for both home and outdoor use is also required. Much of the work on falls prevention and footwear style has concentrated on therapeutic or off-the-shelf footwear for outside use with little attention on indoor footwear (16, 17). As falls frequently occur within the home setting, investigating the individual's choice of footwear and safe mobility in the home as well as outdoors may lead to a greater awareness of modifiable factors (18).

Footwear can be classified as standard retail footwear, niche retail (including comfort footwear, as well as extra depth, extra width, and unusual sizes), or specialist therapeutic footwear (9, 10). Whilst protocols to assist in footwear assessment in relation to general health (19), diabetes (20), and falls risk (21) exist, there is little evidence for these within current rheumatological guidelines. However, the general principles are that footwear should be assessed for its construction and 'fit for purpose'. The footwear assessment tool produced by Barton et al. (19) contains six items related to fit, general aspects, general structure, motion control properties, cushioning, wear patterns, and may be a useful assessment guide. Each item has a number of components that can be graded by the clinician and a visual guide is included to aid decision-making (19).

Footwear properties frequently reported as being of particular importance to patients are heel height, friction on the soles of footwear (17, 22), and comfortable fit (9). Further characteristics such as heel collar height, heel and midsole geometry, type of fixation, and sole hardness have also been shown to improve balance and reduce the associated potential to increase the risk of falls (21, 23). Specific styles of shoes are notably linked with displaying suboptimal characteristics and include slippers, high-heeled court shoes, or footwear with limited or absent fixation. Interestingly, a retrospective analysis of factors affecting knee osteoarthritis determined that wearing high heels did not increase the risk of developing joint pathology in this study (24) and, although women wear shoes with a lower heel and broader toe box as they age (25), the long-term effects of wearing high heels were inconclusive (26).

Overall, when assessing footwear, comfort, fit, sole friction, heel height, and fastening are features to note. There is a need to recognize that individuals' choices regarding footwear selection are multi-factorial and these should also be explored as part of the assessment approach.

Screening techniques

Overview of screening techniques available

Screening assessments seek to identify evidence of rheumatic disease that may or may not be symptomatic. The following sections describe both serological (blood-based) and musculoskeletal screening tests, their rationale for use, and common clinical interpretation.

Serological screening assessments

Two main blood tests are used within rheumatology, both of which seek to identify levels of inflammation: 1) erythrocyte sedimentation rate (ESR) (27); and 2) C-reactive protein (CRP) (28). ESR is an assessment of the rate at which red blood cells form sediment in a collected sample over a 1-hour period. An increased sedimentation rate is indicative of increased inflammatory activity. CRP is an assessment of the amount of a specific protein present in a collected blood sample. An increased amount of CRP is indicative of increased inflammatory activity. Owing to the relative rapidity with which CRP levels can change, CRP is largely considered to be the most indicative test of current systemic inflammatory status. There is some evidence to suggest that neither test may be considered sensitive to low-grade disease activity that may persist in the foot; however, to date these remain the main serological markers of inflammation used in clinical practice.

Musculoskeletal screening examinations

The Gait Arms Legs and Spine (GALS) examination is a brief screening assessment of the musculoskeletal system (29). GALS involves inspecting carefully for joint swelling and abnormal posture, as well as assessing the joints for expected movement, as shown in Table 11.1. Detail of the International Musculoskeletal Foot and Ankle Assessment (IMFAA) examination components is shown in Table 11.2.

Assessing joints and movement

Performing an examination of the musculoskeletal foot and ankle system

When a musculoskeletal problem has been identified in the initial history or GALS examination, a regional assessment of the musculoskeletal system (REMS) should be carried out. REMS is a core set of 50 regional musculoskeletal examination skills, developed via a national consensus process involving UK consultants in rheumatology, orthopaedics, and care of the elderly and selected general practitioners (33, 34). The REMS approach was formed to standardize assessment between different clinicians and to provide a basis from which medical students can learn (33). REMS involves the examination of a group of joints, including the hand and wrist, elbow, shoulder, hip, knee, spine, and foot and ankle. The key stages to be completed during REMS assessment are as follows:

- **Look** at the joint
- **Feel** the joint
- **Move** the joint
- **Assess** the function of the joint.

Table 11.1 The Gait Arms Legs Spine (GALS) musculoskeletal assessment

Description of assessment	Evidence of validation	Author
Gait ◆ Observe the patient's gait for symmetry, smoothness, and the ability to turn quickly ◆ Observe: ◆ bulk and symmetry of the shoulder, gluteal, quadriceps, and calf muscles ◆ limb alignment ◆ alignment of the spine ◆ equal level of the iliac crests ◆ ability to extend the elbows and knees fully ◆ popliteal swelling ◆ abnormalities in the feet such as an excessively high or low arch profile, clawing/retraction of the toes and/or presence of hallux valgus	Association with functional impairment in adult rheumatology population Sensitivity and specificity determined in paediatric rheumatology population Appropriate for use by physicians in primary care, in older patients (≥65 years old)	Plant et al. 1993 (30) Foster et al. 2006 (31) Beattie et al. 2008 (32)
Arms ◆ Assess shoulder abduction and external rotation, and elbow flexion ◆ observe the backs of the hands for joint swelling and deformity and the palms for muscle bulk and abnormality ◆ Assess power grip and grip strength, hand and wrist function, and range of movement in the fingers ◆ Assess fine precision pinch ◆ Check for tenderness across the metacarpophalangeal joints		
Legs ◆ Assess full flexion and extension of both knees, feeling for crepitus ◆ Assess internal rotation of each hip in flexion ◆ Perform a patellar tap to check for a knee effusion ◆ Inspect the feet for swelling, deformity, and callosities on the soles ◆ Check for tenderness across the metatarsophalangeal joints to check for tenderness		
Spine ◆ Inspect the spine for evidence of scoliosis, lordosis, or kyphosis ◆ Assess lateral flexion of the neck ◆ Assess forward movement of the spine and palpate for normal movement of the vertebrae		

The IMFAA protocol has also been established specifically to provide a more comprehensive and standardized approach for the assessment of the foot and ankle (35). The IMFAA approach includes a core set of 20 clinical assessment measures specific to the foot and ankle, which were agreed through an international consensus process involving professionals from rheumatology, orthopaedics, physiotherapy, and podiatry backgrounds (35). The measures defined in IMFAA can be used individually according to the presenting history or findings from GALS examination,

Table 11.2 The International Musculoskeletal Foot and Ankle Assessment

Description of assessment	Evidence of validation	Author
Observation *Non-weightbearing* ◆ Observe the morphology of the feet, comparing one with the other for symmetry ◆ Look for swollen joints or digits ◆ Look specifically at the forefoot for nail changes or skin rashes/lesions ◆ Look for alignment of the toes and evidence of hallux valgus of the big toe ◆ Look for clawing of the toes, joint swelling, and callus formation. If there is clawing of the toes, calluses above and below the MTP joints, pain, and restriction of movement, then there is likely to be subluxation (partial dislocation) of the MTP joints ◆ Look at the underside or plantar surface for callus formation *Weightbearing* ◆ Look for normal alignment of the rear foot ◆ Observe the Achilles tendon and look for bursitis, which may present as swelling on either side of the tendon just above the insertion ◆ Observe the midfoot for deformity and arch position ◆ Observe the forefoot for digital retractions and subluxation of the MTP joints ◆ Assess foot posture using individual features of the foot and ankle or as an aggregate	Face validity for adult population (IMFAA)	Gates et al. (2015) (35)
Foot posture index ◆ Talar head palpation ◆ Curves above and below the malleoli ◆ Inversion/eversion of the calcaneus ◆ Bulge at the region of the talonavicular joint ◆ Congruence of the medial longitudinal arch ◆ Abduction/adduction of the forefoot on rearfoot	Concurrent and predictive validity in normal and pathological adult and paediatric populations (FPI)	Redmond et al. (2006) (36) Keenan et al. (2007) (37) Levinger et al. (2010) (38) Cain et al. (2007) (39) Barton et al. (2010) (40) Barton et al. (2011) (41)
Palpation ◆ Assess the temperature over the forefoot, midfoot, and ankle ◆ Check for the presence of a peripheral pulse ◆ Gently squeeze across the MTP joints, watching the patient's face for signs of discomfort ◆ Palpate the toes for dactylitis ◆ Palpate the midfoot, the ankle, and subtalar joints for tenderness ◆ Palpate the Achilles tendon for tenderness on either side of the tendon just above the insertion ◆ Palpate the proximal plantar fascia insertion for tenderness ◆ Palpate along the tibialis posterior tendon—from the medial malleolus to its insertion on the navicular—for tenderness and swelling ◆ Palpate along the peroneal tendons—from the lateral malleolus over the peroneal tubercle on the calcaneus to the base of the fifth metatarsal and onwards—for tenderness and swelling		

(*continued*)

Table 11.2 Continued

Description of assessment	Evidence of validation	Author
Movement **Ankle** ◆ Patient in supine lying position on the couch with knees relaxed and extended ◆ Using the whole hand against the dorsum of the foot, apply a linear force to create a dorsiflexion movement, limiting any potential eversion (supporting the calcaneus with the other hand may limit this) **Rear foot** ◆ Stabilize the lower leg with one hand and grasp the calcaneus with the other ◆ Move the calcaneus through its frontal plane range of motion (inversion–eversion) **Midfoot and midtarsal** ◆ With the patient in supine lying position on the couch, knees extended and feet over the end, move the midfoot/tarsometatarsal joint (where the five metatarsals articulate with the three cuneiforms and cuboid) through all three planes of motion ◆ Transfer both hands proximally to surround and move the midtarsal joint (comprising the talonavicular medially and calcaneocuboid joints laterally) **First MTP joint** ◆ With the patient in supine lying position on the couch, knees extended, and feet over the end, stabilize the first metatarsal shaft with one hand and grasp the proximal phalanx with the other. Dorsiflex and plantar flex the joint		
Muscle tests *Posterior group, i.e., gastrocnemius/soleus:* ◆ Patient in prone lying, with legs extended ◆ Patient attempts to plantar flex the ankle ◆ Examiner applies resistance to the forefoot ◆ Attention must be paid to ensure the patient is not facilitating or substituting plantar flexion with eversion of the foot *Medial group, i.e., tibialis posterior* ◆ Patient in single limb stance ◆ Patient attempts to raise the rearfoot of the weightbearing limb whilst maintaining forefoot contact with the ground ◆ Indicate if the patient is able to, if there is difficulty, or if he or she is completely unable to perform the *single-limb* heel-rise *Lateral group, i.e., peronei* ◆ Patient sitting or supine lying, with legs extended ◆ Clinician supports leg just above ankle ◆ Patient attempts to evert the foot ◆ Resistance is applied on the base of the first metatarsal (to load both longus and brevis) or the fifth metatarsal (to load brevis) and is directed to resist plantar flexion eversion		

Table 11.2 Continued

Description of assessment	Evidence of validation	Author
Anterior group, i.e., tibialis anterior ◆ Patient sitting or supine lying, with legs extended ◆ Clinician supports leg just above ankle ◆ Patient attempts to dorsiflex the ankle and invert the foot ◆ Resistance is applied to the medial dorsal surface of the foot The patient's effort to contract the muscle should be graded the MRC grading system: **Grade 5:** Muscle contracts normally against full resistance **Grade 4:** Strength reduced but muscle contraction can still move joint against resistance **Grade 3:** Strength further reduced such that the joint can be moved only against gravity with the examiner's resistance completely removed **Grade 2:** Muscle can move only if the resistance of gravity is removed **Grade 1:** Only a flicker of movement in the muscle **Grade 0:** No movement observed		

Function
◆ Assess the patient's gait, watching for the normal cycle of heel strike, stance, and toe-off. Indicate the presence of the following gait parameters:
  ◆ Walking aid—including sticks, crutches, frame, ankle–foot orthosis, etc.
  ◆ Lower limb symmetry—similar movement patterns of both lower limbs throughout the three planes of movement
  ◆ Antalgic gait—a limp adopted to avoid pain on weightbearing structures, characterized by a very short stance phase
◆ Observe and discuss patient's footwear and indicate the:
  ◆ Type of shoe with percentage worn in average week
  ◆ Heel height
  ◆ Check for abnormal or asymmetrical wearing of the sole or upper, for evidence of poor fit, or the presence of special insoles
◆ Assess limb length in standing by visually inspecting the height of both ASIS and in supine—measure from the ASIS to the distal tip of the medial malleolus		

ASIS, Anterior superior iliac spines; FPI, Foot Posture Index; IMFAA, International Musculoskeletal Foot and Ankle Assessment; MRC, Medical Research Council; MTP, metatarsophalangeal joint; REMS, regional assessment of the musculoskeletal system.

or can be used in combination with other examinations to provide a useful screening protocol. The key stages of IMFAA are as follows:

- Observation
- Palpation
- Range of motion
- Muscle tests
- Alignment
- Static posture
- Indirect assessment.

Based on the combined priorities of both REMS and IMFAA there are a number of key stages to be completed during a foot and ankle examination. These are harmonized and discussed below in clinical observation, clinical palpation and clinical assessment of movement, with further detail of the screening techniques provided in Table 11.1.

Clinical observation

The examination should always start with a visual inspection of the foot and ankle at rest. Symmetry should be evaluated by comparing one side to the other. Changes in the appearance of skin, muscle bulk, or the presence of erythema (redness), swelling (e.g., encapsulated or diffuse), or deformity (e.g., a notable difference in joint orientations) should be noted.

Clinical observation of standing foot posture can be aided by use of the Foot Posture Index (FPI). This score was developed to overcome the absence of a reliable and validated method for quantifying variation in foot posture in a clinical setting (36). The FPI consists of multiple segment and multiple plane criteria for assessing foot posture. The FPI tool scores the various features of foot posture into one quantifiable result and rates standing foot posture according to a series of predefined criteria for each of its six components, shown in Table 11.1. Each component of the FPI is graded 0 for good alignment, with a minimum score of –2 for signs of supination and +2 for pronation. When the scores are combined, the summated score gives an estimate of the overall foot posture. However, it should be noted that this measure has not been validated for use in patients with inflammatory arthritis to date.

Overall, assessment of the alignment of the rearfoot relative to the lower leg is considered important, as excessive misalignment can be a hallmark feature of progressive disease in a range of rheumatological conditions (42). When observing the midfoot for arch position, an apparent low arch should resolve when standing on tip toes; failure to do so may indicate either bone change or damage to supporting soft-tissue structures, which can also be frequently affected in rheumatic disease (43).

Clinical palpation

Palpation of joint margins, soft-tissue structures (e.g., joint capsules or ligaments) and tendon insertions to identify inflamed or damaged tissues is important. Tissues should be gently palpated to identify areas of point tenderness, skin temperature differences, the nature of swelling (e.g., tense versus boggy), or the nature of osteophytic protrusion. The extent and nature of movement restriction should be assessed for variation and mobility; for example, the hard bony prominences and sudden terminal range of movement associated with osteoarthritis should be distinguished from the soft, rubbery swelling and graduated terminal range of movement associated with rheumatoid arthritis.

Clinical identification of joint synovitis is achieved following the combined assessment of joint tenderness, warmth, and encapsulated tense swelling over the joint margin.

Erythema may or may not be present. Clinical identification of enthesitis is achieved following the combined assessment of tenderness at the tissue attachment site, warmth, and diffuse but localized swelling. In acute enthesitis, erythema is typically noted. Clinical identification of tendinitis is achieved following the combined assessment of tenderness over the area of affected tendon; there may or may not be palpable interruption of the tendon fibres, warmth, and diffuse but localized swelling. In cases of tenosynovitis, palpable swelling may appear as encapsulated with clear endpoints coinciding with the termination of the tendon sheath. A frequent challenge when assessing structures of the foot and ankle in rheumatology is differentiating between localized tissue trauma, symptoms of generalized disease flare, or, at times, noting a combination of both. Symptoms of generalized flare may include multiple presentations of tender, hot, and swollen joints, morning stiffness lasting longer than 30 minutes, and general malaise. Clinicians are encouraged to continue close working with the patient's multidisciplinary team where possible, and if flare is suspected patients should be referred immediately for further review.

Palpation of the blood vessels of the foot and ankle can also be a useful indicator of vascular status. The posterior tibial and dorsalis pedis arteries are commonly assessed and considered indicative of peripheral arterial function. An inability to palpate the arteries indicates a need for further assessment using a hand-held Doppler. Vascular complications are a leading cause of morbidity and mortality in patients with inflammatory arthropathy and, as such, palpation of the pedal arteries should be undertaken at every clinical opportunity.

Developing rigidity of the skin and underlying tissues, commonly associated with connective tissue diseases, can also be identified following palpation of the skin. Reduced elasticity and plasticity of the skin, in addition to signs of calcium deposition (harder areas tissue, often appearing white in colour), could be considered indicative of progressing disease and may warrant further investigation or treatment.

Clinical assessment of movement

The full range of joint movement should be assessed. The expected range of motion for normal and pathological joints is not confidently confirmed and has been repeatedly shown as difficult to measure precisely under clinical conditions; therefore, comparing sides for symmetry is likely to be most useful. Active range of movement (patient-led) is assessed and then passive range of movement (clinician-led) is completed. If there is a loss of active movement, but passive movement is unaffected, this may suggest a problem with the muscles, tendons, or nerves rather than in the joints, or it may be an effect of unmanaged pain. Loss of movement can be recorded as none, mild, moderate, or severe. The quality of movement should also be recorded, with reference to abnormalities such as increased muscle tone or the presence of crepitus (crunching within the joint during movement).

There are a number of techniques for assessing muscles of the foot and ankle; however, it is difficult to ensure the isolation of individual muscles and thus the validity of clinical findings. Selection of the specific muscle is not always necessary and the assessment may be directed toward the muscle groups; for example, ankle 'dorsiflexors' or 'plantar flexors' and foot 'inverters' or 'everters'. Examples of muscle testing techniques within each major group are given in Table 11.2. These techniques do not guarantee isolation of that muscle, and careful attention should be given to control opposing movements of the joint to limit the effect of muscles that may facilitate movement or be substitute aids for movement in the case of pathology. The patient's effort to contract the muscle should be graded on a standardized format such as the Medical Research

Council (MRC) grading system, as given in Table 11.2. The validity of manual muscle tests varies considerably, depending upon the muscle being tested, the experience of the examiner, the age of the patient, and the condition being tested. For further details of manual muscle tests for specific lower limb muscles, the reader is directed to Hislop et al. (2013) (44).

Assessing pain

Pain is a complex phenomenon and is recognized as being multi-factorial. Assessing foot pain is further complicated in that feet comprise multiple joints, thus pinpointing specific regions is important when considering rheumatological conditions. It is important to have a good awareness of the range of pain sensations (e.g., aching, burning, tingling, prickling, electric shocks), patterns (e.g., constant, episodic, constant with episodes of increased intensity), or regional affectations (single joint, multiple joints, or whole foot regions) that patients with rheumatic disease can experience.

Historically, understanding the nature of foot pain reported by patients with rheumatic disease has arguably been difficult because of the varied and range of definitions of pain used. However, three key themes related to the definition of foot pain appear to be consistently reported by researchers of foot and ankle health: 1) 'generalized foot pain'—this is often reported without further differentiation when reported alongside pain from other areas of the body; 2) 'foot joint pain'—which tends to be reported as 'joint symptoms' and is often presented as an undifferentiated overview of the foot; and 3) 'global foot pain'—which refers to pain in specific locations of the foot but may encompass ranging tissues such as muscle, skin, or nail (Table 11.3).

Primarily it is important for clinicians to understand the patient's description of pain and to start to determine if this is related to systemic rheumatic flare, a localized flare of disease, a specific foot problem unrelated to disease, or a specific foot problem that is exacerbated by the patient's rheumatic disease. The visual analogue scale (VAS) is a well-established measure that is easy to use at the chair-side in clinical practice (52). Likert scales and various small hand-held devices with sliding scales are also available to assist the patient to define the severity of their pain. Specific descriptions of pain such as severity (e.g., using VAS), type (e.g., throbbing or tingling), and duration (e.g., acute or chronic) will direct the clinician toward likely causes and therefore potential targets for treatment.

As many patients with rheumatological conditions may have manifestations impacting throughout the whole musculoskeletal system, it is important to check for referred pain because of nerve entrapment or neurological damage from areas such as the lower spine or, more locally

Table 11.3 Varied case definitions of pain related to the foot used by researchers

Investigators	Type of assessment of pain
Hill et al., 2008 (45)	Generalized foot pain
Garrow et al., 2004 (46)	Generalized foot pain; global foot pain; foot joint pain (non-specific)
Dufour et al., 2009 (47)	Generalized foot pain; global foot pain
Thomas et al., 2004 (48)	Generalized foot pain
Badlissi et al., 2005 (49)	Generalized foot pain; global foot pain (limited); foot joint pain
Menz et al., 2006 (50)	Generalized foot pain
Gay et al., 2014 (51)	Foot joint pain

to the foot and ankle, the tarsal tunnel. A neurological assessment, including evaluation of specific reflex or motor nerve function, dermatome or plantar weightbearing area sensation, or clinical signs of autonomic neuropathy (e.g., rapid capillary refill) is an important step when interpreting pain history and clinical assessment findings. There is some evidence that patients with systemic lupus erythematosus may experience an increase in neuropathic symptoms (53); however, the prevalence of neurological complications affecting the foot and ankle in rheumatic disease is largely poorly understood to date.

There are a growing number of examples of multi-domain-validated questionnaires that seek to assess pain that are relevant to the musculoskeletal status of the foot. These include the Foot Function Index (FFI) (54), the Foot Health Status Questionnaire (FHSQ) (55), the Manchester Foot Pain Disability Index (MFPDI) (56), the Foot Impact Scale (FIS) (57), the Bristol Foot Score (BFS) (58), and The Salford Arthritis Foot Evaluation (SAFE) (59).

Interestingly, the FHSQ, MFPDI, and BFS were developed for general populations (55–57), yet the FFI and FIS appear to be the most ultilized instruments with positive ratings (60). The FFI was developed to measure the impact of foot pathology on function, in terms of pain, disability, and activity restriction, for assessment of surgical interventions (54). The investigators did not intend it to be used specifically in people with rheumatoid arthritis, although the test subjects all had a definitive diagnosis of rheumatoid arthritis (54). The FIS was developed specifically for patients living with rheumatoid arthritis to measure foot pain and disability at all stages, including early- and late-stage disease (57).· SAFE was also developed specifically for rheumatoid arthritis (59). The difference in this tool was that a clinimetric strategy was used in its development to reflect variables of interest and importance to clinicians.

Both the FHSQ and FFI are criticized as being developed by expert professionals (57), whereas MFPDI, BFS, and FIS were all developed with qualitative methodological approaches that involved a series of patient questioning so that the more recently validated instruments are patient-facing (57, 58, 61). SAFE is still under development, is essentially clinician-driven, and is yet to be reported on in clinical investigations (59).

For osteoarthritis the MFPDI appears to be the most utilized outcome measure. Although primarily used to measure 'disabling foot pain', the tool has been used as a basis for defining 'foot pain' through differing criteria (48, 62, 63). Whilst there are yet to be any validated instruments that are specific to other rheumatological conditions, those that are validated do add to the picture in relation to the impact of foot problems for people living with rheumatological conditions.

It is clear that the emphasis is shifting from measurement of the biomechanical aspects of gait and foot function alone toward developing patient-orientated measures based on the patient's own experience of their foot disease. Most people with rheumatic disease may not be in a steady state, and disease progress may vary greatly from one individual to another. Spending time evaluating the patient's musculoskeletal pain status can provide useful information when aligned with a clinical examination that will help guide clinical decision-making and evaluate long-term impact of clinical interventions.

Using patient-reported outcome measures

As discussed in the previous section (Assessing pain), a range of patient-reported outcome measures (PROMS) have been created for use with people with musculoskeletal or rheumatological conditions. PROMS can be a useful aid when trying to determine, in a repeatable way, the nature of foot health complications experienced by people and the impact that they are having. Table 11.4 details a range of PROMS validated for use in rheumatological populations.

Table 11.4 Patient-reported outcome measures (PROM) appropriate for people with rheumatic or musculoskeletal conditions

PROM name	Author	Intended use
The Foot Impact Scale	Helliwell et al. (2005) (57)	Assesses the foot with rheumatoid arthritis with a focus upon the qualitative aspects of pain, stiffness, and biopsychosocial experiences arising from the foot with rheumatoid arthritis. A strong emphasis is placed upon the importance of footwear
The Manchester Foot Pain and Disability Index (MFPDI)	Garrow et al. (2000) (56)	Measures pain specifically related to a foot disability over the past month
The Podiatry Health Questionnaire	Macran et al. (2003) (64)	Assesses foot-related health-related quality of life of podiatry patients and the effectiveness of foot interventions
The Bristol Foot Score	Barnett et al. (2005) (58)	Assesses the impact of foot problems on health-related quality of life over 2 weeks
The Foot Health Status Questionnaire	Bennett et al. (1998) (55).	Assesses foot health status of patients both pre- and post-surgery, over a period of 1 week, and the efficacy of non-surgical interventions
The Rowan Foot Pain Assessment Questionnaire	Rowan (2001) (65)	Evaluates the multi-dimensional aspects of chronic foot pain, including sensory, affective, and cognitive pain dimension
The Revised Foot Function Index—Long & Short Form	Budiman-Mak et al. (2006) (54)	Measures health-related foot function in terms of pain, function, and psychosocial consequences
The Foot and Ankle Ability Measure	Martin et al. (2005) (66)	Assessment of physical performance of individuals with musculoskeletal conditions affecting their foot, ankle, and lower limb
The Manchester-Oxford Foot Questionnaire (MOXFQ)	Dawson et al. (2006) (67)	Assesses how foot problems impair health-related quality of life in clinical trials involving foot surgery

Future research

Whilst many continue to debate whether clinical assessment of the foot and ankle is an art or a science, one aspect that is clear is that computers and interactive technologies are set to dominate the future of clinical assessments. As healthcare becomes increasingly global, new classification systems for assessment of foot and ankle musculoskeletal status will also emerge. These systems will facilitate standardized data collection for both research and clinical purposes with validated variations that span the whole range of diversity in populations and multicultural aspects.

Nanotechnology, the speed with which computers can analyse data and their increasing capacities for storing and processing large amounts of information that are beyond the capacities of the individual clinician, will enable vast amounts of musculoskeletal foot health status data to be collected. Technological advances will ensure that, in the foot care clinical environment, there is likely to be increased uptake of:

- Use of SMART technologies to embed assessment chips in footwear; e.g., temperature changes as a red flag for skin changes related to ulceration.

- Hand-held devices used for instant video links to experts/diagnostic information.
- Immediate transfer of clinical test results online to central diagnostics records.
- Use of SMART technologies to facilitate patient self-assessment with more rapid information and access to clinical assessment and quicker diagnoses.

To achieve this, it is imperative that new ways of assessing the musculoskeletal status of the foot are robustly and systematically validated and tested against traditional clinician-led assessments.

Conclusion

Clinical assessment of the foot and ankle in people who have rheumatic disease should be systematic, thorough, and, where possible, follow standard evidence-informed protocols. It is important to note that people living with rheumatic conditions experience constant changes in both general and foot health. Accurate assessment of changing patient needs is essential to providing tailored and timely healthcare.

References

1. **Keefe FJ, Bonk V.** Psychosocial assessments of pain in patients having rheumatic conditions. *Rheum Dis Clin N Am.* 1999;**25**(1):81–103.
2. **Keefe FJ, Smith SJ, et al.** Recent advances and future directions in the biopsychosocial assessment and treatment of arthritis. *J Cons Clin Psychol.* 2002;**70**(3):640–55.
3. **Hauser W, Thieme K, Turk DC.** Guidelines on the management of fibromyalgia syndrome. *Eur J Pain.* 2010;**14**:5–10.
4. **ARMA.** (2004). Standards of Care for People with Musculoskeletal Foot Health Problems, from http://www.prcassoc.org.uk/standards-project. Accessed 01.08.15
5. **Zhang W, Moskowitz RW, et al.** OARSI recommendations for the management of hip and knee osteoarthritis, Part II: OARSI evidence-based, expert consensus guidelines. *Osteoarthritis Cartilage.* 2008;**16**(2):137–62.
6. **National Institute for Health and Clinical Excellence.** *Rheumatoid Arthritis: The Management of Rheumatoid Arthritis in Adults: Clinical Guidance 79.* London: National Institute for Clinical Excellence, UK; 2009.
7. **Williams AE, Meacher K.** Shoes in the cupboard: the fate of prescribed footwear? *Prosthetics Orthotics Int.* 2001;**25**(1):53–9.
8. **Johnson M, Newton P, et al.** Patient and professional perspectives on prescribed therapeutic footwear for people with diabetes: a vignette study. *Patient Education Council.* 2006;**64**(1–3):167–72.
9. **Silvester RN, Williams AE, et al.** 'Choosing shoes': a preliminary study into the challenges facing clinicians in assessing footwear for rheumatoid patients. *J Foot Ankle Res.* 2010;**3**:24.
10. **Williams AE, Nester CJ.** Patient perceptions of stock footwear design features. *Prosthetics Orthotics Int.* 2006;**30**(1):61–71.
11. **Goodacre LJ, Candy FJ.** 'If I didn't have RA I wouldn't give them house room': the relationship between RA, footwear and clothing choices. *Rheumatology.* 2011;**50**(3):513–17.
12. **Gutweniger S, Kopp M, et al.** Body image of women with rheumatoid arthritis. *Clin Exp Rheumatol.* 1999;**17**(4):413–417.
13. **Williams AE, Rome K, et al.** A clinical trial of specialist footwear for patients with rheumatoid arthritis. *Rheumatology.* 2007;**46**(2):302–7.
14. **Williams AE, Nester CJ, et al.** Rheumatoid arthritis patients' experiences of wearing therapeutic footwear—a qualitative investigation. *BMC Musculoskel Dis.* 2007;**8**:104.

15. **Naidoo S, Anderson S, et al.** 'I could cry, the amount of shoes I can't get into': a qualitative exploration of the factors that influence retail footwear selection in women with rheumatoid arthritis. *J Foot Ankle Res.* 2011;**4**:21.
16. **Kelsey JL, Procter-Gray E, et al.** Footwear and falls in the home among older individuals in the MOBILIZE Boston Study. *Footwear Science.* 2010;**2**(3):123–9.
17. **Spink MJ, Menz HB, et al.** Effectiveness of a multifaceted podiatry intervention to prevent falls in community dwelling older people with disabling foot pain: randomised controlled trial. *Br Med J.* 2011;**342**:d3411.
18. **Menz HB, Morris ME, et al.** Footwear characteristics and risk of indoor and outdoor falls in older people. *Gerontology.* 2006;**52**(3):174–80.
19. **Barton C, Bonanno D, et al.** Development and evaluation of a tool for the assessment of footwear characteristics. *J Foot Ankle Res.* 2009;**2**:10.
20. **Nancarrow S.** Footwear suitability scale: a measure of shoefit for people with diabetes. *Aus J Podiatric Med.* 1999;**33**:57–62.
21. **Menz HB, Sherrington C.** The Footwear Assessment Form: a reliable clinical tool to assess footwear characteristics of relevance to postural stability in older adults. *Clin Rehabil.* 2000;**14**(6):657–64.
22. **Menant JC, Steele JR, et al.** Effects of footwear features on balance and stepping in older people. *Gerontology.* 2008;**54**(1):18–23.
23. **Menant JC, Steele JR, et al.** Optimizing footwear for older people at risk of falls. *J Rehabil Res Devices.* 2008;**45**(8):1167–81.
24. **Dawson J, Thorogood M, et al.** The prevalence of foot problems in older women: a cause for concern. *J Pub Health Med.* 2002;**24**(2):77–84.
25. **Menz HB, Roddy E, et al.** Epidemiology of shoe wearing patterns over time in older women: associations with foot pain and hallux valgus. *Gerontology.* 2016;**1**:4.
26. **Riskowski J, Dufour AB, et al.** Arthritis, foot pain and shoe wear: current musculoskeletal research on feet. *Curr Opin Rheumatol.* 2011;**23**(2):148–55.
27. **Westergren A.** Diagnostic tests: the erythrocyte sedimentation rate range and limitations of the technique. *Triangle.* 1957;**3**(1):20–5.
28. **Pepys MB, Hirschfield GM.** C-reactive protein: a critical update. *J Clin Invest.* 2003;**111**(12):1805–12.
29. **Doherty M, Dacre J, et al.** The 'GALS' locomotor screen. *Ann Rheum Dis.* 1992;**51**:1165–9.
30. **Plant MJ, Linton S, et al.** The GALS locomotor screen and disability. *Ann Rheum Dis.* 1993;**52**:886–90.
31. **Foster HE, Kay L, et al.** Musculoskeletal screening examination (pGALS) for school-age children based on the adult GALS screen. *Arthritis Care Res.* 2006;**55**(5):709–16.
32. **Beattie KA, Bobba R, et al.** Validation of the GALS musculoskeletal screening exam for use in primary care: a pilot study. *BMC Musculoskel Dis.* 2008;**9**:115.
33. **Coady D, Walker D, Kay L.** Regional Examination of the Musculoskeletal System (REMS): a core set of clinical skills for medical students. *Rheumatology.* 2004;**43**:633–9.
34. **Foster H, Kay L, et al.** Pediatric regional examination of the musculoskeletal system: a practice- and consensus-based approach. *Arthritis Care Res.* 2011;**63**(11):1503–10.
35. **Gates LS, Bowen CJ, Arden NK.** Clinical measures of musculoskeletal foot and ankle assessment: an international consensus statement. *Int J Health Sci Res.* 2015;**5**(2):91–105.
36. **Redmond AC, Crosbie J, Ouvrier RA.** Development and validation of a novel rating system for scoring standing foot posture: the Foot Posture Index. *Clin Biomech.* 2006;**21**:89–98.
37. **Keenan A, Redmond AC, et al.** The Foot Posture Index: Rasch analysis of a novel, foot-specific outcome measure. *Arch Phys Med Rehabil.* 2007;**88**(1):88–93.
38. **Levinger P, Menz H, et al.** Foot posture in people with medial compartment knee osteoarthritis. *J Foot Ankle Res.* 2010;**3**(1):29.
39. **Cain LE, Nicholson LL, et al.** Foot morphology and foot/ankle injury in indoor football. *J Sci Med Sport.* 2007;**10**(5):311–19.

40. **Barton C, Bonanno D, et al.** Foot and ankle characteristics in patellofemoral pain syndrome: a case control and reliability study. *J Orthop Sports Phys Ther.* 2010;**40**(5):286–96.
41. **Barton C, Menz HB, Crossley KM.** The immediate effects of foot orthoses on functional performance in individuals with patellofemoral pain syndrome. *Br J Sports Med.* 2011;**45**(3):193–7.
42. **Woodburn J, Helliwell PS, Barker S.** Three-dimensional kinematics at the ankle joint complex in rheumatoid arthritis patients with painful valgus deformity of the rearfoot. *Rheumatology.* 2002;**41**(12):1406–12.
43. **Semple R, Murley GS, et al.** Tibialis posterior in health and disease: a review of structure and function with specific reference to electromyographic studies. *J Foot Ankle Res.* 2009;**2**:24.
44. **Hislop H, Avers D, Brown M.** *Daniels and Worthingham's Muscle Testing,* 9th edn. Missouri: Elsevier Saunders; 2013.
45. **Hill CL, Gill TK, et al.** Prevalence and correlates of foot pain in a population-based study: the North West Adelaide health study. *J Foot Ankle Res.* 2008;**1**(1):2.
46. **Garrow AP, Silman AJ, et al.** The Cheshire Foot Pain and Disability Survey: a population survey assessing prevalence and associations. *Pain.* 2004;**110**(1–2):378–84.
47. **Dufour AB, Broe KE, et al.** Foot pain: is current or past shoe wear a factor? *Arthritis Rheum.* 2009;**61**(10):1352–8.
48. **Thomas E, Peat G, et al.** The prevalence of pain and pain interference in a general population of older adults: cross-sectional findings from the North Staffordshire Osteoarthritis Project (NorStOP). *Pain.* 2004;**110**(1–2):361–8.
49. **Badlissi F, Dunn JE, et al.** Foot musculoskeletal disorders, pain, and foot-related functional limitation in older persons. *J Am Ger Soc.* 2005;**53**(6):1029–033.
50. **Menz HB, Tiedemann A, et al.** Foot pain in community-dwelling older people: an evaluation of the Manchester Foot Pain and Disability Index. *Rheumatology.* 2006;**45**(7):863–7.
51. **Gay A, Culliford D, et al.** Associations between body mass index and foot joint pain in middle-aged and older women: a longitudinal population-based cohort study. *Arthritis Care Res.* 2014;**66**(12):1873–9.
52. **Wolfe F, Michaud K.** Assessment of pain in rheumatoid arthritis: minimal clinically significant difference, predictors, and the effect of anti-tumor necrosis factor therapy. *Rheumatology.* 2007;**34**(8):1674–83.
53. **Cherry L, Alcacer-Pitarch B, Hopkinson N, et al.** The prevalence of self-reported lower limb and foot health problems experienced by participants with systemic lupus erythematosus: Results of a UK national survey. *Lupus.* 2017;**26**(4):410–16.
54. **Budiman-Mak E, Conrad KJ, et al.** The Foot Function Index: a measure of foot pain and disability. *J Clin Epidemiol.* 1991;**44**(6):561–70.
55. **Bennett PJ, Patterson, C, et al.** Development and validation of a questionnaire designed to measure foot-health status. *J Am Podiatric Med Assoc.* 1998;**88**(9):419–28.
56. **Garrow AP, Papageorgiou AC, et al.** Development and validation of a questionnaire to assess disabling foot pain. *Pain.* 2000;**85**(1–2):107–13.
57. **Helliwell P, Reay N, et al.** Development of a foot impact scale for rheumatoid arthritis. *Arthritis Rheum.* 2005;**53**(3):418–22.
58. **Barnett S, Campbell R, Harvey I.** The Bristol Foot Score: developing a patient-based foot-health measure. *J Am Podiatric Med Assoc.* 2005;**95**(3):264–72.
59. **Walmsley S, Ravey M, et al.** Development of a patient-reported outcome measure for the foot affected by rheumatoid arthritis. *J Clin Epidemiol.* 2012;**65**(4):413–22.
60. **van der Leeden M, Steultjens MP, et al.** A systematic review of instruments measuring foot function, foot pain, and foot-related disability in patients with rheumatoid arthritis. *Arthritis Rheum.* 2008;**59**(9):1257–69.
61. **Helliwell P, Woodburn J, et al.** *The Foot and Ankle in Rheumatoid Arthritis: A Comprehensive Guide.* London: Elsevier Churchill Livingstone; 2007.

62. **Buchman AS, Shah RC, et al.** Musculoskeletal pain and incident disability in community-dwelling older adults. *Arthritis Care Res.* 2010;**62**(9):1287–93.
63. **Laslett LL, Quinn SJ, et al.** A prospective study of the impact of musculoskeletal pain and radiographic osteoarthritis on health related quality of life in community dwelling older people. *BMC Musculoskel Dis.* 2012;**13**(168):1–8.
64. **Macran S, Kind P, et al.** Evaluating podiatry services: testing a treatment specific measure of health status. *Quality Life Res.* 2003;**12**(2):177–88.
65. **Rowan K.** The development and validation of a multi-dimensional measure of chronic foot pain: the Rowan Foot Pain Assessment Questionnaire (ROFPAQ). *Foot Ankle Int.* 2001;**22**(10):795–809.
66. **Martin RL, Irrgang JJ, et al.** Evidence of validity for the Foot and Ankle Ability Measure (FAAM). *Foot Ankle Int.* 2005;**26**(11):968–83.
67. **Dawson J, Coffey J, et al.** A patient-based questionnaire to assess outcomes of foot surgery: validation in relation to surgery for hallux valgus. *Quality Life Res.* 2006;**15**:1211–22.

Chapter 12

Imaging of arthritis in the foot and ankle

Emma Rowbotham, Richard Wakefield, and Andrew Grainger

Introduction

Imaging of rheumatological disease in the foot and ankle has become increasingly more sophisticated. While conventional radiographs remain the mainstay for radiological investigation of these conditions, the foot and ankle have a complex 3D morphology that makes imaging challenging, particularly when visualizing the overlapping bones and joints of the hindfoot and midfoot. This means that cross-sectional imaging has an important role to play. Computerized tomography (CT) shows exquisite bone structure and its cross-sectional nature enables outstanding visualization of the joints of the foot; however, poor soft-tissue contrast limits its role in the investigation of soft-tissue abnormality and it is here that magnetic resonance imaging (MRI) and ultrasound are pre-eminent. Routine bone scintigraphy is extremely sensitive to bone and joint disease but suffers from poor specificity and resolution. More sophisticated nuclear medicine techniques are now available, ensuring a continuing role for these techniques.

In this chapter we review the imaging modalities available for investigating rheumatological conditions in the foot and ankle, discussing their strengths and weaknesses and highlighting important imaging findings.

Conventional radiology

Although ultrasound and MRI are more sensitive for imaging inflammatory arthropathy compared to conventional radiographs, particularly for identifying early disease (1), there is still a role for baseline and follow-up plain film imaging. Joint involvement within the foot and ankle is a relatively common feature of many forms of arthritis and therefore a view of both feet, along with both hands and wrists, is often included in the initial imaging screening of patients with a suspected arthritis.

The subtle changes seen in early inflammatory arthritis require high-quality radiographs, which also need to be viewed in optimal lighting conditions. Digital radiography is now commonplace and has been shown to be beneficial to the reader (2). A systematic approach to viewing plain film radiographs is necessary and includes:

- Joint space assessment
- Bone appearance
  - Osteopenia
  - Erosion
  - Enthesopathy
- Soft-tissue shadows and calcification.

The distribution of disease is also extremely important when establishing a differential diagnosis from the imaging findings. Although not considered necessary for diagnosis, weightbearing views are required to assess bone and joint alignment, particularly when planning surgical intervention.

Joint space assessment

Destruction of the articular cartilage leading to loss of joint space is a feature common to many joint diseases. In inflammatory arthropathy the joint space loss is typically uniform across the joint; this is in contrast to joint space loss in osteoarthritis, which is usually non-uniform (Figure 12.1). Detection of joint space loss means that there has been irreversible damage caused to the joints in question. Preservation of joint space is also important to recognize and is a feature of both gout (until the late stages of the disease) and amyloid arthropathy.

In severe arthropathy there may by bony ankylosis across joint spaces, which may be either fibrous or bony in nature. This is most commonly described in spondyloarthropathy and also in juvenile arthritis and represents end-stage disease. Rarely, widening of the joint space may occur secondary to a tense effusion distending the joint space.

Osteopenia

This is a common finding in patients with arthritis, although subtle osteopenic change in early disease may be difficult to detect. Comparison with other joints is a helpful way to assess for these early changes, although this may be misleading in cases where there is also an element of more generalized disuse osteopenia. Periarticular osteopenia in particular is a well-recognized feature of rheumatoid arthritis (RA).

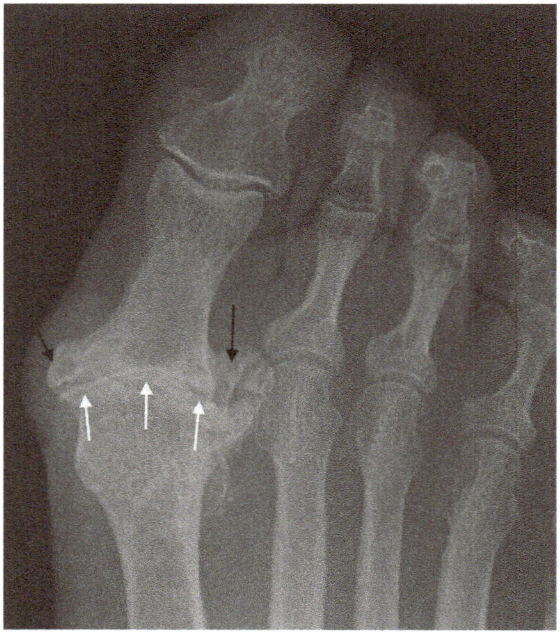

Figure 12.1 Osteoarthritis of the first metatarsophalangeal joint: dorsoplantar radiograph showing a moderate hallux valgus deformity with marked loss of joint space (white arrows), extensive osteophyte formation (black arrows), and subchondral sclerosis.

Erosions

Bone erosions are a characteristic feature of inflammatory arthritis and indicate that significant and usually irreversible joint damage has occurred. Proliferative erosions are associated with new bone formation and are classically a feature of entheseal disease; non-proliferative erosions are a feature of seropositive RA. Erosions may also be described in terms of their position relative to the joint:

- Marginal erosions are a classic feature of RA and affect the exposed bone between the edge of the articular cartilage and the joint capsule (Figure 12.2).
- Juxta-articular erosions occur at a distance slightly further away from the joint and are commonly seen in gout (Figure 12.3).

Detection of erosions on plain film radiography is relatively insensitive compared with both ultrasound and MRI (3); a cortical break is not always appreciated on a radiograph and erosions may be impossible to distinguish from small subcortical cysts using this imaging modality.

Enthesopathy

Enthesitis is the term used to describe inflammation at tendon, ligament, or joint capsule insertions and is classically seen in spondyloarthropathy, including ankylosing spondylitis, reactive arthritis, and psoriatic arthritis. Within the foot and ankle both the Achilles tendon insertion and the plantar fascia origin are common sites of entheseal disease (Figure 12.4). In terms of distribution, prominent peripheral involvement within the foot is more common in both psoriasis and reactive arthritis than in ankylosing spondylitis.

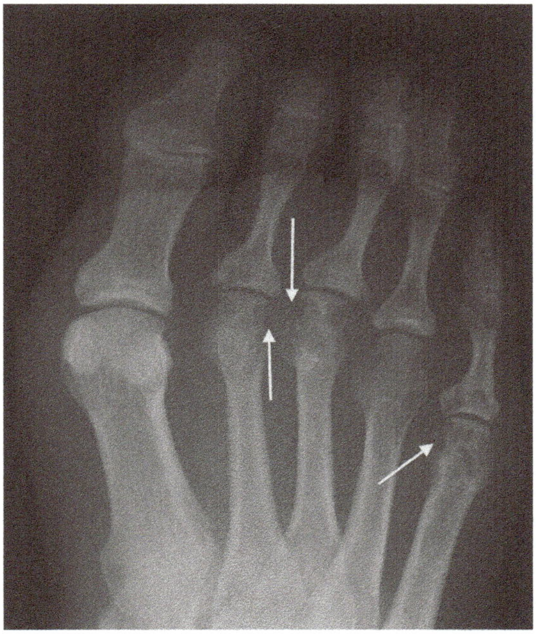

Figure 12.2 Rheumatoid arthritis: dorsoplantar radiograph of the foot in a patient with established rheumatoid arthritis. There is extensive marginal erosive change (white arrows) affecting the second, third, and fifth metatarsal heads and also the second and fifth proximal phalanges.

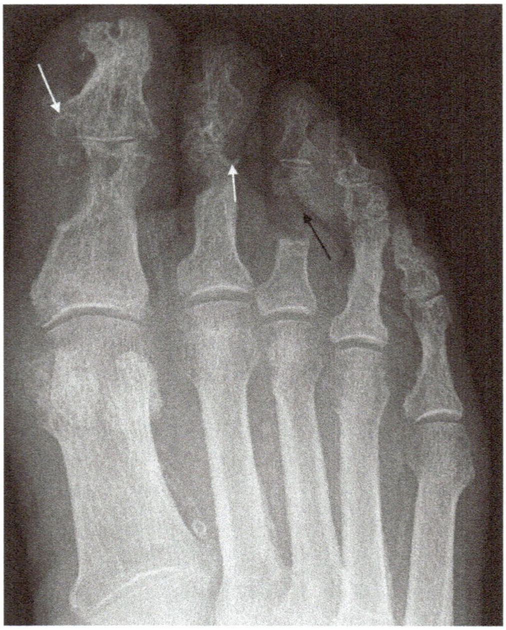

Figure 12.3 Gout: dorsoplantar radiograph of the forefoot showing numerous areas of erosive change in a predominantly juxta-articular distribution (white arrows). These erosions have overhanging sclerotic margins. In addition, there is a punched-out bone lesion affecting the third proximal phalanx (black arrow).

Soft-tissue shadows and calcification

Soft-tissue swelling is a very early sign of inflammatory arthropathy on plain film imaging. This represents a combination of synovial hypertrophy, soft-tissue oedema, and joint effusion. Evaluation of the fat planes adjacent to the joints is useful in assessing for pathological soft-tissue swelling. Calcification within the soft tissues has a variety of causes, including crystal deposition,

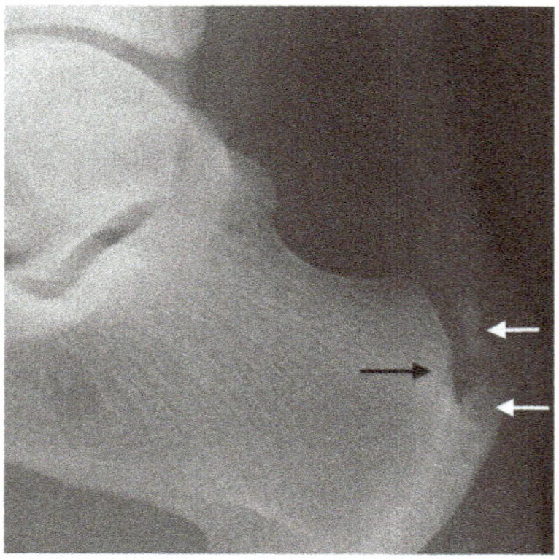

Figure 12.4 Inflammatory arthritis: there is entheseal disease present at the calcaneal insertion of the Achilles tendon in this patient with ankylosing spondylitis. There is calcification within the soft tissues adjacent to the site of insertion (white arrows) with adjacent soft-tissue swelling. In addition, there is a subtle area of erosive change affecting the posterior calcaneus (black arrow).

vascular calcification, or as an association of enthesitis. Other causes of soft-tissue calcification include systemic sclerosis and hyperparathyroidism; plain film imaging in these cases is often very helpful in delineating the calcification, which may be less evident on ultrasound and MRI.

Plain film appearances in common conditions

Osteoarthritis

Plain film imaging is usually sufficient to confirm a clinical diagnosis of osteoarthritis. The classic features of osteoarthritis, including non-uniform joint space loss, subchondral cyst formation, sclerosis, and osteophyte formation, are all readily identifiable on this imaging modality. Osteoarthritis in the foot is most commonly seen within the first metatarsophalangeal (MTP) joint (Figure 12.1) but is also frequently seen within the tarsometatarsal joints of the midfoot.

Rheumatoid arthritis

The characteristic conventional radiographic features of RA are soft-tissue swelling, periarticular osteopenia, joint space loss, erosion, and malalignment. The first sign to be apparent is often periarticular soft-tissue swelling secondary to synovitis and/or a joint effusion. Tenosynovitis may also contribute to the degree of soft-tissue swelling in the foot. Osteopenia also occurs early in the disease process and is seen originally in a periarticular distribution but progresses in chronic disease to become more generalized secondary to disuse. Erosive change predominantly affects the MTP joints with a predilection for the fourth and fifth metatarsal heads (Figure 12.2).

Spondyloarthropathy

This group of conditions is characterized by involvement of entheses with inflammation classically seen at the bony insertions of tendons and ligaments.

Psoriatic arthritis: the most common pattern of distribution is distal disease affecting the distal interphalangeal joints. Soft-tissue swelling is an early, but non-specific, feature of psoriatic arthritis; global swelling of a digit is characteristic of this condition. Terminal tuft resorption is a characteristic finding, as are marginal erosions associated with fluffy new bone formation both at and adjacent to the site of erosion (Figure 12.5).

Reactive arthritis: involvement of the posterior and plantar aspects of the calcaneus is a common feature of this condition (Figure 12.6) frequently associated with retrocalcaneal bursitis and poorly defined calcaneal erosions. Within the foot there may be asymmetric involvement of the MTP and interphalangeal joints, which may eventually lead to severe deforming arthropathy with potential ankylosis of the joints.

Ankylosing spondylitis: although clinical symptoms in the foot are relatively uncommon in patients with this condition, it has been shown that radiological findings in the foot are prevalent and include erosions, enthesophyte formation, joint effusion, joint space narrowing, and subchondral sclerosis (4).

Gout

Gout is the most common depositional disease to affect the foot; this results from deposition of monosodium urate crystals within the joint itself but also within the synovial fluid and the periarticular soft tissues (Figure 12.3). The erosions associated with gout are usually well-defined, punched-out lesions with sclerotic margins and overhanging edges. Soft-tissue swelling adjacent to the joint with preservation of the joint space are the typical imaging findings. The great toe MTP joint is classically affected, although almost all joints within the foot may be affected.

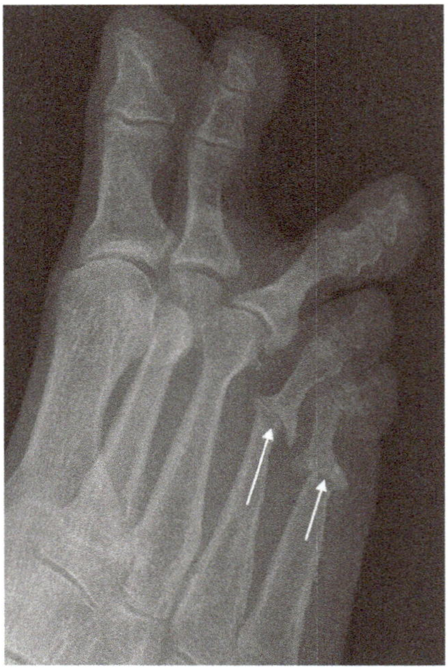

Figure 12.5 Psoriatic arthropathy: oblique plain film of the forefoot showing a pencil in cup deformity of the fourth and fifth metatarsophalangeal joints (white arrows). This appearance results from progressive periarticular erosions and bone resorption.

Diabetic foot

It has been recognized that 90% of cases of pedal osteomyelitis occur as a result of contiguous spread from foot ulcers (5). However, often areas of ulceration are not conspicuous on plain film imaging. Diffuse soft-tissue swelling and periosteal reaction may be detected on plain films in the diabetic foot. Swelling corresponds to soft-tissue oedema on MRI (6). With progression of infection, findings will develop to show cortical disruption and medullary involvement.

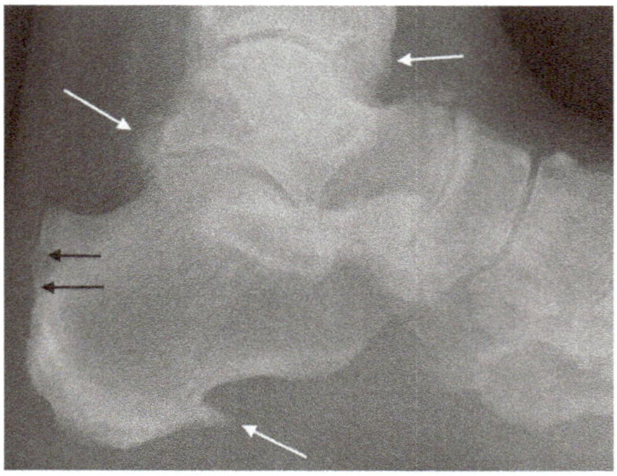

Figure 12.6 Reactive arthritis: fluffy periosteal areas of bone proliferation are seen on this lateral ankle radiograph affecting the tibial plafond, the anterior and posterior aspects of the talus, and the plantar calcaneal spur (white arrows). There is also cortical irregularity affecting the posterior aspect of the calcaneus (black arrows).

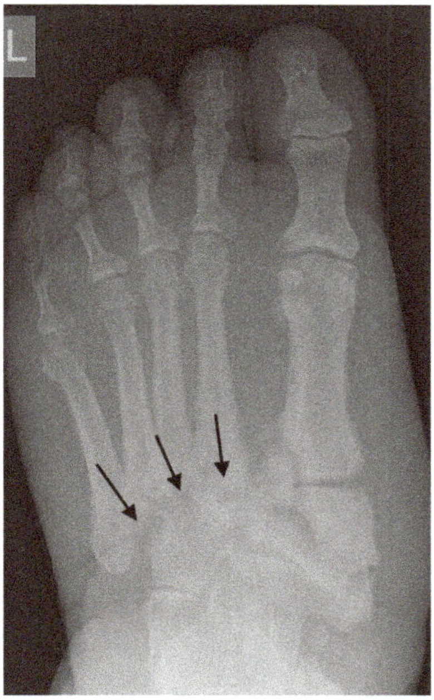

Figure 12.7 Charcot foot: DP radiograph of the foot where there is extensive deformity with marked separation of the bases of the first and second metatarsal bases and lateral drift of the second–fifth metatarsals. There is loss of the joint spaces across the tarsometatarsal joints with small areas of debris seen throughout the Charcot joint (black arrows).

Diabetic neuropathic arthropathy most commonly affects the Lisfranc joint (tarsometatarsal joint) within the foot (7) but may occur at any joint. In the acute setting radiographs may reveal only soft-tissue swelling and joint effusion. Any malalignment across the Lisfranc joint should raise concern for neuropathic disease; the earliest feature may be widening of the distance between the first and second metatarsal bases. In the more subacute stage, plain film radiography will demonstrate the collapse and fragmentation of the articular surface, subchondral cysts, and marginal erosions. In the chronic phase, the neuropathic foot shows joint subluxations and dislocations as well as bone destruction and fragmentation (Figure 12.7). In the late stage of the disease the bones may become necrotic and collapse (8).

Reflex sympathetic dystrophy

Imaging findings in this complex group of conditions have been shown to be only approximately 60% sensitive and specific; bone scan has been shown to have greater sensitivity and specificity than both plain film and MRI (9). The plain film findings in reflex sympathetic dystrophy include patchy periarticular osteopenia, soft-tissue swelling with eventual soft-tissue atrophy, and subperiosteal bone resorption; the joint spaces are preserved (Figure 12.8).

Computerized tomography

CT, like conventional radiography, utilizes X-rays to generate an image, relying on the differing attenuation of the X-ray beam by the different tissues to provide contrast. As with conventional radiographs, soft-tissue contrast is relatively poor, but the technique is able to provide unparalleled visualization of bony structures.

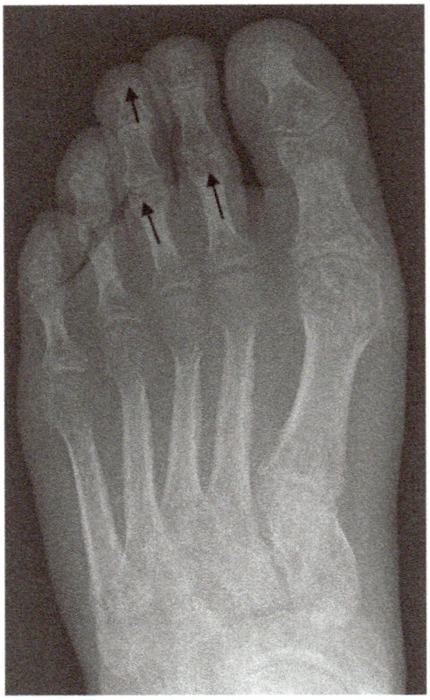

Figure 12.8 Reflex sympathetic dystrophy: dorsoplantar radiograph of the foot with severe patchy osteopenia in a periarticular distribution. There are numerous areas of subperiosteal bone resorption (black arrows). The joint spaces are preserved throughout the forefoot, which is a characteristic finding of reflex sympathetic dystrophy.

At its simplest CT produces cross-sectional images of the body part being scanned and on early machines cross-sections were produced in a single plane. However, CT technology has developed immeasurably over the past 20 years and modern systems allow the acquisition of a contiguous high-resolution volume of data that can then be reconstructed in multiple planes for analysis. The acquisition of such data also allows 3D reconstruction of images using computer-generated surface rendering techniques. These do not offer any additional information over conventional multiplanar sectional views; indeed, the post-processing techniques involved can artefactually deteriorate the image, but 3D reformatting can be useful to aid understanding of the anatomy for those less familiar with interpreting cross-sectional anatomy. Other recent advances include techniques to minimize metal artifact and the advent of dual and multi-energy CT, which is starting to find applications in rheumatological imaging.

Information from the soft tissues can be improved through the use of intravenous contrast medium. Contrast medium can also be injected into joints to allow CT arthrography, which may be useful for the assessment of articular cartilage and the presence of loose bodies, although for the majority of situations involving imaging of soft tissues and intra-articular structures, ultrasound and MRI are the techniques of choice. Consequently, the primary use for CT in the musculoskeletal system is the assessment of bone, and it remains pre-eminent for the detection of bone trauma. Within the field of rheumatology, it has uses that generally rely on its advantages over conventional radiographs for the detailed assessment of bone.

Specific roles for computerized tomography in rheumatological imaging of the foot and ankle

Assessment of complex bone anatomy

The foot has a complex 3D anatomy that is not well suited for assessment with conventional radiographs where the resultant image comprises multiple overlapping shadows from the bones. The joints of the hindfoot and midfoot do not lie in standard orthogonal planes and in many joints curved articular surfaces contribute to difficulty in evaluation using conventional radiographs. Added to this the alignment of joints is affected by joint deformities and subluxations commonly seen in rheumatological conditions, further complicating the 3D anatomy.

Using CT, cross-sections can be obtained through the joints to assess their congruence, joint space, the presence or absence of erosions, and subchondral bone change and osteophyte formation (Figure 12.9). CT can also be useful when looking for congenital coalitions of the tarsal bones or acquired ankylosis.

An important application for CT is the investigation of bone and joint disease in patients who are unable to tolerate MRI or cannot undergo MRI owing to the presence of a contraindication (e.g., a pacemaker). For instance, although CT does not provide the soft-tissue detail that can be seen with MRI it can still provide useful information in cases of suspected foot sepsis if MRI is not possible (10).

Evaluation of fine bone detail

Although many of the advantages CT brings are also seen with MRI and ultrasound, which show superior soft-tissue contrast, for the evaluation of fine bone detail CT remains unparalleled. CT shows significant advantages over other imaging modalities for the detection of subtle erosion (11). In clinical practice ultrasound and MRI are more commonly utilized for detecting erosions

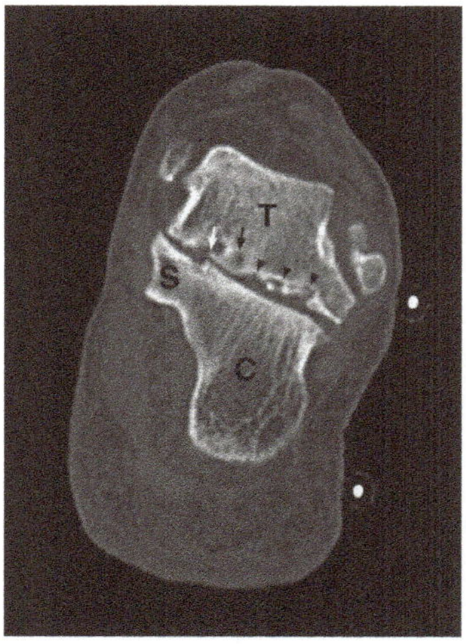

Figure 12.9 Osteoarthritis: coronal oblique reconstruction of hindfoot computerized tomography through the subtalar joint. There is osteoarthritis of the posterior subtalar joint with subchondral bone irregularity (arrowheads), subchondral cyst formation (black arrow), and osteophyte (white arrow). Note also the irregular joint space narrowing. C, Calcaneus; S, sustentaculum; T, talus.

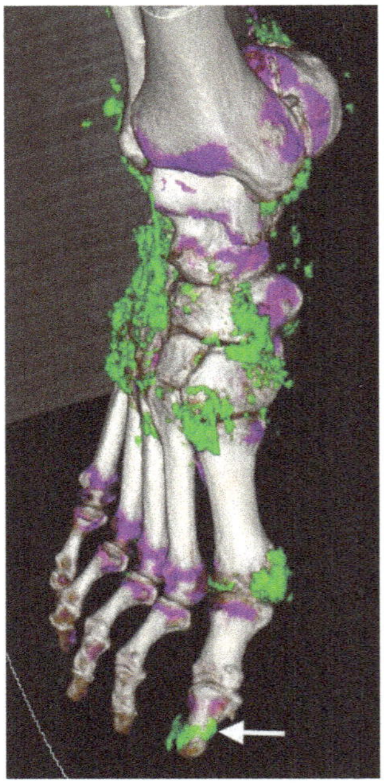

Figure 12.10 Dual energy computerized tomography scan, 3D reconstruction: patient with multiple gouty tophi. The image is processed to code urate deposits as green. The study shows one of the recognized artifacts seen with this technique whereby the patient's toenail has also coded as green (arrow).

Image courtesy of Dr PL Munk MD, Department of Radiology, Vancouver General Hospital, Canada.

not seen on conventional radiographs owing to their ability also to show soft-tissue changes relating to joint disease.

Demonstration of urate deposition in crystal arthropathy

A relatively new application for CT in the investigation of foot and ankle rheumatological disease makes use of CT systems with two or more X-ray sources with different energies. This technique is known as dual energy CT (DECT) or multi-energy CT. The technique was first conceived in the 1970s and has proved useful in evaluating renal calculi (12). It also has emerging applications in the evaluation of cardiovascular and pulmonary disease (13–15). DECT exploits the variation in attenuation of X-rays of differing energies by different tissues. This technique can accurately be used to detect the presence of urate crystals in the soft tissues, joints, and bones (16–18) (Figure 12.10). Special CT equipment is required to undertake this type of imaging and, although it is becoming more widely available, not all radiology departments have these systems available. Understanding of the technique is evolving but it is important to recognize that there are a number of pitfalls and artifacts to be aware of when interpreting these images (19).

Nuclear medicine

With the development and improvement of cross-sectional imaging techniques, radionuclide imaging for the diagnosis of rheumatological conditions is now less commonly used, but in certain situations it can be helpful.

Two-phase radionuclide bone scintigraphy

Conventional two-phase radionuclide bone scanning involves the intravenous injection of a radiopharmaceutical, usually a polyphosphonate labelled with radioactive technetium-99m (^{99m}Tc), which is then taken up in proportion to the metabolic activity of the bone. Gamma rays emitted by the ^{99m}Tc can then be detected by gamma cameras, producing an image representing the distribution of the radiopharmaceutical. Two-phase scanning involves obtaining images approximately 5 minutes following injection of the radiopharmaceutical, representing an early blood pool phase providing information relating to the vascular and extravascular distribution of the radiopharmaceutical. Subsequently, 3–4 hours following injection the bone phase imaging shows the uptake of the radiopharmaceutical in bone; the degree of uptake will relate to the level of bone turnover (Figure 12.11a, b).

^{99m}Tc bone scintigraphy is extremely sensitive to the detection of increased bone turnover and changes in the vascular distribution of isotope. However, a huge disadvantage is the lack of specificity of the imaging test, with many different pathologies giving rise to increased tracer uptake and therefore similar scintigraphy findings. A further disadvantage of the technique is the relatively poor spatial resolution for localizing sites of tracer uptake. A technique known as single positron emission computed tomography (SPECT) utilizes rotating gamma cameras to localize the location of activity in three dimensions, considerably improving the localization of sites of uptake. Advancements in technology now allow the combination of SPECT with conventional CT imaging to produce a hybrid image with the radiopharmaceutical tracer uptake shown on the CT image, allowing for better localization of uptake (Figure 12.11c).

Other nuclear medicine techniques

While ^{99m}Tc bone scintigraphy remains the most common nuclear medicine investigation undertaken in the foot and ankle, its lack of specificity remains a problem and many applications for its use have now been superseded by other cross-sectional imaging techniques such as MRI. However, more specific radionuclide techniques have developed. These are based on the use of different radiopharmaceuticals, which are more specific in their sites of uptake. Radiolabelled white cells may be used to investigate infection and other techniques exist for investigating arthritis, including the use of radiolabelled antibodies (20–23). More recently, 18F-fluorodeoxyglucose positron emission tomography (FDG-PET) imaging has become more widely available and is principally used in oncology. However, applications in arthritis are starting to emerge, particularly for monitoring disease activity in RA, although these have not yet found their way into clinical practice (24–27).

Clinical applications of radionuclide imaging in rheumatology

Osteoarthritis

The lack of specificity means that scintigraphy has a very limited role in the diagnosis of osteoarthritis. However, it is important to recognize that osteoarthritis is a cause of increased periarticular tracer uptake when interpreting bone scintigraphy, to avoid confusion with other pathologies. Unsurprisingly in the foot and ankle, increased uptake at the first MTP joint is a frequent finding. A further problem with using bone scintigraphy to identify sites of osteoarthritis in the foot and ankle is the relatively poor spatial resolution, which limits the ability of the test to identify specific joints in the midfoot, although localization is possible using SPECT or SPECT-CT (Figure 12.11).

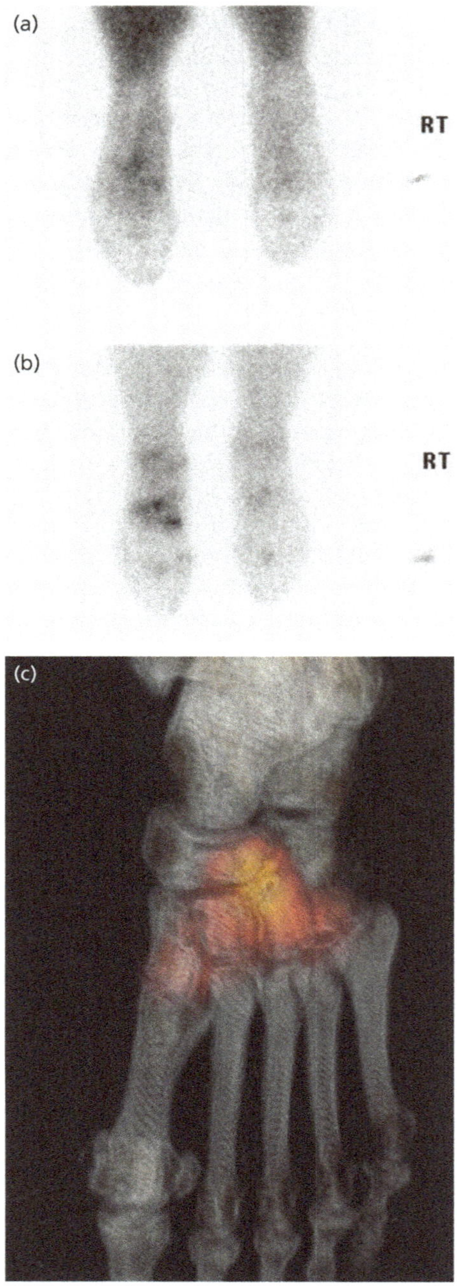

Figure 12.11 (a) Blood pool. (b) Delayed plantar view ^{99m}Tc scintigrams demonstrate increased uptake in the region of the left midfoot. On these images alone, the location of the uptake is difficult to determine. (c) Hybrid single positron emission computerized tomography-computerized tomography (CT) image using a 3D CT reconstruction locates the increased tracer uptake to the joint between the navicular and lateral and intermediate cuneiforms. The increased uptake represents osteoarthritis in this case.

Images courtesy of Dr S Vaidyanathan, Department of Radiology, Leeds Teaching Hospitals, UK.

Inflammatory arthritis

Two-phase bone scintigraphy shows uptake on both blood phase and delayed images. Again, appearances are non-specific but the distribution of joint disease in the foot and ankle is well shown, and knowledge of the pattern of joint involvement may help in identifying the underlying diagnosis. For instance, distal interphalangeal joint involvement would point towards psoriatic arthritis rather than RA. The excellent accuracy that ultrasound and MRI show for identifying synovitis and erosions means that bone scintigraphy has very little role to play in investigating inflammatory arthritides in current practice. Alternative radiopharmaceuticals have been used for the assessment of inflammatory arthritis, but these have not found their way into routine clinical practice.

The diabetic foot

In common with other arthritides, neuropathic arthropathy, seen in patients with diabetic neuropathy, results in increased tracer uptake on bone scintigraphy. As expected, the test is highly sensitive but shows very poor specificity (reportedly as low as 0%) (28). Other modalities offer many advantages over bone scintigraphy, which has largely been replaced for this indication. However, when investigating the presence of osteomyelitis in the diabetic foot, radionuclide imaging may be more useful. A frequent problem in the foot and ankle is the distinction between soft-tissue infection and osteomyelitis. Bone scintigraphy has been used for this in the past, and a negative bone scan strongly excludes the probability of osteomyelitis. High sensitivities and specificities for the diagnosis of osteomyelitis can be achieved by combining isotope-labelled white cell scintigraphy with conventional scintigraphy, and this technique has the advantage of being effective even in the presence of neuropathic joint disease, which may present problems for the diagnosis of osteomyelitis using other modalities (29, 30). Again, MRI has largely taken over this role and has been shown to have a higher sensitivity and specificity than bone scans for detecting osteomyelitis in diabetic patients (31).

Reflex sympathetic dystrophy

Reflex sympathetic dystrophy is often included under the umbrella term of bone marrow oedema syndrome and, seen in the foot and ankle, is associated with increased radionuclide uptake on early- and late-phase bone scintigraphy. Although very sensitive, the findings will precede the radiographic demonstration of osteopenia, and bone scintigraphy shows very poor specificity for detecting bone marrow oedema syndrome, so the findings must be interpreted within the correct clinical context (32, 33). Typically, in reflex sympathetic dystrophy uptake will be in a periarticular distribution.

Magnetic resonance imaging

MRI is increasingly employed in the investigation of pathology in the foot and ankle owing to its high soft-tissue contrast and resolution and the ability to image in any plane. Many of the features of arthritis seen on radiographs, such as joint space loss, erosions, and subluxations occur late in the disease process when irreparable damage has already occurred. It is possible to detect much earlier features of these disease processes on MRI, making this an invaluable imaging entity. A precise clinical history and indication of differential diagnosis is crucial in ensuring that the correct sequences are performed and the correct anatomical area is covered.

Synovium

MRI scanning is currently the gold standard modality for imaging synovitis and tenosynovitis in patients with inflammatory arthritis (34). Inflamed synovium within the joints or tendon sheaths is seen as thickened intra-articular intermediate signal tissue on T1-weighted (T1W) imaging, which appears high signal on T2-weighted (T2W) imaging and, importantly, shows enhancement following intravenous contrast. Studies have shown a high degree of correlation between the degree of inflammation of the synovium and vascularity of synovium obtained at biopsy and post-contrast enhancement on matching dynamic MRI scans (35).

Soft-tissue pathology

Tendon pathology may be broadly divided into tendinosis or tendinopathy and inflammatory enthesitis. Tendon abnormality in spondyloarthropathy tends to be closely related to the fibrocartilaginous enthesis. There will be increased vascularity within the tendon (36) and the normal entheseal architecture is disrupted with defects at the bone–fibrocartilage interface. There may be erosions at the site of tendon insertion. MRI of the abnormal tendons will reveal increased intrinsic signal and thickening of the tendons (37).

Tenosynovitis is common in RA and has been postulated to be the first manifestation of this condition (38); it is also associated with other forms of arthropathy, including gout and pseudogout. On MRI, tenosynovitis is characterized by the demonstration of fluid and synovitis in the tendon sheath.

In the neuropathic foot the earliest MRI features will include diffuse soft-tissue oedema (39). As this condition progresses and the Lisfranc joint becomes affected, axial MRI can be useful in depicting the Lisfranc ligament. Signal change within the bone marrow, low T1W signal and high T2W signal, is similar in appearance to the changes seen in osteomyelitis.

Plantar plate pathology in patients with RA has been shown to be related to other abnormal imaging findings, including synovitis, bone marrow oedema, and bone erosion. As opposed to plantar plate pathology in other groups of patients, involvement of the fourth and fifth MTP joints is the most common location in patients with RA (40).

Bone marrow oedema (bone oedema)

MRI-depicted bone oedema occurs in various forms of inflammatory and non-inflammatory arthritis and probably represents a cellular infiltrate within bone (41). Subchondral bone oedema is commonly seen in patients with osteoarthritis, transient osteoporosis (42), and both infectious and inflammatory arthropathies (43), amongst other conditions. In RA the presence of bone oedema is associated with progressive erosive disease and is related to poor functional outcome.

In spondyloarthropathy MRI will not only demonstrate tendon or ligament changes, but it is also able to demonstrate bone marrow oedema at the insertion sites.

The diagnosis of osteomyelitis on MRI is based upon identifying an abnormal bone marrow pattern (Figure 12.12). Infection within the bone results in loss of the normal fatty marrow signal with bone with oedema seen on water-sensitive sequences and enhancement on T1W post-gadolinium sequences (44). Although these findings in a non-subchondral location have a high sensitivity for infection, many other pathologies such as fracture, tumour, neuropathic disease, or severe inflammatory arthritis will have similar imaging findings.

Erosions

Bone erosion is a central feature of RA and is associated with disease severity and poor functional outcome (45). Alongside synovitis and bone oedema, erosions are important indicators of disease in this condition and MRI has been shown to be more sensitive than plain film for detection of erosions. T1W imaging is used for imaging of erosions where there is loss of marrow signal. Erosions are demonstrated on MRI as breaks in the bone cortex filled with synovial tissue

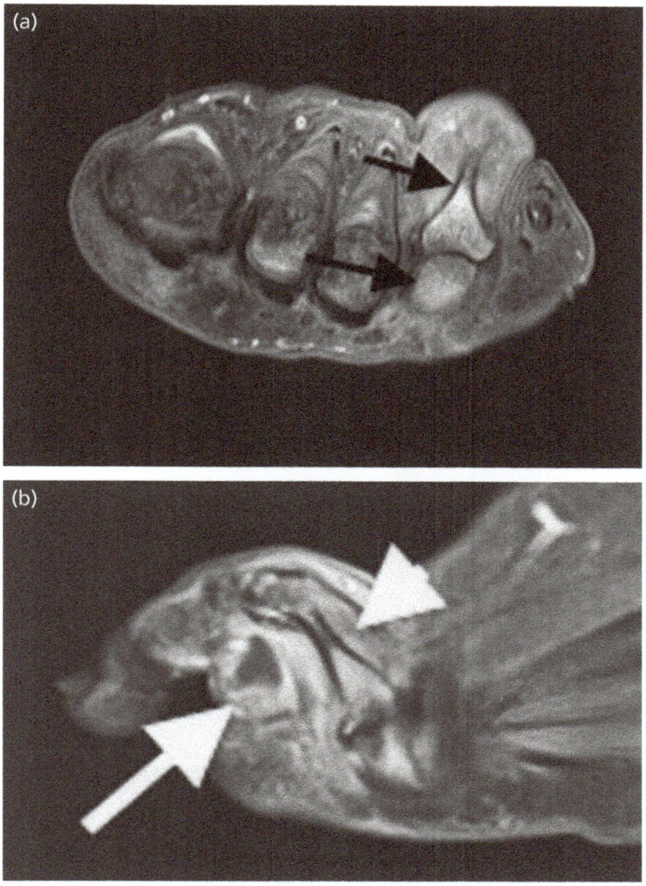

Figure 12.12 (a) Diabetic foot magnetic resonance imaging: axial image through the forefoot showing marked bone oedema within the fourth metatarsal head and also within the fourth toe proximal phalanx (black arrows). There is also soft-tissue oedema adjacent to the proximal phalanx extending along the fourth toe. This patient had osteomyelitis of the fourth metatarsal and phalanges secondary to an ulcer on the dorsal aspect of the fourth toe. (b) Sagittal image through the fourth toe in the same patient. This image shows the extensive bone oedema within the fourth toe (white arrowhead) but also a small fluid collection within the plantar soft tissues (white arrow), in keeping with an associated soft-tissue abscess.

(Figure 12.13). Crucially, erosions must be appreciated in two planes to be considered true erosions; 3D imaging, which can then be reformatted, is extremely useful when imaging for the presence of erosions as this avoids the need to perform imaging in different planes.

MRI may also reveal RA changes within the feet when imaging of the hands is normal. In terms of location, bone erosions in RA are most commonly detected on the plantar aspect of the metatarsal heads (46). Bone erosions are also the most common radiological finding in patients with ankylosing spondylitis and are detectable on MRI in up to 90% of patients with this condition (4).

Erosions associated with gout have a characteristic 'rat bite' configuration, with overhanging edges and sclerotic margins (Figure 12.14). The associated gouty tophi are usually isointense on T1 imaging with enhancement post-gadolinium and hypointense on T2.

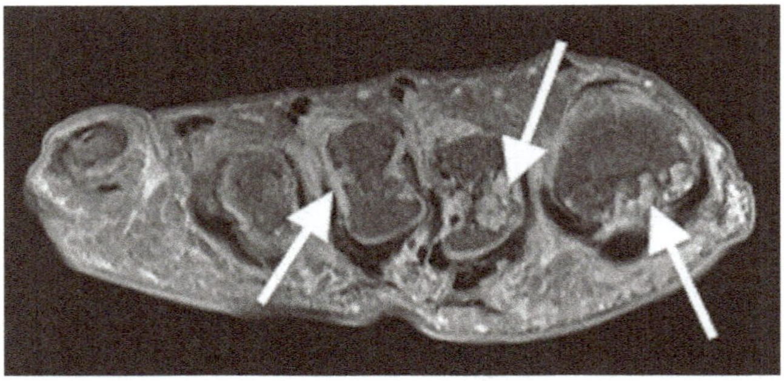

Figure 12.13 Rheumatoid arthritis: axial post-gadolinium magnetic resonance imaging through the level of the metatarsal heads. There is extensive erosive change seen affecting the first, second, and third metatarsal heads (white arrows) with synovitis seen within the areas of erosive change.

Ultrasound

In recent years, ultrasound imaging has become an established technique for the investigation of foot symptoms in rheumatology patients. Its major strength lies with the fact that it can be performed in real time (enabling direct correlations of scan findings with symptoms in addition to the guidance of interventions) and its ability to evaluate both bone and soft tissues dynamically. Its limitations, however, relate to its need for an acoustic window and its inability to see below the bone cortex (hence it is unable to see bone marrow oedema as MRI can). It is also more

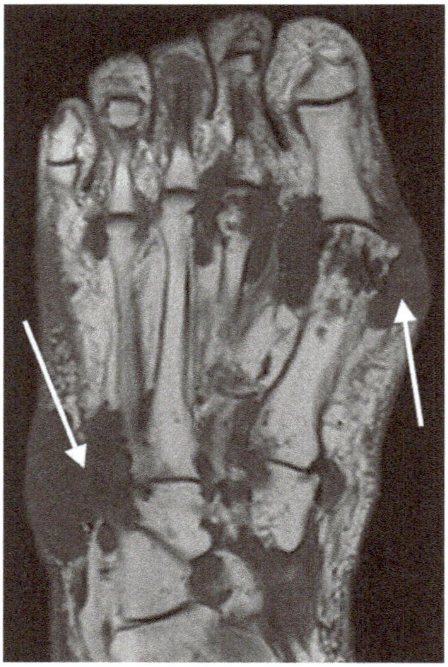

Figure 12.14 Gout: T1-weighted coronal magnetic resonance imaging. There is global erosive change seen throughout the foot in this patient with gout. There is marked associated low-signal soft tissue in keeping with gouty tophi (white arrows).

operator-dependent than other techniques and so a good level of technical skill and anatomical knowledge is required. The increasing accessibility of ultrasound equipment as a result of falling costs and improved ease of use has opened the doors for the technique to be performed by a wide range of non-radiology health professionals, such as rheumatologists, orthopaedic surgeons, sports physicians, podiatrists, and physiotherapists. It has been recommended that anyone from a non-traditional training setting who performs ultrasound undertakes a recognized formal training programme (47).

In rheumatology, much interest lies with the need to identify features associated with inflammation as early as possible. Clinicians commonly adopt a 'treat-to-target' approach where treatment with disease-modifying agents is tightly titrated against the degree of inflammation. Improved patient outcomes of this approach have been demonstrated in patients with RA (48) and psoriatic arthritis (49). Typical features that can be seen on ultrasound suggestive of active disease include synovitis/synovial hypertrophy, tenosynovitis, and/or enthesitis, whilst the presence of bone erosion, subluxation, and osteophytosis suggests the structural consequences of inadequately treated inflammation.

Synovium

The synovial membrane is usually not seen on ultrasound unless there is synovial proliferation and associated effusion. Synovial proliferation is most commonly associated with inflammatory joint diseases but may also be seen in joints with degenerative changes or those under excessive mechanical stress. The thickened synovial membrane is usually noted to be more hypoechoic (darker) in appearance on B-mode (greyscale) scanning when compared to adjacent dermal soft tissue (50) (Figure 12.15). It may be partially compressed by the overlying transducer. It may also exhibit increased blood flow secondary to vasodilation and/or neoangiogenesis (new vessel growth), which may be detected by Doppler (Figure 12.16). The presence of Doppler flow is widely considered to be the hallmark of active inflammation and a strong predictor of disease persistence and future structural damage.

Ultrasound may be used to detect synovitis in all foot joints. In early RA, synovitis is most commonly seen in the tibiotalar joints, talonavicular joints, subtalar, and MTP joints. It may be subclinical and not exhibit symptoms. Subclinical inflammation found on ultrasound, especially if associated with Doppler, has been shown to result in subsequent bone damage (51). Later, the tarsometatarsal joints and midfoot joints are more likely to be involved, often with associated secondary degenerative joint changes. In osteoarthritis, synovitis is most commonly seen in the

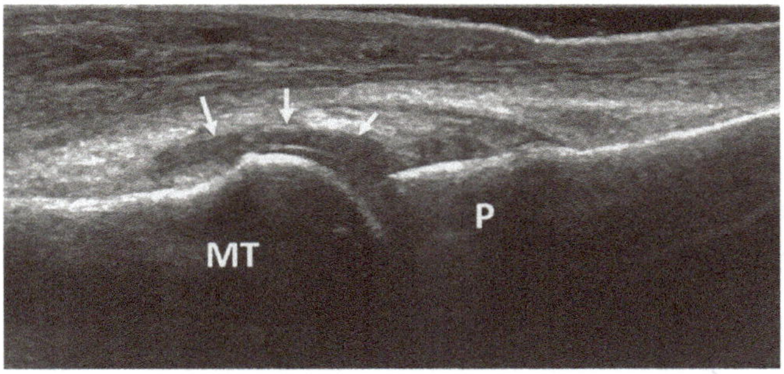

Figure 12.15 Greyscale synovitis. Longitudinal dorsal view through an metatarsophalangeal joint. The normal smooth profile of the bones is noted as a bold white line. Hypoechoic synovial thickening is seen consistent with mild/moderate synovitis. MT, metatarsal; P, phalanx.

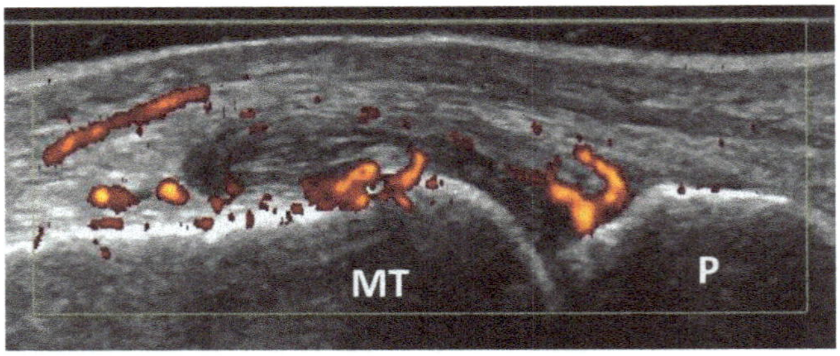

Figure 12.16 Doppler-associated synovitis. Longitudinal dorsal view through a metatarsophalangeal joint of a patient with rheumatoid arthritis. There is a moderate degree of Doppler signal within the distended joint capsule. There is also some extracapsular Doppler signal noted. MT, metatarsal; P, phalanx.

midfoot area or first MTP joint. In gout, synovitis is most often seen in the first MTP joint or ankle. In psoriatic arthritis, synovitis may be observed in any joint, but the distribution of joint involvement is not as symmetrical as in RA.

Tendon and ligament pathology

The tendons of the foot may be considered in four compartments. Those around the medial (posterior tibialis tendon, flexor digitorum longus, and flexor hallucis longus), lateral (peroneal longus and brevis), and anterior aspects (tibialis anterior, extensor digitorum longus, and extensor hallucis longus) of the foot are surrounded by a synovial-lined tendon sheath. Posteriorly, the Achilles tendon does not have a synovial-lined sheath, only a paratenon. Ultrasound lends itself well to the assessment of tendon disease as the majority of tendons are superficial and therefore high frequency (better resolution) can be used. Ultrasound may identify features of tendinopathy (thickening, loss of fibrillar pattern, and increased vascularity) and tears, as well as thickening of the tendon sheath/paratenon, again with increased vascularity (52) (Figure 12.17). A smaller transducer is sometimes preferred to examine the tendons in the perimalleolar area because of improved transducer access. Ligaments have a similar ultrasound appearance to tendons and may be susceptible to the same changes seen in tendons. They are often not the primary focus in rheumatology unless there is a specific history of trauma.

Enthesitis

An enthesis is a point of union between a tendon or ligament or joint capsule and bone. Inflammatory rheumatological diseases (e.g., the seronegative spondyloarthropathies) have a predilection for these sites, but enthesitis may also occur in other inflammatory joint diseases (e.g., RA) and also secondary to mechanical stress (e.g., occupational). In the foot, the two commonest sites for observing enthesitis are the insertions of the Achilles tendon and the origin of the plantar fascia into the calcaneum (Figure 12.18). The Outcome Measure in Rheumatology (OMERACT) group have suggested that the ultrasound features of hypoechogenicity, increased Doppler signal at the insertion (within 2–3 mm), and tendon/ligament thickening should be considered features of active disease, whilst bone erosions, enthesophytes, and soft-tissue calcifications are features of structural damage (53). Enthesitis may also be noted at other sites, such as the insertion of peroneal brevis into the base of the fifth metatarsal or the posterior tibialis tendon into the navicular bone.

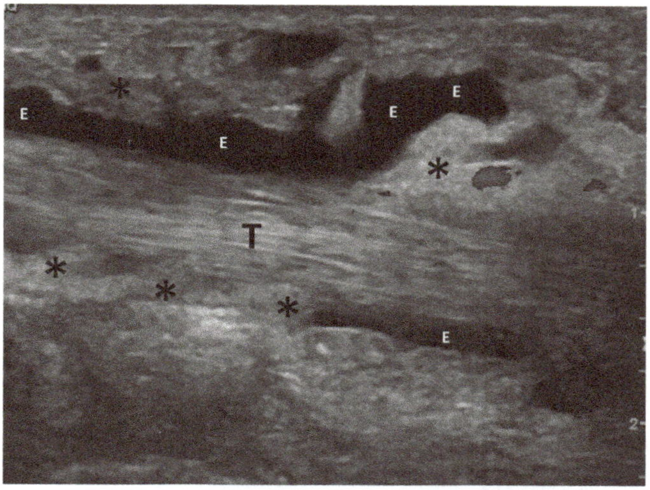

Figure 12.17 Tenosynovitis. Longitudinal view through the posterior tibialis tendon (T) of a patient with rheumatoid arthritis. There is marked synovial proliferation (*), effusion (E), and increased Doppler in the tendon sheath consistent with tenosynovitis.

Bone erosions

Bone erosions are defects of the surface of the bone cortex. The OMERACT definition of an ultrasound erosion is a break in the bone cortex seen in more than one imaging plane (50) (Figure 12.19a, b). Although there is no official size limit for a 'break' to be called an erosion, the larger they are the more specific they are for an underlying pathological process such as RA (54). As with other imaging techniques, as the resolution of images continues to improve, smaller bone defects are now being visualized, some of which may be pathological, but some may also be physiological; for example, marking an entry point of a nutrient vessel entering the bone. A knowledge of your machine and normal ultrasound anatomy is therefore important to determine what is significant. Bone erosions associated with synovial-based diseases such as RA, psoriatic arthritis, and gout tend to be intra-articular. They usually have a similar appearance

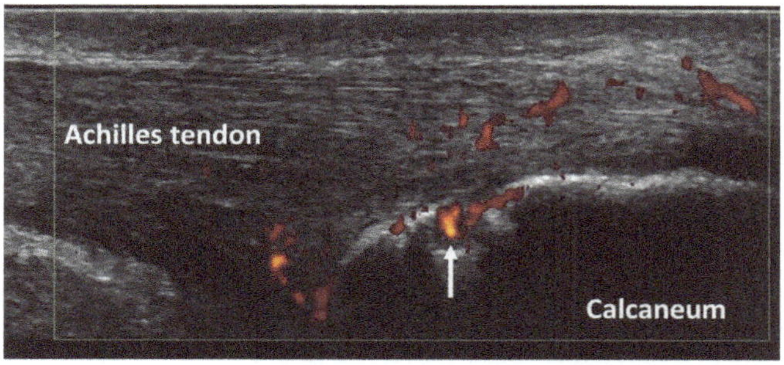

Figure 12.18 Enthesitis. Longitudinal view through the Achilles tendon of a patient with psoriatic arthritis. There is thickening of the tendon toward the insertion and increased Doppler activity. The closer the Doppler signal is to the bone surface, the more specific it is for a spondyloarthropathy. The white arrow depicts insertional Doppler and erosive bone changes in this case.

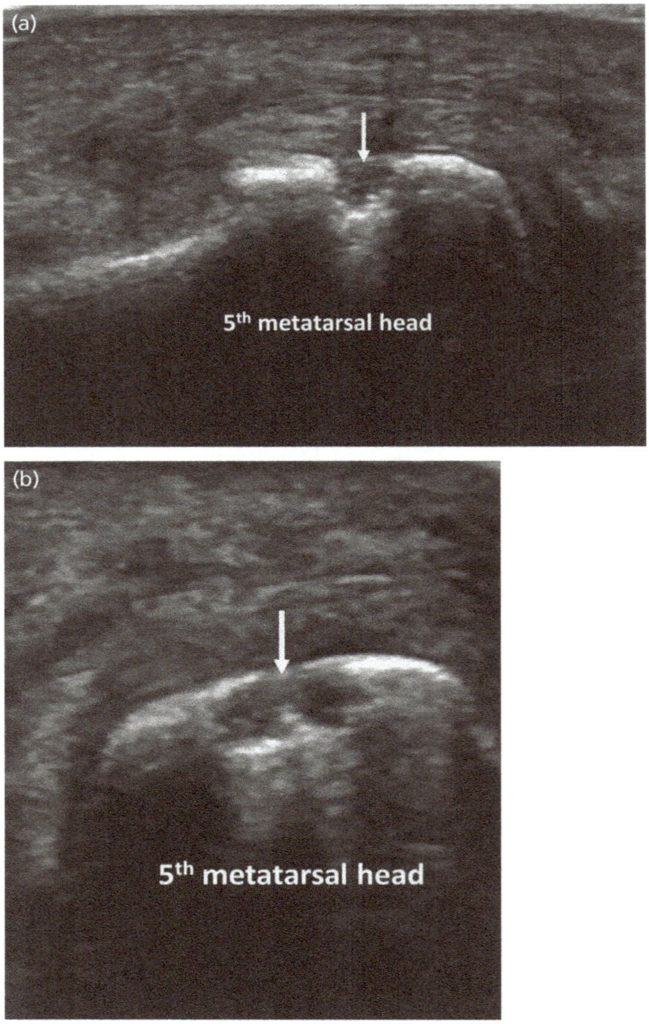

Figure 12.19 (a) Synovial-based bone erosion: longitudinal view through the lateral aspect of a fifth metatarsal head in a patient with rheumatoid arthritis (RA). A discontinuity or break in the bone cortex is seen (arrow). The fifth metatarsal head is an important early site to check for bone erosion in RA. They are frequently seen on ultrasound when they are not on radiographs. (b) Synovial-based bone erosion; the same erosion as seen in Figure 12.19a. Here it is confirmed in a transverse plane.

and can occur in similar sites; however, gouty erosions may sometimes be very large with overhanging edges. In early disease, especially RA, erosions may be seen on the lateral side of the fifth metatarsal head; they later appear on the underside of the metatarsal head. Erosions on the medial aspect of the first metatarsal head are less specific for inflammatory diseases and occur commonly in association with osteoarthritis and hallux valgus. Bone erosions may also occur at entheseal sites—as with synovial-based erosions, small ones may be seen in normal individuals or after trauma, whilst larger ones are more suggestive of a primary inflammatory disease (Figure 12.20a, b).

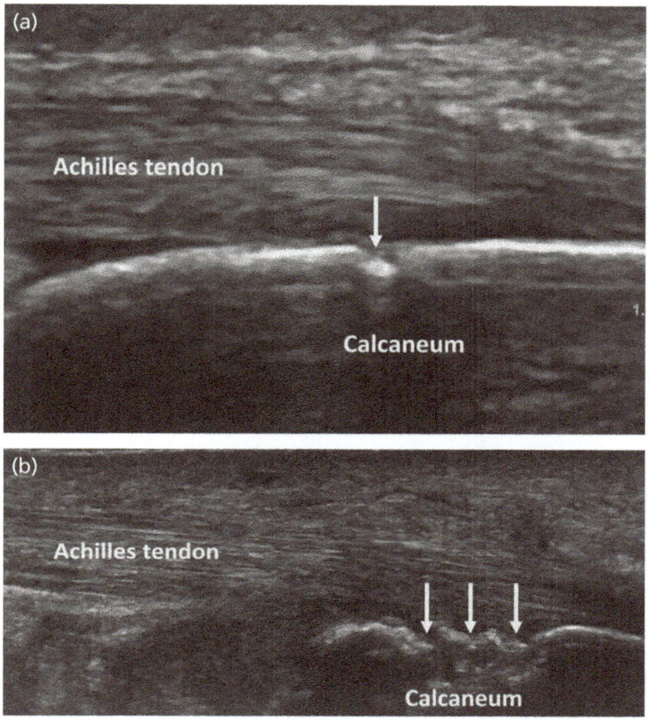

Figure 12.20 (a) Small entheseal bone erosions. Longitudinal view through the distal insertion of the Achilles tendon into the calcaneum in a normal asymptomatic person. There is a small bone erosion; at this size they are non-specific and non-diagnostic. (b) Large entheseal bone erosions. Longitudinal view through the distal insertion of the Achilles tendon of a patient with psoriatic arthritis. There are large erosions (arrows) noted at the insertion. Assuming that there is no history of previous trauma or surgery, then the likelihood of an underlying inflammatory arthritis such as a spondyloarthropathy (psoriatic arthritis in this case) is high.

Osteophytes and enthesophytes

Osteophytes are upward projections of the bone surface (55). They are markers of degenerative arthritis and are easily identified on ultrasound. In the feet they are most commonly seen in the first MTP joint (Figure 12.21) and midfoot area. Joints with osteophytosis are often associated with greyscale synovitis and sometimes increased Doppler signal suggestive of an inflammatory component. Enthesophytes are similar to osteophytes in appearance but occur at the entheses. They are common in patients with spondyloarthropathies but are also seen in normal asymptomatic people, making them a non-specific finding. Their positions are thought to relate to lines of force created by mechanical stress (56).

In addition to identifying inflammatory-related pathology, ultrasound is commonly used to investigate other soft-tissue and bony abnormalities.

Bursitis

Bursae are common in the feet and bursitis is an important cause of foot symptoms (57). They are most commonly seen between the metatarsal heads (intermetatarsal bursae) (Figure 12.22a)

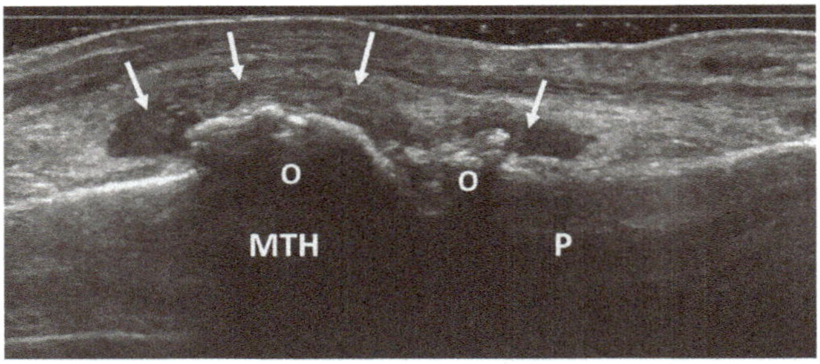

Figure 12.21 Osteoarthritis. Longitudinal view through a first metatarsophalangeal joint demonstrating osteophytes (O) of the metatarsal head (MTH) and phalanx (P) in a patient with osteoarthritis. There is also associated greyscale synovitis (white arrows).

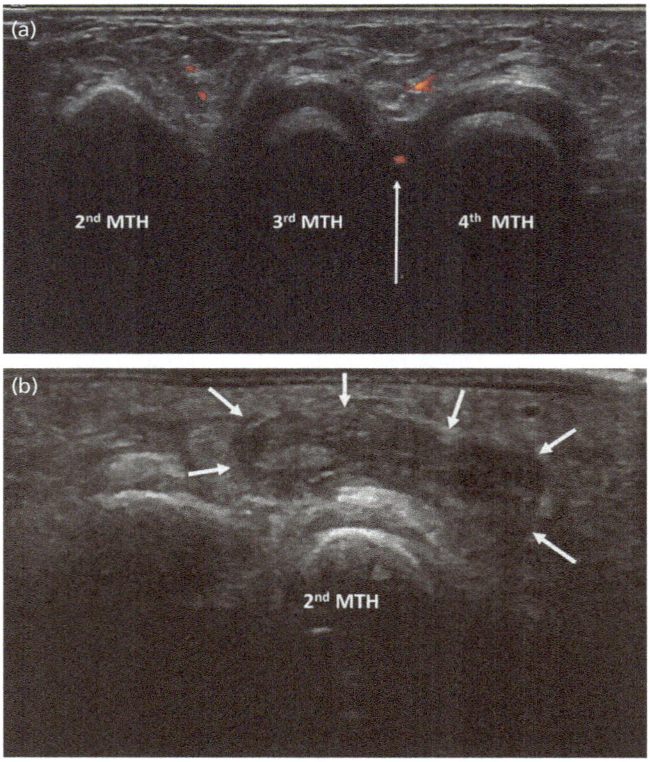

Figure 12.22 (a) Intermetatarsal bursitis. Transverse view through second to fifth metatarsophalangeal joints. Hypoechoic soft tissue is seen between the third and fourth metatarsal heads (white arrow). There is also evidence of Doppler flow. These features are suggestive of an intermetatarsal bursitis. (b) Submetatarsal bursitis. Transverse view under the second metatarsal head demonstrating a large adventitial submetatarsal bursa. These are often associated with subluxed metatarsal heads.

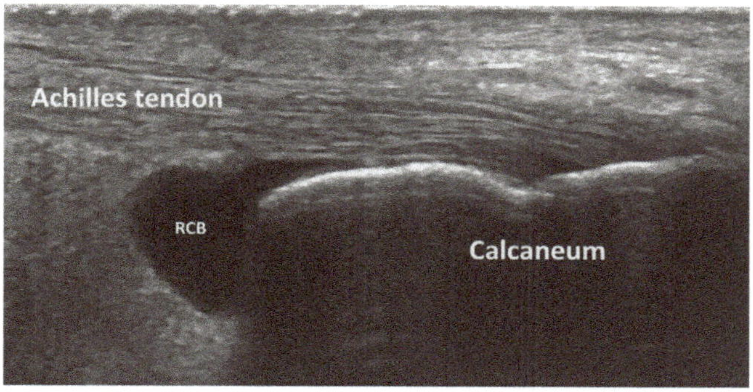

Figure 12.23 Retrocalcaneal bursitis. Longitudinal view through the Achilles tendon. Although the tendon appears normal, there is a large hypoechoic collection of fluid seen in the retrocalcaneal bursa (RCB). Small fluid-filled bursae are common in normal patients. As the bursae are synovial-lined, in more severe cases there is often visible synovial proliferation and increased Doppler signal seen.

or under the metatarsal heads (Figure 12.22b). They may also be seen on the medial aspect of the first metatarsal head or lateral aspect of the fifth metatarsal head, both of which may relate to footwear. In a similar way, bursae may occur on the dorsal midfoot if shoes are tight or are rubbing. Ultrasound is often used to identify and guide injections into the retrocalcaneal bursae (Figure 12.23). These are synovial-lined cavities that lie between the Achilles tendon and calcaneum. They may be symptomatic, especially if large, and exhibit Doppler signal. They are often associated with enthesitis, but also may be lone findings or associated with mechanical/degenerative Achilles disorders. They are therefore not core features of the ultrasound definition of a spondyloarthropathy.

Achilles tendinopathy/mechanical plantar fasciitis

Tendinopathy of the Achilles tendon is typically noted in the midportion of the Achilles tendon halfway between the musculotendinous junction and the enthesis (Figure 12.24). (58). It sometimes extends down to the enthesis. It is the author's experience that entheseal tendon

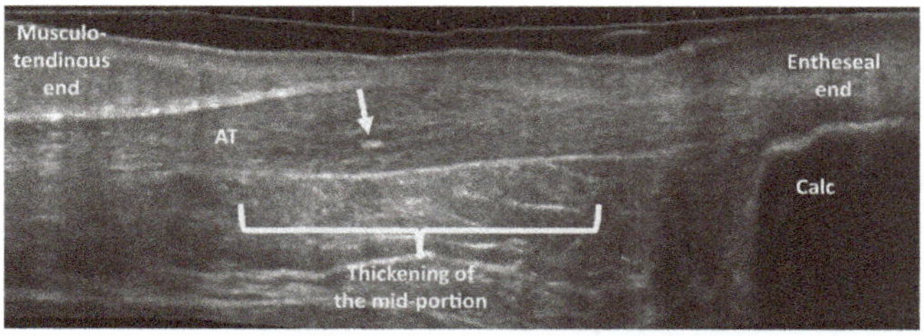

Figure 12.24 Degenerate Achilles tendinopathy. Longitudinal view through a degenerate Achilles tendon (AT). There is fusiform swelling noted in the midportion of the tendon with relative normal tendon proximally (toward the musculotendinous junction) and distally (at insertion). A small hyperechoic focus (arrow) is seen within the substance of the tendon, which possibly reflects a small calcification. Calc, calcaneum.

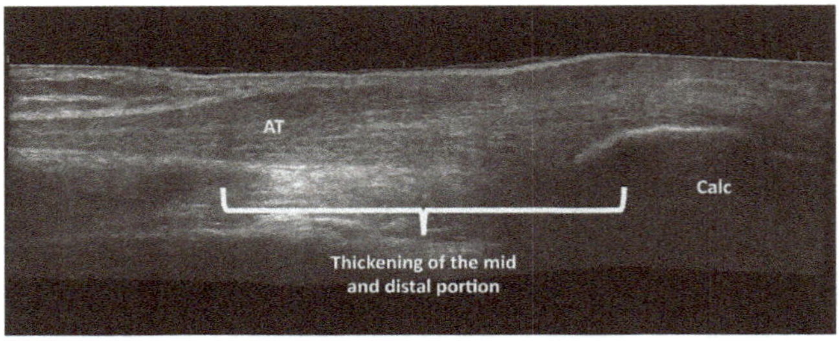

Figure 12.25 Longitudinal view of a degenerative Achilles tendon (AT). Rather than being only localized to the midportion, there are changes extending distally to the insertion into the calcaneum (Calc).

abnormalities rarely extend proximally and, therefore, if both are seen then the likely cause is primarily a tendinopathy (Figure 12.25). The ultrasound features of tendinopathy have been noted in the section on 'Tendon and ligament pathology' but can sometimes be seen to have intrasubstance tears which can extend to full thickness and rupture (Figure 12.26). The vascularity of the Achilles tendon is often associated with pain (Figure 12.27a). It is rarely seen in the plantar fascia (Figure 12.27b), either because of an inflammatory or mechanical cause.

Dactylitis

This is a clinical term used to describe a diffusely swollen digit. It is commonly observed in patients with psoriatic arthritis but may also be seen in gout, sarcoidosis, or even infection. The features seen on ultrasound include soft-tissue oedema (often with increased Doppler signal), tenosynovitis, and joint synovitis (59) (Figure 12.28).

Cartilage and joint space

Normal hyaline cartilage is seen as a hypoechoic rim over the articular bone surface. Because of the lack of an acoustic window, ultrasound is unable to visualize the whole cartilage surface, but even a limited view may provide an indication of the state of the cartilage elsewhere. Crystals may be deposited on the surface of the cartilage in gout, producing what is known as the double contour sign (60). This is typically seen in the first MTP joint but may be seen in other MTP joints and foot joints as well (Figure 12.29). Other features of gout may be observed concomitantly, such as echogenic microaggregates within the adjacent synovium consistent with tophi.

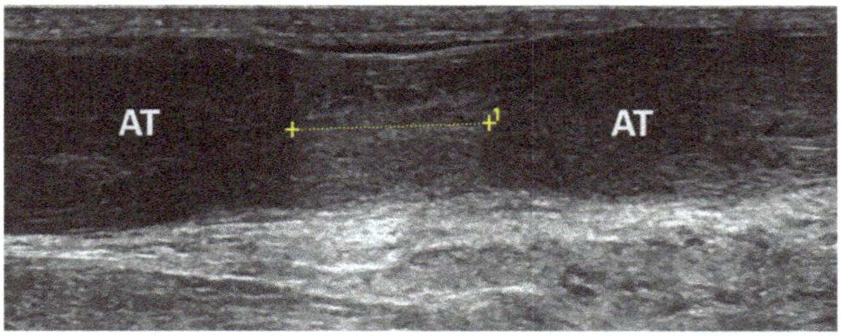

Figure 12.26 Longitudinal scan through a degenerate Achilles tendon (AT) that has torn. The tendon is hypoechogenic and thickened. There is a gap noted, suggesting a retracted full thickness tear.

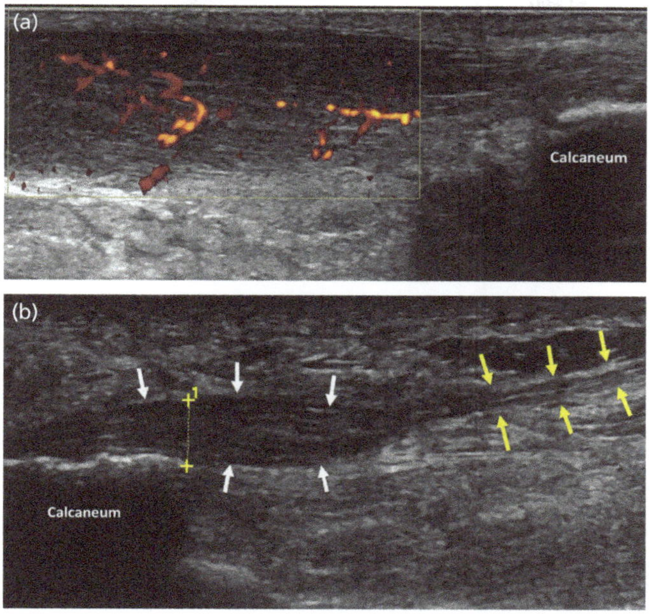

Figure 12.27 (a) Longitudinal section through the Achilles tendon of a patient with midportion–distal tendinopathy, likely to be secondary to degenerative causes. There is thickening of the tendon, in addition to marked vascularity. The enthesis appears relatively normal. (b) Longitudinal view through the plantar fascia of a patient with heel pain when weightbearing. The insertion of the fascia at the calcaneum is thickened (white arrows) and hypoechoic but does not exhibit any Doppler. The fascia thickness is normally thinner as it spreads out towards the toes (yellow arrows), but the proximal part is abnormally thick. The normal upper limit of thickness is <5 mm; here it was 6.3 mm (here measured using electronic calipers; yellow dotted line).

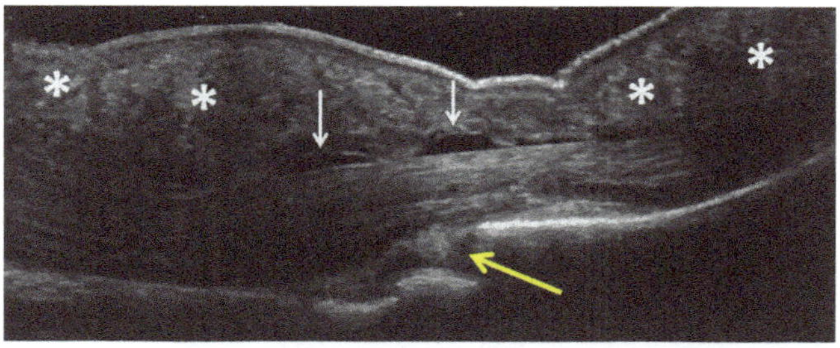

Figure 12.28 Longitudinal view through the plantar aspect of a toe with dactylitis from a patient with psoriatic arthritis. There is marked subcutaneous oedema/thickening (*), which on Doppler studies is frequently very vascular (not shown in this image). The white arrows represent fluid in the flexor tendon sheath, which is commonly seen in tenosynovitis. A small degree of greyscale synovitis is also seen in the joint (yellow arrow).

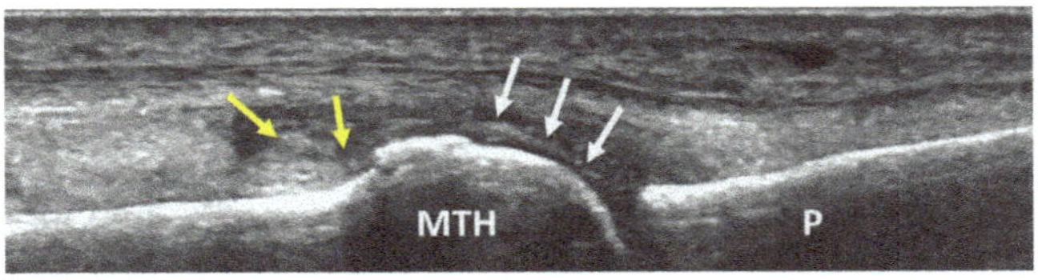

Figure 12.29 Longitudinal view through a first metatarsophalangeal joint. The white arrows demonstrate a double contour sign consistent with gout. There are also some additional hyperechoic foci in the joint space consistent with microaggregates of uric acid crystals. MTH, Metatarsal head; P, phalanx.

Alongside a loss of cartilage is a loss of joint space, which is a surrogate marker of the former. Ultrasound can provide an estimation of a loss of joint space (as well as directly visualizing the cartilage), but this has not been standardized for research.

Bone fractures

Although not common in rheumatology, stress fractures, especially of the metatarsals, may be seen. There is usually a history of mechanical stress but not always. The foot will usually be swollen on the dorsal aspect and very painful in the initial stages. A fracture may be seen as a discontinuity of the bone cortical surface (Figure 12.30); later, callus formation is seen. There is often a local soft-tissue inflammatory response with increased Doppler signal noted in the vicinity.

Morton's neuroma

Both ultrasound and MRI can be used to identify a Morton's neuroma. It has been suggested that they need to be at least 5 mm in diameter before they can be seen on ultrasound. They can be difficult to distinguish from an intermetatarsal bursae. Both conditions have been noted to occur simultaneously as they probably have a similar aetiology of mechanical stress (61).

Interventions

A significant benefit of ultrasound is its ability to direct a needle for aspirating a lesion, administrating treatments such as corticosteroids and local anaesthetic, or performing procedures such as biopsies or dry needling of tendons (62). Needle guidance can be either indirect (where the skin is marked after an ultrasound, but the needle is placed without the ultrasound)

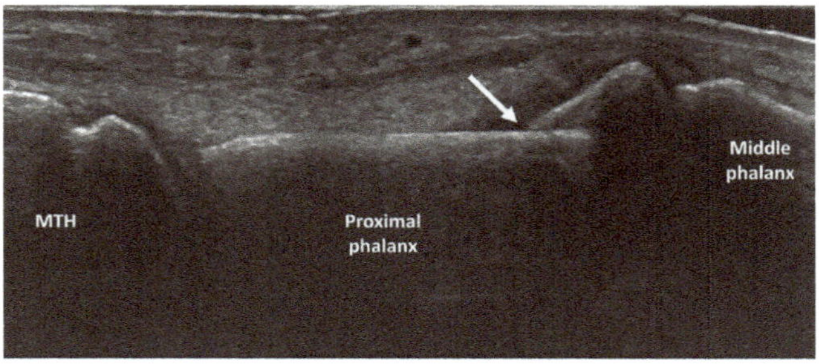

Figure 12.30 Longitudinal dorsal view through a toe demonstrating a displaced fracture of the distal middle phalanx. The fracture is shown as a discontinuity of the bone surface (white arrow). There is no callus formation, suggesting it is quite recent. MTH, Metatarsal head.

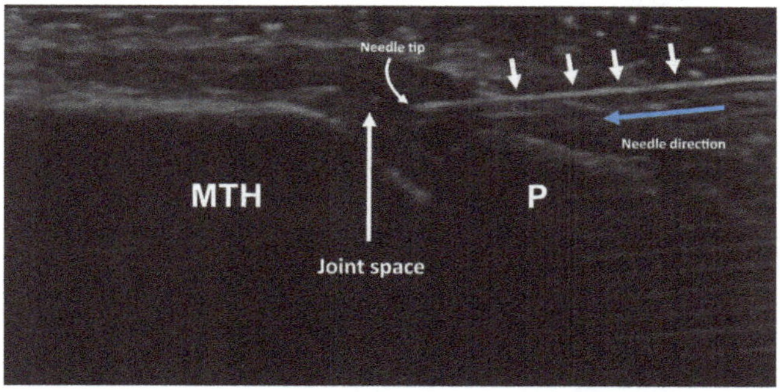

Figure 12.31 Longitudinal scan through a metatarsophalangeal joint. The needle (white arrows) is advanced so that the tip is accurately placed within the joint space. MTH, Metatarsal head; P, phalanx.

or directly under guidance (Figure 12.31). The preferred method is to use direct guidance as the needle can be observed throughout the process from skin surface to target region, thereby reducing the risk of hitting a neurovascular structure. With the indirect approach, it is possible that the patient may move, thus changing the relationship of the skin mark with the target.

Conclusion

In conclusion, imaging provides an additional means to investigate a wide range of foot and ankle disorders but should always be used in the context of the clinical history and examination. The techniques can assist in diagnosis and monitoring of rheumatic disease as well as enabling the guidance of interventions. Each modality has its own strengths and weaknesses, and use is dependent on the question being asked.

References

1. **Foley-Nolan D, et al.** Magnetic resonance imaging in the assessment of rheumatoid arthritis—a comparison with plain film radiographs. *Br J Rheumatol.* 1991;**30**(2):101–6.
2. **Paskins Z, Rai A.** The impact of Picture Archiving and Communication Systems (PACS) implementation in rheumatology. *Rheumatology (Oxford).* 2006;**45**(3):354–5.
3. **Chen TS, et al.** Magnetic resonance imaging is more sensitive than radiographs in detecting change in size of erosions in rheumatoid arthritis. *J Rheumatol.* 2006;**33**(10):1957–67.
4. **Erdem CZ, et al.** MR imaging features of foot involvement in ankylosing spondylitis. *Eur J Radiol.* 2005;**53**(1):110–19.
5. **Gold RH, et al.** Imaging the diabetic foot. *Skeletal Radiol.* 1995;**24**(8):563–71.
6. **Goodwin DW, et al.** Plantar compartments of the foot: MR appearance in cadavers and diabetic patients. *Radiology.* 1995;**196**(3):623–30.
7. **Cofield RH, Morrison MJ, Beabout JW.** Diabetic neuroarthropathy in the foot: patient characteristics and patterns of radiographic change. *Foot Ankle.* 1983;**4**(1):15–22.
8. **Clouse ME, et al.** Diabetic osteoarthropathy. Clinical and roentgenographic observations in 90 cases. *Am J Roentgenol Radium Ther Nucl Med.* 1974;**121**(1):22–34.
9. **Cappello ZJ, Kasdan ML, Louis DS.** Meta-analysis of imaging techniques for the diagnosis of complex regional pain syndrome type I. *J Hand Surg Am.* 2012;**37**(2):288–96.
10. **Johnson PT, Fayad LM, Fishman EK.** CT of the foot: selected inflammatory arthridites. *J Comp Assisted Tom.* 2007;**31**(6):961–9.

11. **Perry D, et al.** Detection of erosions in the rheumatoid hand; a comparative study of multidetector computerized tomography versus magnetic resonance scanning. *J Rheumatol.* 2005;**32**(2):256–67.
12. **Primak AN, et al.** Noninvasive differentiation of uric acid versus non-uric acid kidney stones using dual-energy CT. *Acad Radiol.* 2007;**14**(12):1441–7.
13. **Kang M-J, et al.** Dual-energy CT: clinical applications in various pulmonary diseases 1. *Radiographics.* 2010;**30**(3):685–98.
14. **Ruzsics B, et al.** Dual-energy CT of the heart for diagnosing coronary artery stenosis and myocardial ischemia—initial experience. *Eur Radiol.* 2008;**18**(11):2414–24.
15. **Thieme SF, et al.** Dual energy CT for the assessment of lung perfusion—correlation to scintigraphy. *Eur J Radiol.* 2008;**68**(3):369–74.
16. **Gerster JC, et al.** Imaging of tophaceous gout: computed tomography provides specific images compared with magnetic resonance imaging and ultrasonography. *Ann Rheum Dis.* 2002;**61**(1):52–4.
17. **Girish G, Glazebrook KN, Jacobson JA.** Advanced imaging in gout. *AJR Am J Roentgenol.* 2013;**201**(3):515–25.
18. **Nicolaou S, et al.** Dual-energy CT as a potential new diagnostic tool in the management of gout in the acute setting. *AJR Am J Roentgenol.* 2010;**194**(4):1072–8.
19. **Mallinson PI, et al.** Artifacts in dual-energy CT gout protocol: a review of 50 suspected cases with an artifact identification guide. *AJR Am J Roentgenol.* 2014;**203**(1):W103–W109.
20. **Jamar F, et al.** Inflammatory arthritis: imaging of endothelial cell activation with an indium-111-labeled F(ab')2 fragment of anti-E-selectin monoclonal antibody. *Radiology.* 1995;**194**(3):843–50.
21. **Jamar F, et al.** A comparison between ^{111}In-anti-E-selectin mAb and ^{99}Tcm-labelled human non-specific immunoglobulin in radionuclide imaging of rheumatoid arthritis. *Br J Radiol.* 1997;**70**(833):473–81.
22. **Tumeh SS.** Scintigraphy in the evaluation of arthropathy. *Radiol Clin North Am.* 1996;**34**(2):215–31, ix.
23. **Barrera P, et al.** Scintigraphic detection of tumour necrosis factor in patients with rheumatoid arthritis. *Ann Rheum Dis.* 2003;**62**(9):825–8.
24. **Beckers C, et al.** ^{18}F-FDG PET imaging of rheumatoid knee synovitis correlates with dynamic magnetic resonance and sonographic assessments as well as with the serum level of metalloproteinase-3. *Eur J Nuc Med Mol Imag.* 2006;**33**(3):275–80.
25. **Chaudhari AJ, et al.** High-resolution ^{18}F-FDG PET with MRI for monitoring response to treatment in rheumatoid arthritis. *Eur J Nuc Med Mol Imag.* 2010;**37**(5):1047.
26. **Goerres GW, et al.** F-18 FDG whole-body PET for the assessment of disease activity in patients with rheumatoid arthritis. *Clin Nucl Med.* 2006;**31**(7):386–90.
27. **dos Anjos DA, et al.** Extra-articular inflammatory sites detected by F-18 FDG PET/CT in a patient with rheumatoid arthritis. *Clin Nucl Med.* 2010;**35**(7):540–1.
28. **Aliabadi P, Nikpoor N, Alparslan L.** Imaging of neuropathic arthropathy. *Semin Musculoskelet Radiol.* 2003;7(3):217–25.
29. **Poirier JY, et al.** Diagnosis of osteomyelitis in the diabetic foot with a ^{99m}Tc-HMPAO leucocyte scintigraphy combined with a ^{99m}Tc-MDP bone scintigraphy. *Diabetes Metab.* 2002;**28**(6 Pt 1):485–90.
30. **Schauwecker DS, et al.** Combined bone scintigraphy and indium-111 leukocyte scans in neuropathic foot disease. *J Nucl Med.* 1988;**29**(10):1651–5.
31. **Yuh WT, et al.** Osteomyelitis of the foot in diabetic patients: evaluation with plain film ^{99m}Tc-MDP bone scintigraphy and MR imaging. *AJR Am J Roentgenol.* 1989;**152**(4):795–800.
32. **Genant HK, et al.** The reflex sympathetic dystrophy syndrome. A comprehensive analysis using fine-detail radiography photon absorptiometry and bone and joint scintigraphy. *Radiology.* 1975;**117**(1):21–32.
33. **Korompilias AV, et al.** Bone marrow edema syndrome. *Skeletal Radiol.* 2009;**38**(5):425–36.
34. **McQueen FM.** The MRI view of synovitis and tenosynovitis in inflammatory arthritis: implications for diagnosis and management. *Ann N Y Acad Sci.* 2009;**1154**:21–34.

35. **Tamai K, et al.** Dynamic magnetic resonance imaging for the evaluation of synovitis in patients with rheumatoid arthritis. *Arthritis Rheum.* 1994;**37**(8):1151–7.
36. **McGonagle D, et al.** Histological assessment of the early enthesitis lesion in spondyloarthropathy. *Ann Rheum Dis.* 2002;**61**(6):534–7.
37. **Hodgson RJ, O'Connor PJ, Grainger AJ.** Tendon and ligament imaging. *Br J Radiol.* 2012;**85**(1016):1157–72.
38. **Eshed I, et al.** Tenosynovitis of the flexor tendons of the hand detected by MRI: an early indicator of rheumatoid arthritis. *Rheumatology (Oxford).* 2009;**48**(8):887–91.
39. **Marcus CD, et al.** MR imaging of osteomyelitis and neuropathic osteoarthropathy in the feet of diabetics. *Radiographics* 1996;**16**(6):1337–48.
40. **Siddle HJ, et al.** MRI identifies plantar plate pathology in the forefoot of patients with rheumatoid arthritis. *Clin Rheumatol.* 2012;**31**(4):621–9.
41. **McQueen FM, Ostendorf B.** What is MRI bone oedema in rheumatoid arthritis and why does it matter? *Arthritis Res Ther* 2006;**8**(6):222.
42. **Chowdhury FU, Robinson P, Grainger AJ, Harris N.** Transient regional osteoporosis: a rare case of foot and ankle pain. *Foot Ankle Surg.* 2006;**12**(2):79–83.
43. **Hofmann S, et al.** Painful bone marrow edema of the knee: differential diagnosis and therapeutic concepts. *Orthop Clin North Am.* 2004;**35**(3):321–33, ix.
44. **Morrison WB, et al.** Diagnosis of osteomyelitis: utility of fat-suppressed contrast-enhanced MR imaging. *Radiology.* 1993;**189**(1):251–7.
45. **Schett G, Gravallese E.** Bone erosion in rheumatoid arthritis: mechanisms diagnosis and treatment. *Nat Rev Rheumatol.* 2012;**8**(11):656–64.
46. **Siddle HJ, et al.** Anatomical location of erosions at the metatarsophalangeal joints in patients with rheumatoid arthritis. *Rheumatology (Oxford).* 2014;**53**(5):932–6.
47. **Siddle HJ, et al.** The EULAR points to consider for health professionals undertaking musculoskeletal ultrasound for rheumatic and musculoskeletal diseases. *Ann Rheum Dis.* 2018;**77**:311–13.
48. **Grigor C, et al.** Effect of a treatment strategy of tight control for rheumatoid arthritis (the TICORA study): a single-blind randomised controlled trial. *Lancet.* 2004;**364**:263–9.
49. **Coates L, et al.** Effect of tight control of inflammation in early psoriatic arthritis (TICOPA): a UK multicentre open-label randomised controlled trial. *Lancet.* 2015;**386**:2489–98.
50. **Wakefield RJ, et al.** Musculoskeletal ultrasound including definitions for ultrasonographic pathology. *J Rheumatol.* 2005;**32**:2485–7.
51. **Brown AK, et al.** Presence of significant synovitis in rheumatoid arthritis patients with disease-modifying antirheumatic drug-induced clinical remission: evidence from an imaging study may explain structural progression. *Arthritis Rheum.* 2006;**54**:3761–73.
52. **Alcalde M, et al.** A systematic literature review of US definitions scoring systems and validity according to the OMERACT filter for tendon lesion in RA and other inflammatory joint diseases. *Rheumatology (Oxford).* 2012;**51**:1246.
53. **Terslev L, et al.** Outcome Measures in Rheumatology Ultrasound Task Force Defining enthesitis in spondyloarthritis by ultrasound: results of a Delphi process and of a reliability reading exercise. *Arthritis Care Res (Hoboken).* 2014;**66**:741–8.
54. **Wakefield R, et al.** The value of sonography in the detection of bone erosions in patients with rheumatoid arthritis: a comparison with conventional radiography. *Arthritis Rheum.* 2000;**43**:2762–70.
55. **Hammer HB, et al.** Global ultrasound assessment of structural lesions in osteoarthritis: a reliability study by the OMERACT ultrasonography group on scoring cartilage and osteophytes in finger joints. *Ann Rheum Dis.* 2016;**75**:402–7.
56. **McGonagle D, et al.** Distinct topography of erosion and new bone formation in Achilles tendon enthesitis: implications for understanding the link between inflammation and bone formation in spondyloarthritis. *Arthritis Rheum.* 2008;**58**:2694–9.

57. **Bowen C, et al.** Assessment of the natural history of forefoot bursae using ultrasonography in patients with rheumatoid arthritis: a twelve-month investigation. *Arthritis Care Res (Hoboken).* 2010;**62**:1756–62.
58. **Wijesekera NT, et al.** Imaging in the assessment and management of Achilles tendinopathy and paratendinitis. *Semin Musculoskelet Radiol.* 2011;**15**:89–100.
59. **Bakewell CJ, et al.** OMERACT Ultrasound Task Force Ultrasound and magnetic resonance imaging in the evaluation of psoriatic dactylitis: status and perspectives. *J Rheumatol.* 2013;**40**:1951–7.
60. **Sivera F, et al.** Diagnostic value of clinical laboratory and imaging findings in patients with a clinical suspicion of gout: a systematic literature review. *J Rheumatol Suppl.* 2014;**92**:3–8.
61. **Cohen SL, et al.** Sonography of Morton neuromas: what are we really looking at? *J Ultrasound Med.* 2016;**35**:2191–5.
62. **Yablon CM.** Ultrasound-guided interventions of the foot and ankle. *Semin Musculoskelet Radiol.* 2013;**17**:60–8.

Chapter 13

Pathomechanics and gait analysis

Graham Chapman and Philip Helliwell

Introduction

Gait analysis is the study of human walking and is often used to describe and understand how different musculoskeletal conditions affect lower limb function. Gait analysis techniques can range from very simple to very complex, depending on the requirements of the user and/or the clinical rationale for requiring gait analysis in understanding the relationship between pathology and function. This chapter will describe the two-way interaction between biological processes of the human body and lower limb mechanics and link these processes to functional/mechanical changes that are evident in musculoskeletal diseases by describing disease-specific changes to foot/ankle function. We will provide a detailed overview of the different techniques used for gait analysis and highlight how different musculoskeletal conditions of the foot and ankle affect how we walk; each technique is critiqued to highlight which technique is best depending on what the user/clinician requires. Finally, we will discuss how clinicians can use (bio)mechanical information within a clinical setting.

At Leeds, the gait laboratory houses a full range of equipment that allows us to understand the complex relationship between biological processes associated with musculoskeletal disease and mechanics of the foot and ankle, as well as other lower limb joints. This laboratory is designed to allow for greater insight and understanding of how rheumatic and musculoskeletal disease affects joints and how patients may adapt their gait due to pain and/or disease states during activities of daily living. We can also use this equipment to understand the impact of musculoskeletal disease on foot/ankle function, understand how treatment affects function, and also provide clinicians with greater detail of how a patient might function via a referral process.

Pathomechanics of gait are linked to pathology

Most of the work in this area has been done in rheumatoid arthritis (RA) (1). In the rearfoot, excessive and prolonged eversion is the hallmark motion pattern in patients with progressive pes planovalgus (2, 3). It is characterized by progressive shift towards eversion as the subtalar joint becomes unstable. Woodburn et al. found evidence to support early motion changes (disease duration ~5 years) in patients with active peritalar disease: abnormal eversion of the calcaneus at heel-strike, everted subtalar alignment through the entire stance phase of gait, and insufficient inversion motion during propulsion to establish a neutral or inverted subtalar joint alignment (2).

The subtalar joint has a 'torque converter' role, which couples subtalar joint inversion with external leg rotation, and eversion with internal leg rotation. Therefore, the pronated foot is associated with compensatory proximal and distal adaptations such that, in the pes planovalgus foot, the ankle joint complex fails to reach a neutral or inversion alignment, resulting in the lower leg failing to reach a neutral or externally rotated alignment under the barefoot walking condition

(3). As a potential injury mechanism, valgus heel and knee deformities are frequently observed together in RA.

RA is primarily a synovial disease, but articular inflammation will extend to the periarticular region and cause inflammation of the capsule and surrounding ligaments. Further, major tendons are enclosed in a sheath lined with synovium. The medial ankle (e.g., deltoid ligament) and tarsal joint ligaments have important stabilizing functions, and tibialis posterior is considered the major muscle maintaining the medial longitudinal arch. Persistent or repeated inflammation at these sites leads to collapse of the arch (pes planus) or valgus of the hindfoot (pes valgus) or both (pes planovalgus) depending on the patterns of joint and soft-tissue involvement. Under physiological loads, the largest tarsal joint rotations are found at the talonavicular joint, especially in the frontal plane, and this joint is frequently inflamed in RA (4). This joint remains stable because the inferior calcaneonavicular (the spring ligament) and the superomedial calcaneonavicular ligaments are load-bearing and resist medial and plantar displacement of the talar head, assisted by the expansive insertion and blending of the tibialis posterior to the tuberosity of the navicular. However, persistent inflammation will weaken these structures and eventually result in 'collapse of the medial arch'.

In the forefoot, persistent inflammation of metatarsophalangeal (MTP) joints is a hallmark of RA and may be the first clinical feature of disease. Synovitis results in localized pain and swelling so that a patient may change their gait to accommodate the symptoms—hence slower cadence (reduces ground reaction forces, and reluctance to 'toe-off') and increased double support time. Persistent inflammation leads to joint and ligament damage, resulting in stretching and weakening of the capsular distensions and loss of integrity of the stabilizing structures, such as the collateral ligaments and plantar plate. As a consequence, first subluxation and eventually dislocation of the MTP joints occurs. The plantar fat pad, which usually lies beneath the MTP joints, is pulled distally, exposing the metatarsal heads to increased pressure. In addition to the plantar metatarsal effects, the subluxation and dislocations of the MTP joints create an imbalance between the intrinsic and extrinsic muscles of the foot, resulting in progressive hammer or claw toe deformities and pressure lesions on the dorsum of the interphalangeal joints. The result is loss of toe weightbearing and increased pressure under the metatarsal heads, clinically demonstrated by the development of skin callosities and bursae. The hallux also loses its capsular integrity and deviates laterally from the long axis of the metatarsal into a valgus position.

The eventual result is a combination of forefoot, midfoot, and rearfoot disease. The identifiable pes planovalgus deformity of the midfoot and rearfoot in RA is manifested by flattening of the medial longitudinal arch, valgus deformity of the calcaneus, and tibialis posterior dysfunction. The medial arch collapse is demonstrable by plantar pressure measurements. Initially the foot remains mobile, but the incidence of rigid flatfoot increases with disease duration. Varus deformity has also been described in a minority of patients: the mechanism may be related to an attempt to avoid loading the metatarsal heads by walking on the outside of the foot (1).

Measuring mechanical change and pathomechanics in musculoskeletal diseases

There are a number of different techniques that can be used to analyse gait to understand foot/ankle function in healthy individuals and those with different musculoskeletal conditions. Over the years, gait analysis has developed from simply observing a patient in clinic through to descriptive techniques, and modern, highly complex systems. This section will provide some insight into a range of techniques that can be used (and are used within our gait laboratory) to understand the impact of rheumatic and musculoskeletal disease on foot and ankle function.

Temporal and spatial parameters

Instrumented walkways

Descriptive measurements of gait can be broken down into temporal (timing) and spatial (distance) components defined by the different phases of the gait cycle based on when the foot is in contact with the ground (stance phase) or in the air (swing phase). Double support occurs when both feet are on the ground at the same time whereas single support is when only one foot is on the floor (Figure 13.1).

The simplest method for determining temporal measures such as walking speed or cadence can be determined by using a stopwatch or counting the number of steps to complete a set distance. These measures are, however, very descriptive, prone to user error, and do not detail symmetry or describe how the lower limbs move or durations of how long the foot is in contact with the ground. Simple spatial measures can be collected where individuals walk on paper with marker pens attached to shoes or feet/shoes dipped in ink result in step and/or stride length and width being measured. These techniques are also very time-consuming and subject to human error.

Commercially available instrumented walkways are a common feature in most gait laboratories and in some clinical settings. These walkways consist of either a solid or portable matting with embedded pressure sensors that detect and record each footfall made along the length of the walkway. With the use of dedicated software associated with the instrumented walkway, automated calculations of temporal and spatial measures are obtained, allowing for quick acquisition of data (~5 minutes), which is appealing in research and clinical settings. In our gait laboratory in Leeds, we use a GAITRite™ instrumented walkway (Figure 13.2a) to measure temporal and spatial gait parameters. This system is portable, easy to use, and can collect data on patients barefoot or shod, and also when patients require/use assistive walking devices. It is well established that the GAITRite™ system is valid, reliable (5, 6), and can detect gait differences between musculoskeletal conditions and healthy individuals (7). Figure 13.2b depicts an output from the GAITRite™

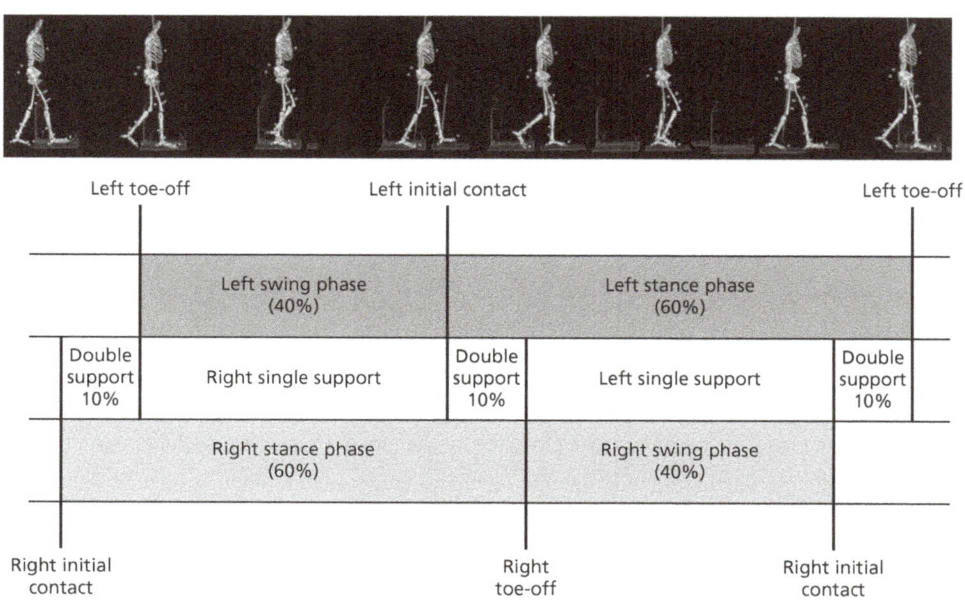

Figure 13.1 A schematic diagram of the different phases of the gait cycle.

(a)

(b)

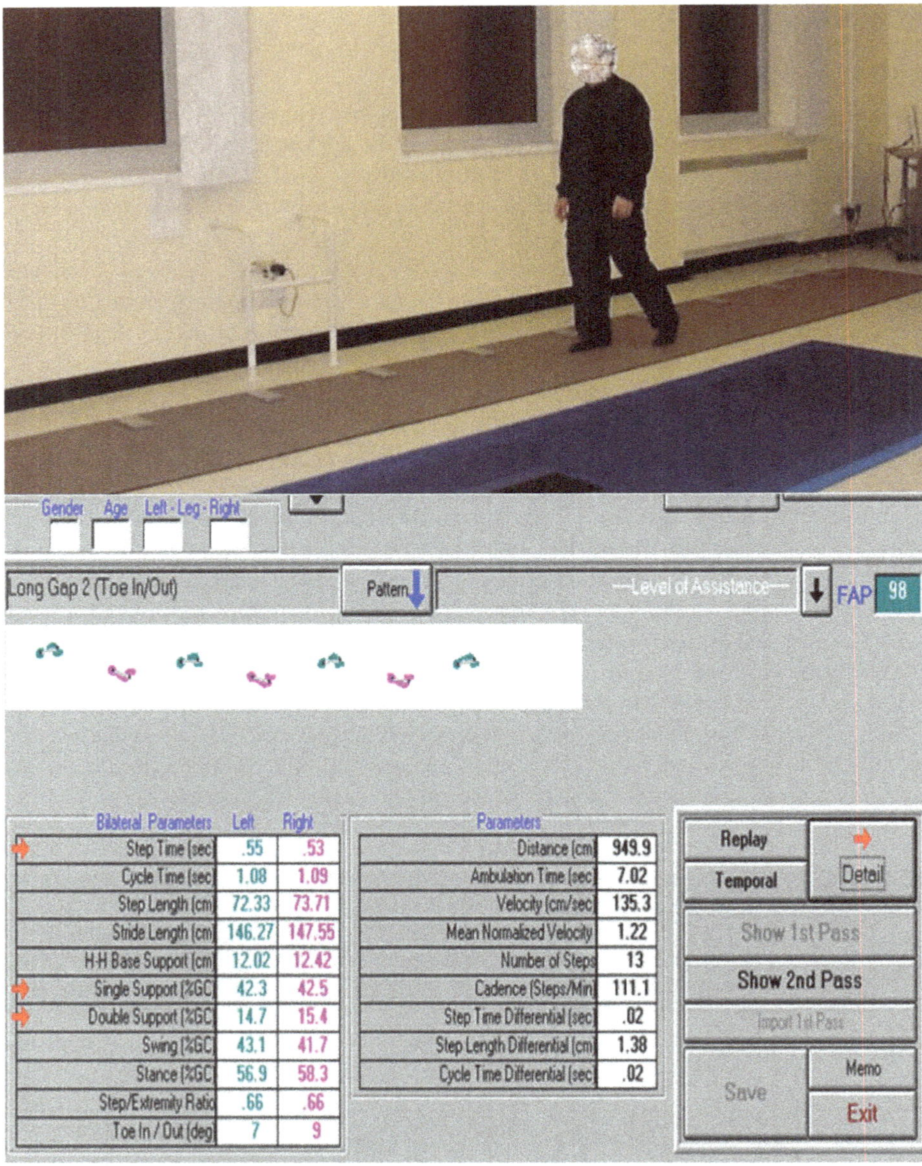

Figure 13.2 (a) A patient walking along the GAITRite™ instrumented walkway. (b) An example of a data output from the GAITRite™ instrumented walkway.

system and illustrates the large number of temporal and spatial variables available based on the footfall patterns acquired from the walkway. Variable outputs can be quantified in absolute units (i.e., seconds or centimetres) or as a percentage of the gait cycle and can be split into unilateral or bilateral outputs.

Studies examining the effect of musculoskeletal conditions on patients' gait typically select a number of temporal and spatial variables that provide a good descriptor of how the patient population is functioning. Patients with RA, for example, typically walk more slowly, with reduced cadence, shorter stride length, and longer durations spent in double support compared to healthy individuals (see Carroll et al. [8] for more details). These temporal spatial gait parameters suggest that patients with RA adopt an antalgic gait to avoid pain in the foot and ankle. Such gait adaptations could be caused by a number of disease-related factors, including severity of disease and/or foot/ankle pain associated with foot deformity. A recent study highlighted the importance of ensuring that repeat measures are conducted at the same time of day in people with an inflammatory condition with known diurnal variation in symptomatology. Backhouse et al. (9) used the GAITRite™ to demonstrate that patients with RA were slower and produced a smaller stride length early in the morning compared to improved gait parameters later on in the day. These findings suggest that, if clinicians and/or future studies aim to collect repeated measures of gait parameters of RA patients, these measures should be conducted at the same time of day to exclude diurnal variation.

The main disadvantage of using instrumented walkways (or other temporal/spatial techniques), however, is that they do not provide any detailed information on how different body segments move with respect to each other (for example, shank or thighs) during gait. Therefore, the user must be cautious regarding the conclusions made when using temporal and spatial parameters in isolation owing to the complex interactions between the disease state, deformity, pain status, and ongoing treatment effect. Overall, however, the ease of data collection and analysis of instrumented walkways (i.e., GaitRite™) makes them an ideal piece of equipment that could assist clinicians in more objective input into clinical decision-making.

Plantar pressure measurements

As already highlighted in Chapter 3, plantar pressure measurements can be acquired in the form of a platform-based system (e.g., Emed SF [Novel GmbH, Munich, Germany]), which is predominantly used for barefoot walking, or an insole-based system (e.g., Pedar [Novel GmbH, Munich, Germany]), which is placed within patients' shoes. Both systems are used at Leeds gait laboratory and are easy to set up; data acquisition is relatively quick (~10 minutes) and easy (compared to 3D gait analysis). Our Emed system consists of 6080 capacitive sensors housed within a sensing area of a 700 × 403-mm plate, similar in appearance to a force plate (Figure 13.3). Similarly, the Pedar system consists of flexible insoles embedded with pressure-sensitive sensors (Figure 13.4). As a result, both systems accurately detect the contact areas of the plantar surface with the sensor plate/insole, the location of the centre of foot pressure (COFP), and the vertical ground reaction force (vGRF) during the stance phase (Figure 13.4b, c). With the known location and magnitude of vGRF and the contact area, plantar pressure can be calculated using the formula, plantar pressure = force/contact area, and is often reported in kPa. The platform system provides the advantage of offering a greater resolution (one or four sensors/cm^2) for barefoot walking compared to the in-shoe system. The in-shoe system, however, allows for more 'real-world' data collection during activities of daily living, i.e., stair ascent or descent or investigating how orthoses change plantar pressure and forces acting on the foot.

For analysis purposes, both systems provide detailed numeric and visual plantar pressure information across the entire plantar surface, allowing for quick feedback/educational tool in a clinical setting (Figure 13.3). Both systems are widely used in research and clinical settings to demonstrate pathological changes over time and/or due to disease severity (Figure 13.5) or response to therapy (Figure 13.6).

The accompanying analysis software (Novel-win program) associated with these systems allows the user to mask predefined regions of the foot (Figure 3.7a, b). In a recent randomized controlled

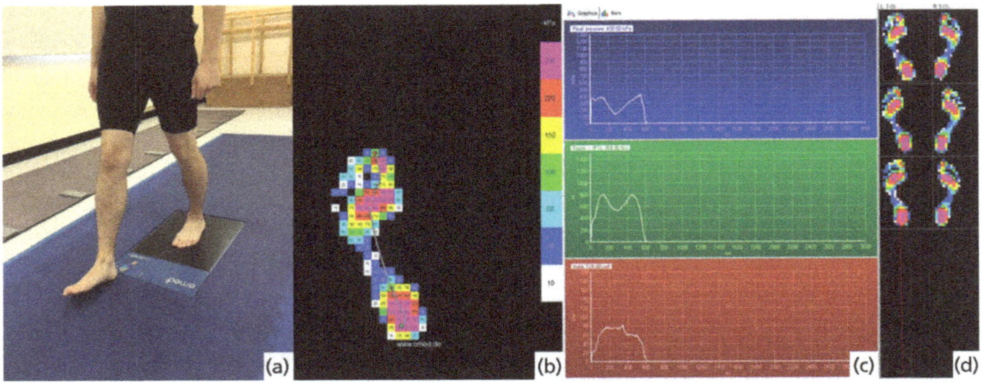

Figure 13.3 (a) An individual walking over the Emed platform. (b) A typical 'footprint' output from Emed illustrating the parts of the foot that have made contact with the platform. The different colours represent the difference in pressure, with white representing low pressure, increasing to pink representing high pressure. The line running through the 'footprint' represents the centre of foot pressure. (c) Graphical output illustrating peak pressure (kPa), force (N), and area (cm^2) during the stance phase on the platform. (d) Number of 'footprints' collected.

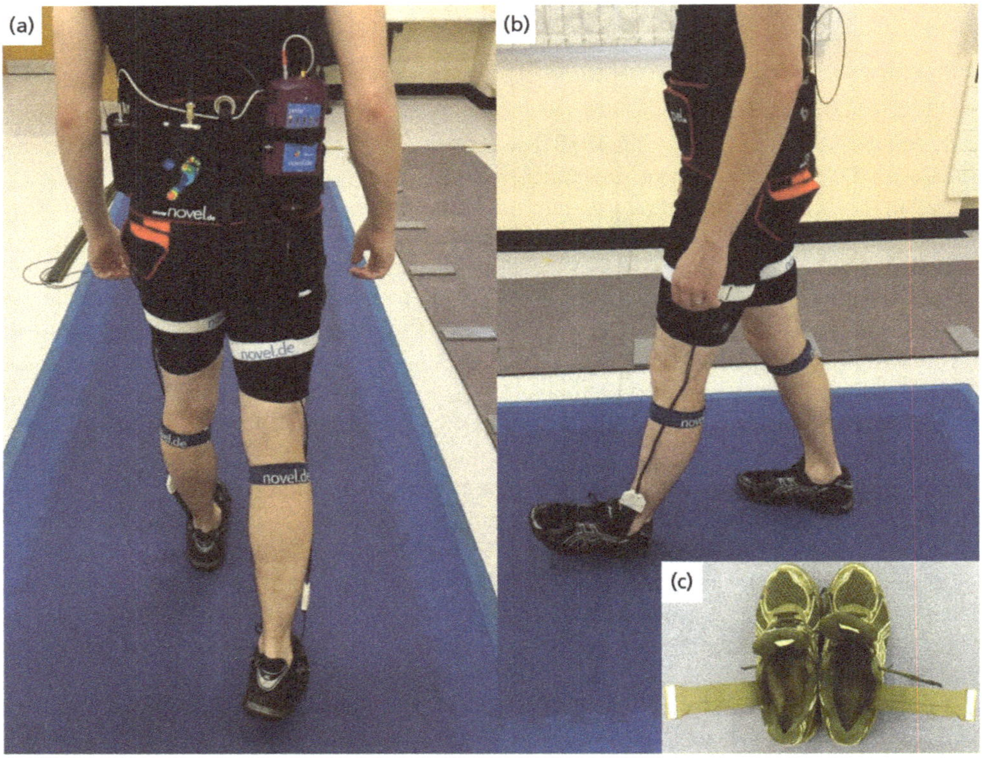

Figure 13.4 (a) Posterior view and (b) sagittal view of a patient walking whilst wearing the Pedar pressure system. (c) Pedar insoles in patient's footwear.

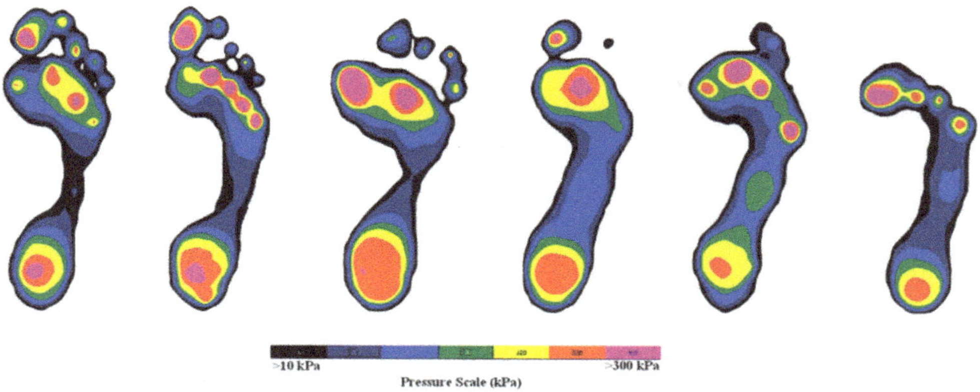

Figure 13.5 Peak pressure distribution profiles of six different patients with rheumatoid arthritis with increasing (left to right) severity of pes planovalgus.

feasibility trial, Halstead et al. (10) used the Pedar in-shoe system to examine the effect of a functional foot orthosis (FFO) compared to a sham orthosis for improving pain and function in symptomatic midfoot osteoarthritis (OA) patients during a 3-month feasibility randomized controlled trial. For the analysis of the plantar pressure data, Halstead et al. (10) used the predefined percentage mask dividing the foot into three regions: hindfoot, midfoot, and forefoot (Figure 13.7a). Results demonstrated that those symptomatic midfoot OA patients assigned to wear an FFO for 12 weeks showed improvements in pain, plantar pressure, and biomechanical measures compared to those assigned to wear a sham orthosis. In an ancillary analysis, Chapman et al. (11) increased the number of regions of interest (Figure 13.7b) to examine the mechanism of action of the FFO and sham used in Halstead et al's. (10) study. This study demonstrated that the same FFO worn for 12 weeks decreased hindfoot and forefoot maximum force and peak pressure, whilst increasing maximum force and contact area under the midfoot. The sham orthosis yielded plantar pressures similar to the shoe-only condition (Figure 13.6).

The number of masked regions can be increased if the user is interested in individual toes or metatarsal heads, for example. Figure 13.7c illustrates a 12-region mask that was used to investigate the plantar pressures of the forefoot in patients with psoriatic arthritis compared to controls (12). Despite Wilkins et al. (12) suggesting that plantar pressures do not differ between groups, this is a good example of how detailed plantar pressures, such as individual toes, can be examined for small regions of the foot.

The software also allows the user to define their own masks for analysing specific areas of clinical interest or to analyse deformed feet. However, questions around the validity of customized plantar pressure masks may arise based on whether the masks accurately represent the anatomical regions of interest. Therefore, care must be taken to ensure their accuracy whether they are intended to be used in clinical practice or research.

One of the main disadvantages of plantar pressure measurements is the lack of information on foot/ankle joint function. The combination of plantar pressure and force/vGRF data allows the user to postulate how foot deformity or orthoses change foot function. However, neither system provides any information on how the ankle or foot joints move during gait. In addition, the Pedar system is a little cumbersome and, despite this system being telemetry-based, a number of wires attached from the insoles to the record on the belt are required (Figure 13.4). Despite these drawbacks, both plantar pressure systems are easy to use and provide quick results, and could be a

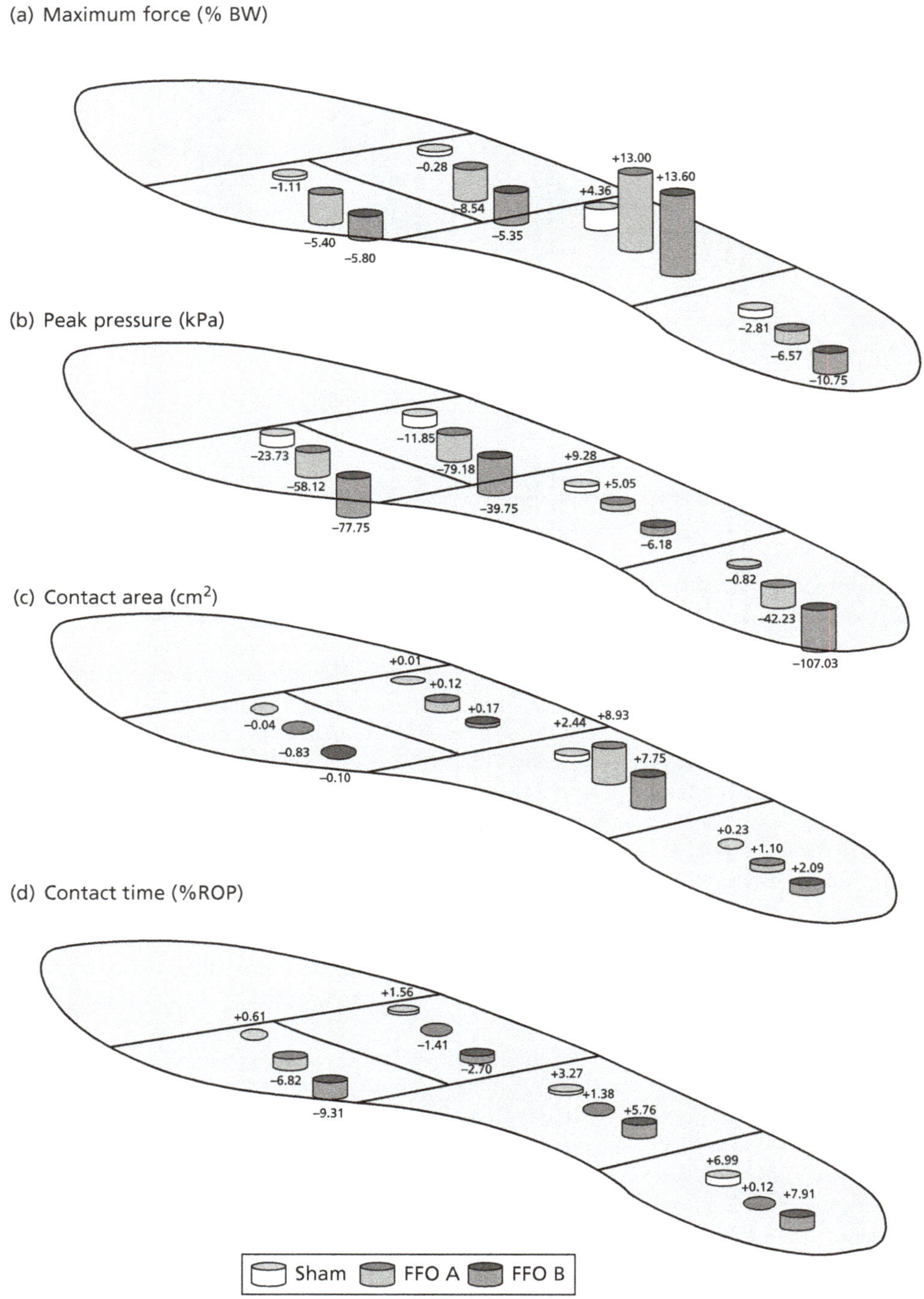

Figure 13.6 Mean change in maximum force (a), peak pressure (b), contact area (c) and contact time (d) under three different insole conditions; sham, functional foot orthosis A (FFO A) and functional foot orthosis B (FFO B). BW, Body weight; %ROP, percentage of rollover process.

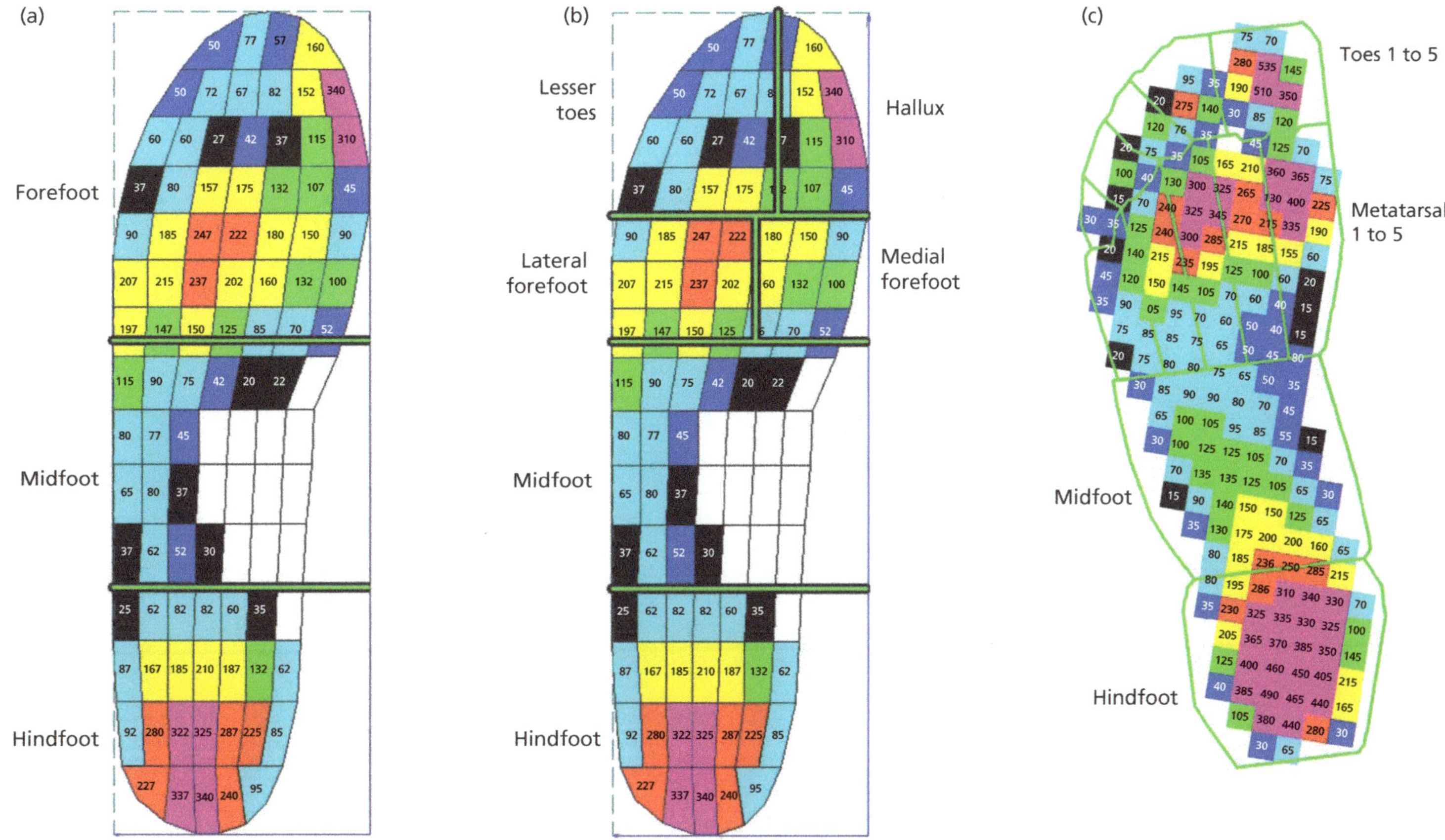

Figure 13.7 (a) Predefined percentage mask dividing the foot into three regions: hindfoot (31%), midfoot (33%), and forefoot (36%) as used by Halstead et al. (10). (b) Predefined percentage mask dividing the foot into six regions: hindfoot (30%), midfoot (30%), medial and lateral forefoot (15%), hallux (25% [length] and 35% [width]) and lesser toes (25% [length] and 65% [width]), as used by Chapman et al. (11); (c) Predefined 12 masked region for examining plantar pressures of the toes.

useful addition in the clinical setting, if available, especially when used as an educational/feedback tool for patients.

Kinematics

For gait analysis purposes, the lower limbs are split into different segments, including the pelvis, thighs, shanks, and feet (Figure 13.8), and kinematics describes, in detail, how one segment moves with respect to an adjoining, distal segment. At least three markers are required on each segment to report the motions in three planes: sagittal, frontal, and transverse, thereby allowing descriptions of flexion/extension, abduction/adduction, and internal/external rotations, respectively.

A common method for collecting accurate and reliable kinematics is through a 3D motion capture system. These systems are quite rare within clinical settings but are often associated with gait laboratories in a research environment. The Leeds gait laboratory houses a 10-camera Vicon motion capture system (Vicon MX, Oxford Metrics, UK) (Figure 13.9) that uses retro-reflective markers that are attached to the participant/patient's skin or placed on non-orthogonal

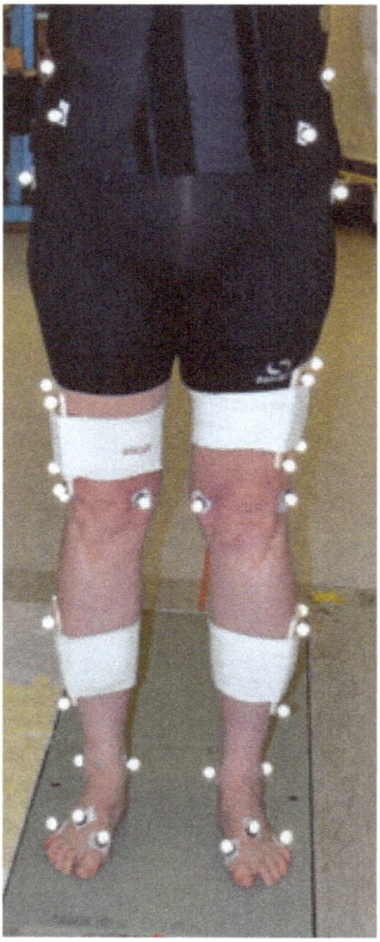

Figure 13.8 The location of retroreflective markers on a patient.

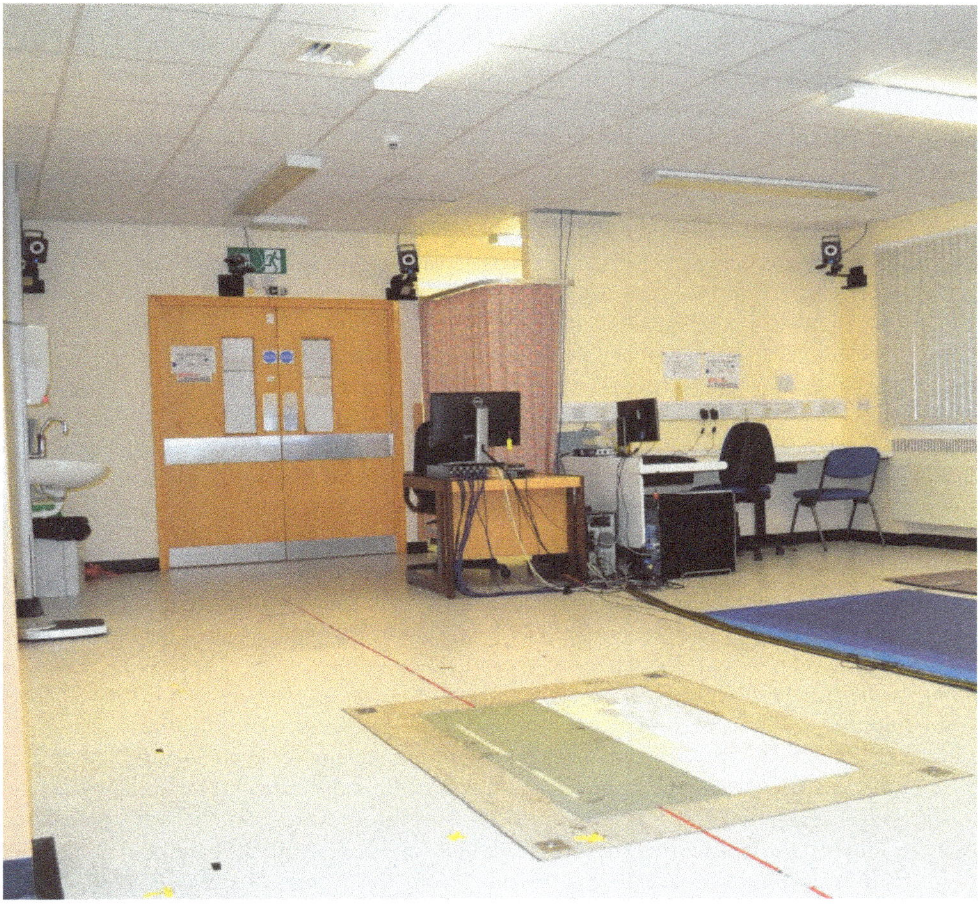

Figure 13.9 The gait laboratory at Chapel Allerton Hospital, Leeds.

pads (Figure 13.8). Other motion capture systems are commercially available and either use the same technology (for example, Qualisys) or are based on 'active' marker systems (for example, Codamotion), in which markers/sensors emit their own signal back to the camera and therefore require less post-processing than retroreflective marker systems. The main disadvantages with 'active' sensor systems stem from the wires that are attached to the markers and the fact that the data capture frequency must be reduced as the number of active sensors increases due to limitations in the hardware.

Typically for gait analysis, these systems collect kinematic data between 60 Hz and 120 Hz; this frequency, however, can be increased depending on the speed of the actions being performed by the subject/patient. To obtain movement data from an individual, retroflective markers need to be attached to the individual. A combination of individual retroreflective markers and orthogonal tracking pads are used. The individual markers are placed on bony, anatomical landmarks, to define joint centres, and non-orthogonal tracking pads track the moving segments with respect to the relative joint centres. These are initially captured during a static, calibration trial at the beginning of the session (Figure 13.8). Data is then collected on the patient/individual walking, normally collecting between three and five trials. Post-processing involves filtering the raw data and selecting the appropriate part of the walking trials, i.e., from heel-strike on the force plate to the following heel-strike of the same limb. This data is then exported to a third-party piece of software called Visual3D (C-Motion, Rockville, Maryland, USA), which is a user-friendly biomechanical analysis tool that allows the user to create and view biomechanical models and provides all the necessary tools to analyse biomechanical data. At Leeds, we create reports that allow us to view the kinematic data for quality assurance purposes before extracting the relevant data; for example, minimum/maximum joint angles or joint range of motion (Figure 13.10).

Whilst this biomechanical model produces repeatable kinematic data, the user, however, needs a good anatomical knowledge to identify the correct locations for the anatomical markers. Another source of error can come from soft-tissue artifact, whereby movement of excessive skin and subcutaneous adipose tissue independent of the underlying bones leads to measurement error. In the Leeds gait laboratory, we attempt to overcome this potential limitation by using non-orthogonal tracking pads that are tightly attached to the individual's thighs and shank (Figure 13.8).

There are a number of biomechanical models that can be used to obtain ankle/foot kinematics. The simplest model defines the foot as a single segment with four markers placed on the first and fifth metatarsal heads, one positioned on the midfoot and one positioned on the posterior calcaneus (Figure 13.8). This model provides basic information on how the ankle complex moves in all three planes, therefore giving such information as ankle plantar flexion/dorsiflexion, inversion/eversion, and foot abduction/adduction. Figure 13.10 depicts data from all lower limb joints, with the bottom row depicting kinematics of the ankle joint complex. During a normal gait cycle, the stance phase can be split into three subphases based on the sagittal motion of the ankle (Figure 13.11): 1) the heel rocker; 2) the ankle rocker; and 3) the forefoot rocker. The heel rocker begins at heel-strike, where the ankle is in a slight plantar flexed position pivoting around the calcaneus (the continuation of plantar flexion) until the end of the heel rocker when the foot is flat on the ground. The ankle rocker is where the ankle moves from plantar flexion to dorsiflexion, during which the shank (tibia and fibula) rotate forward around the ankle, allowing forward progression of the body. During the forefoot rocker, the foot rotates around the forefoot, starting when the calcaneus lifts off the ground, evident by the ankle beginning to plantar flex and continuing until maximum plantar flexion is achieved at toe-off. During the swing phase the ankle dorsiflexes, enabling the foot to clear the ground and avoiding stumbling/tripping, before returning to slight plantar flexion at heel-strike. In the frontal plane, for the majority of individuals, inversion occurs at heel-strike, and progresses to eversion during mid-stance phase, allowing the heel to rise and push off into swing. This basic biomechanical foot model allows the user/clinician to understand how musculoskeletal conditions affect gross foot/ankle motion. The main disadvantage is the simplicity of the model in that it does not allow the tracking of all the bones/joints in the foot and ankle.

For those clinicians and/or researchers wishing to understand how the foot/ankle moves in more detail there are a number of biomechanical models that can be used. The two most common are the Oxford Foot Model (OFM) (13) (Figure 13.12) and Rizzoli Foot Model (14, 15) (Figure 13.13). These biomechanical models split the foot into different functional segments to understand how the foot and/or pathology affects movements. The OFM, for example, divides the foot/ankle into four segments: the shank, the hindfoot, the forefoot, and the hallux. The Rizzoli Foot Model goes into slightly more detail by including a midfoot segment in addition to those of the OFM. Both of these models have been shown to be able to distinguish between 'normal' and pathological conditions (15–18).

The main disadvantages of these two-foot models for the clinician is that the foot is being partitioned into functional segments rather than individual bones or joints owing to the limitations in accurately tracking all bones in the foot. Another possible downside is the number of markers

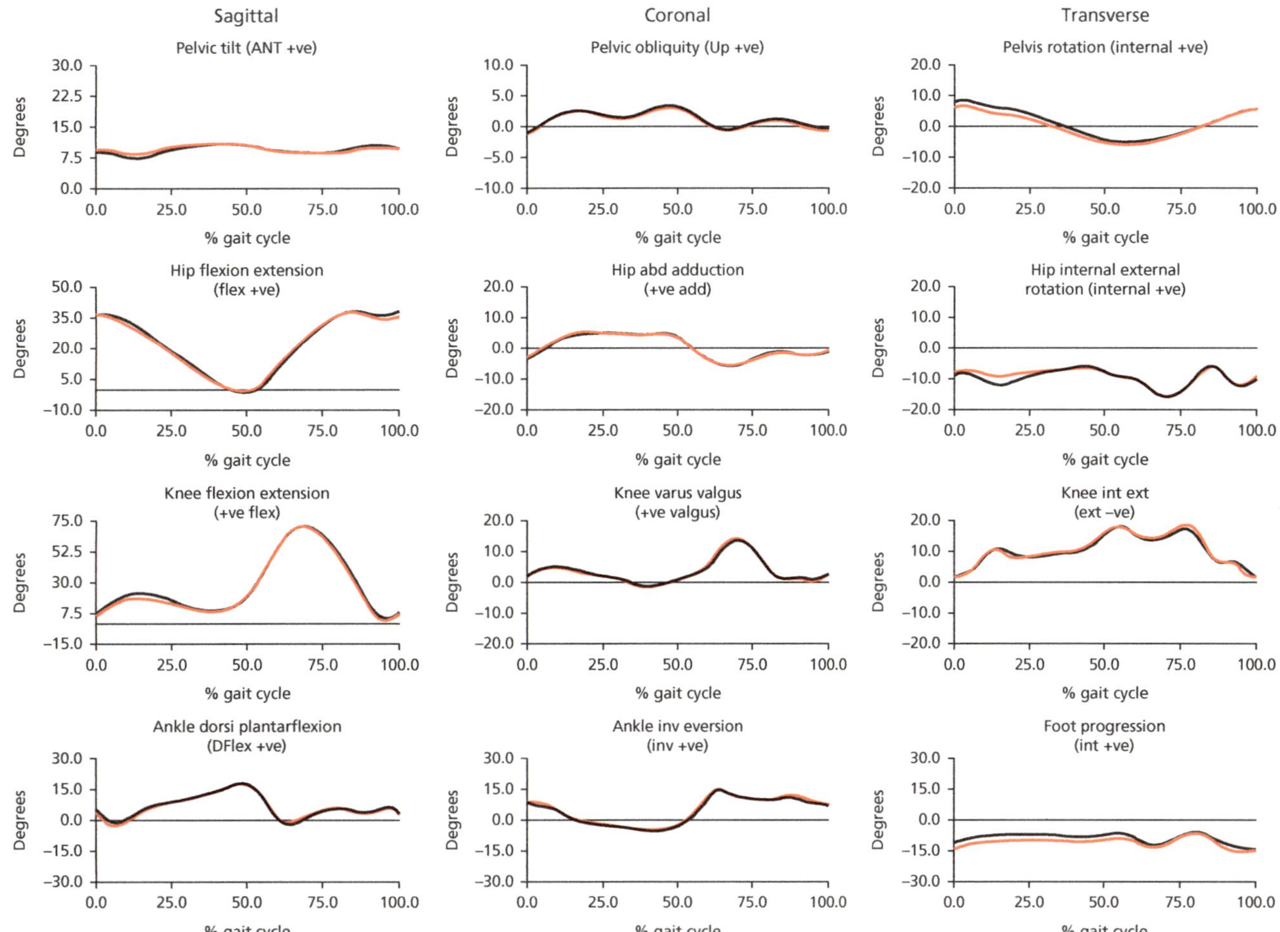

Figure 13.10 An example of pelvis, hip, knee, and ankle kinematics (top to bottom), for all three anatomical planes: sagittal, coronal, and transverse (left to right). Red and black lines correspond to right and left foot, respectively.

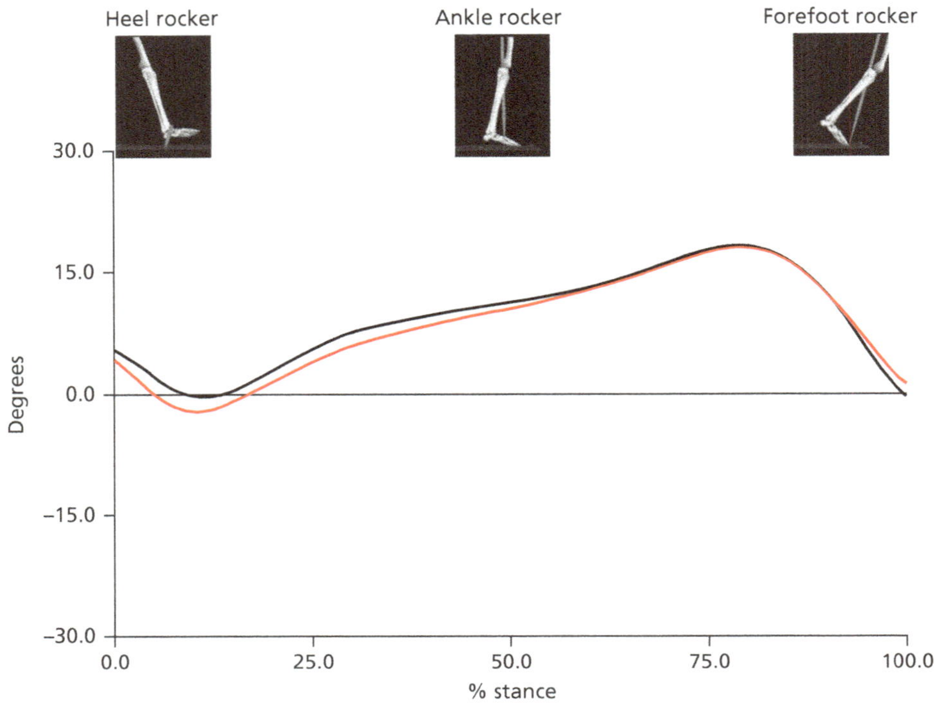

Figure 13.11 Ankle joint complex sagittal kinematics for the stance phase (enlarged from Figure 13.8) in conjunction with each ankle rocker. Red and black lines correspond to right and left foot, respectively.

needing to be placed directly onto the skin, making it difficult to measure in-shoe kinematics, which clinicians/researchers are likely to want to know if they are researching how a newly designed shoe and/or insole changes foot kinematics. One method around this issue is to cut 'windows' into shoes for the skin-mounted markers to protrude through the shoe for the cameras to see the markers. It could be argued, however, that the structural integrity of the shoe may be

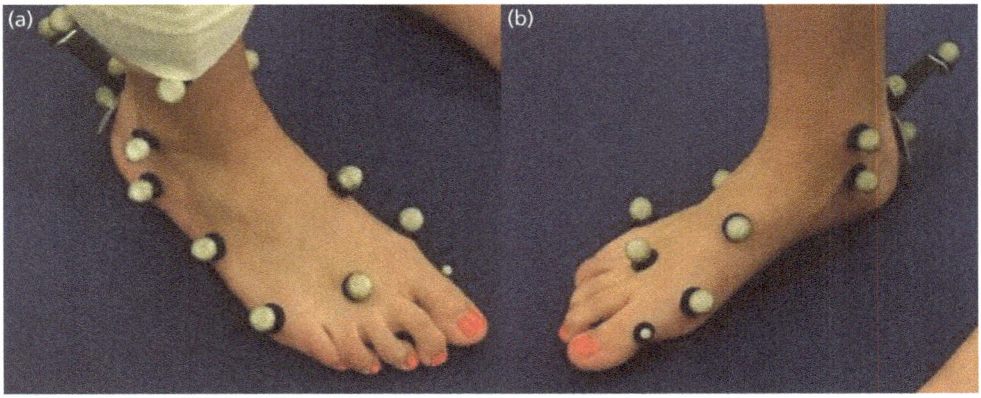

Figure 13.12 (a) The anterior-lateral and (b) anterior-medial view of the Oxford Foot Model.

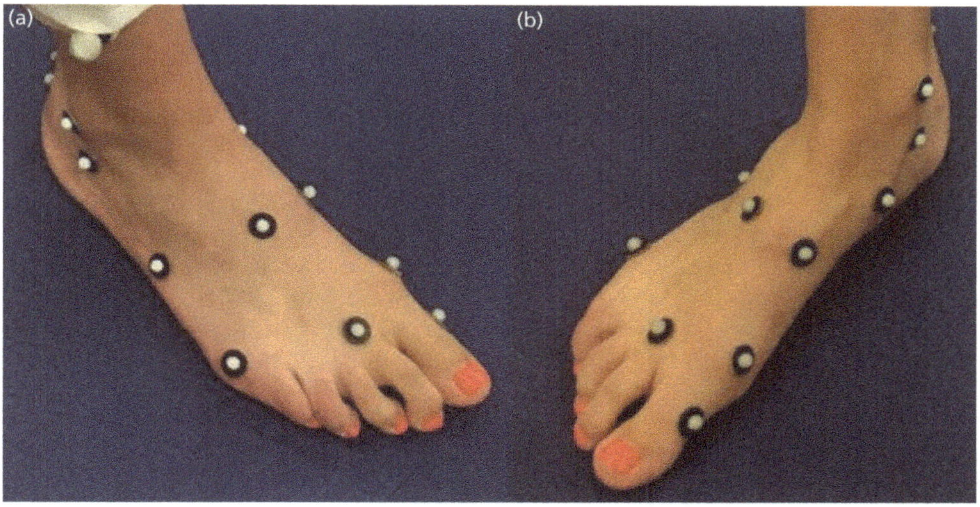

Figure 13.13 (a) The anterior-lateral and (b) anterior-medial view of the Rizzoli Foot Model.

compromised. Recently, Halstead et al. (10) modified the 'window' approach and replaced the window with a mesh in an attempt to maintain the structural integrity of the footwear, whilst still allowing the markers to be tracked. This approach demonstrated that it was possible to determine kinematic differences between healthy control participants and patients with mechanical foot pain.

Within RA, studies have been conducted examining the effect of RA on barefoot kinematics. Results commonly demonstrate that range of motion in all foot segments (shank, rearfoot, forefoot, and hallux) are reduced, potentially owing to joint stiffness and/or deformity. Rearfoot kinematics were consistent with pes planovalgus deformity with increased eversion and external rotation, and navicular height was also reduced (19). In a more recent study, Turner and Woodburn (20) demonstrated, through gait analysis, that it is possible to distinguish RA patients with severe forefoot, rearfoot, or combined deformities. Patients in the rearfoot and combined deformity groups demonstrated excessive rearfoot eversion and midfoot collapse, whereas the forefoot group demonstrated greater forefoot inversion.

Kinetics

The gait cycle can be split into phases: the stance phase and the swing phase (Figure 13.1). The start of the stance phase occurs when the heel/foot strikes the ground, resulting in the foot applying a force on the ground. At the same time, a force from the ground, known as the ground reaction force (GRF), is applied to the individual with the same magnitude but in the opposite direction. To measure the GRF during walking, we use force plates that are flush to the ground and are fundamental to most gait laboratories. Force plates can be made up of strain gauges (AMTI, Watertown, MA, USA or Bertec Corporation, Columbus, USA) or piezo electric transducers (Kistler Instrumentation, Winterthur, Switzerland), but essentially provide the same information.

An advantage of acquiring data from force plates is that, once installed, data is straightforward to collect as long as only one foot lands within the perimeter of the force plate and the other foot does not touch the same force plate. In this instance, careful consideration should be taken when planning the orientation of the force plate or force plates. In the Leeds gait laboratory, we have two AMTI force plates embedded, flush in the ground, allowing the individual/patient to walk across the force plates without changing gait and acquiring sequential forces for both limbs on separate force plates (Figure 13.9). The disadvantage, however, is that, with pathological and/or older patients, step length and/or width may be reduced, therefore complicating data capture. In this instance, the user would ask the individual to adjust their starting position to the left or right so that only one foot is likely to land on the force plate(s). Another consideration is making sure the patient/individual does not 'target' the force plate(s), resulting in an unnatural gait.

Take the example of an individual's foot making a clean contact within the perimeter of a force plate. The force plate records the GRF vector and the point of application on the force plate, known as the centre of pressure, which, in this instance, is the path of the GRF within the area of the foot. Figure 13.14 depicts the force vector for a healthy individual (solid line) and a pathological patient (dashed lines), in all three planes: medial-lateral (Fx, red lines), anterior-posterior (Fy, green lines), and vertical (Fz, blue lines) forces. GRF outputs can be either in newtons (N) or as a percentage of body weight (newtons/body weight). The vertical GRF (Fz) shows a typical 'M-shaped' vertical GRF for a healthy individual (blue solid line) and can be broken down into three parts. Fz1 is the first peak, or maximum weightbearing force, that occurs when the foot makes contact with the ground and relates to the amount the individual is loading that limb. The first peak depicted in Figure 13.14 is in the region of 1.2 times body weight, which is typical for a healthy individual, although this can be higher depending on the individual's walking speed. The 'trough' (Fz2) informs on how fluently the individual is moving over the stance limb. The 'trough' occurs when the body moves over the stance limb and the centre of mass approaches its highest

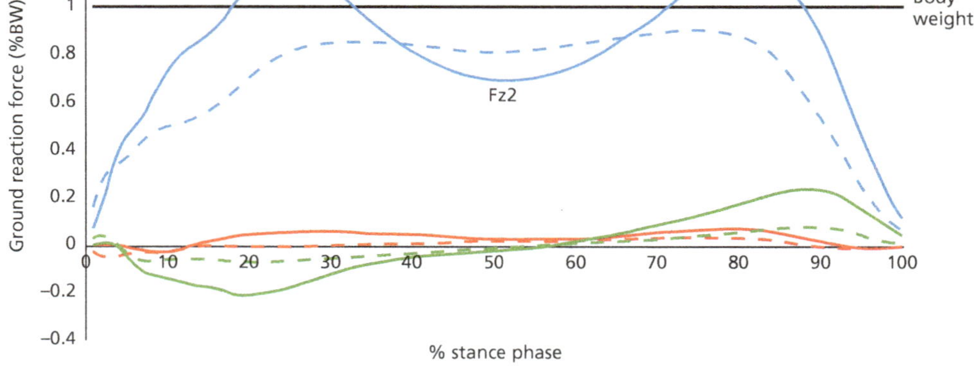

Figure 13.14 The ground reaction forces (GRF) for a healthy individual (solid lines) and a pathological patient (dashed lines). Blue, green, and red lines correspond to vertical, anterior-posterior, and medio-lateral GRFs, respectively. Ankle rockers are included to illustrate how the GRFs correspond to the stance phase. BW, Body weight.

point, with a typical value in the region of 0.7 times body weight. The second peak (Fz3) relates to the amount of vertical propulsion being generated by the foot/ankle joint complex prior to the toe-off/swing phase of gait. In comparison, the dashed blue line depicts a patient's vertical GRF, which is a noticeably different shape to that of the healthy individual in that the first (Fz1) and second (Fz3) vertical peak do not reach or exceed body weight, suggesting reduced load in the stance limb and diminished ability to push off whilst there is a lack of a 'trough' (Fz2). This pattern of vertical GRF is typical for patients suffering with musculoskeletal conditions due to patients often walking more slowly due to pain and/or deformity, which will in turn change the shape of the vertical GRF.

Figure 13.14 shows the anterior-posterior GRF (green lines) and typically shows a negative peak, also known as the maximum posterior loading force, as the foot drives into the force plate during the first half of stance. In the second half of the stance phase, a positive peak or maximum anterior thrusting force can be seen in which the body moves over the foot and drives the body forward, i.e., the propulsion phase. Finally, the medio-lateral GRF (red lines) are typically depicted as a predominant medial force. For the patient's anterior-posterior (green dashed line) and medio-lateral GRF (red dashed line), the shape is similar to that of the healthy individual but to a far less magnitude, potentially because of walking more slowly due to pain and/or deformity.

This chapter has so far described how to collect kinematic and GRF data, both of which can describe how an individual is moving. To understand how major muscle groups act on lower limb joints during the gait cycle, we can calculate internal joint moments by a process called inverse dynamics, which calculates the net turning force caused by muscles and tendons. In its simplest form, internal moments are calculated as the perpendicular distance of the GRF vector away from the axis of rotation (often a joint centre). Joint moments can be a daunting concept to understand but are very useful when trying to understand how different musculoskeletal diseases may affect gait compared to healthy controls.

One limitation of calculating joint moments of the foot/ankle is that, as the foot is often modelled as a single segment, it is difficult/near impossible to track all the motions of the many bones in the foot/ankle. Therefore, for simplicity, many researchers and clinicians often use a single rigid foot to allow for the calculations of the moment and power of the ankle joint complex.

The ankle moment obtained from gait analysis (Figure 13.15) demonstrates a dorsiflexion moment at heel-strike as the dorsiflexors eccentrically control the rotation of the foot onto the ground and prevent the foot from slapping the ground. During the second rocker, there is a plantar flexor moment as the ankle dorsiflexors contract eccentrically to allow forward progression of the shank over the foot. During the third rocker, the plantar flexion moment continues, with the plantar flexors contracting concentrically towards toe-off. Ankle joint moments acquired from gait analysis do not commonly report ankle moments in the coronal or transverse planes owing to the complex nature of movement of the ankle joint complex and the high variability between individuals.

Joint powers allow the clinician/researcher to understand which muscles are contracting during walking. Joint powers are calculated by multiplying the net moment of the force by the angular velocity of the segment. Ankle powers (Figure 13.15) detailed when the major muscles acting on the ankle joint complex are either absorbing (negative values) or generating (positive values) power during gait. The negative values correspond to power absorption from the plantar flexors eccentrically contracting during the heel and ankle rockers. The maximum joint power of the ankle joint complex is generated at approximately 50% of gait cycle during the forefoot rocker, demonstrating the power generation of the plantar flexors required for the lower limb to propel forward towards toe-off.

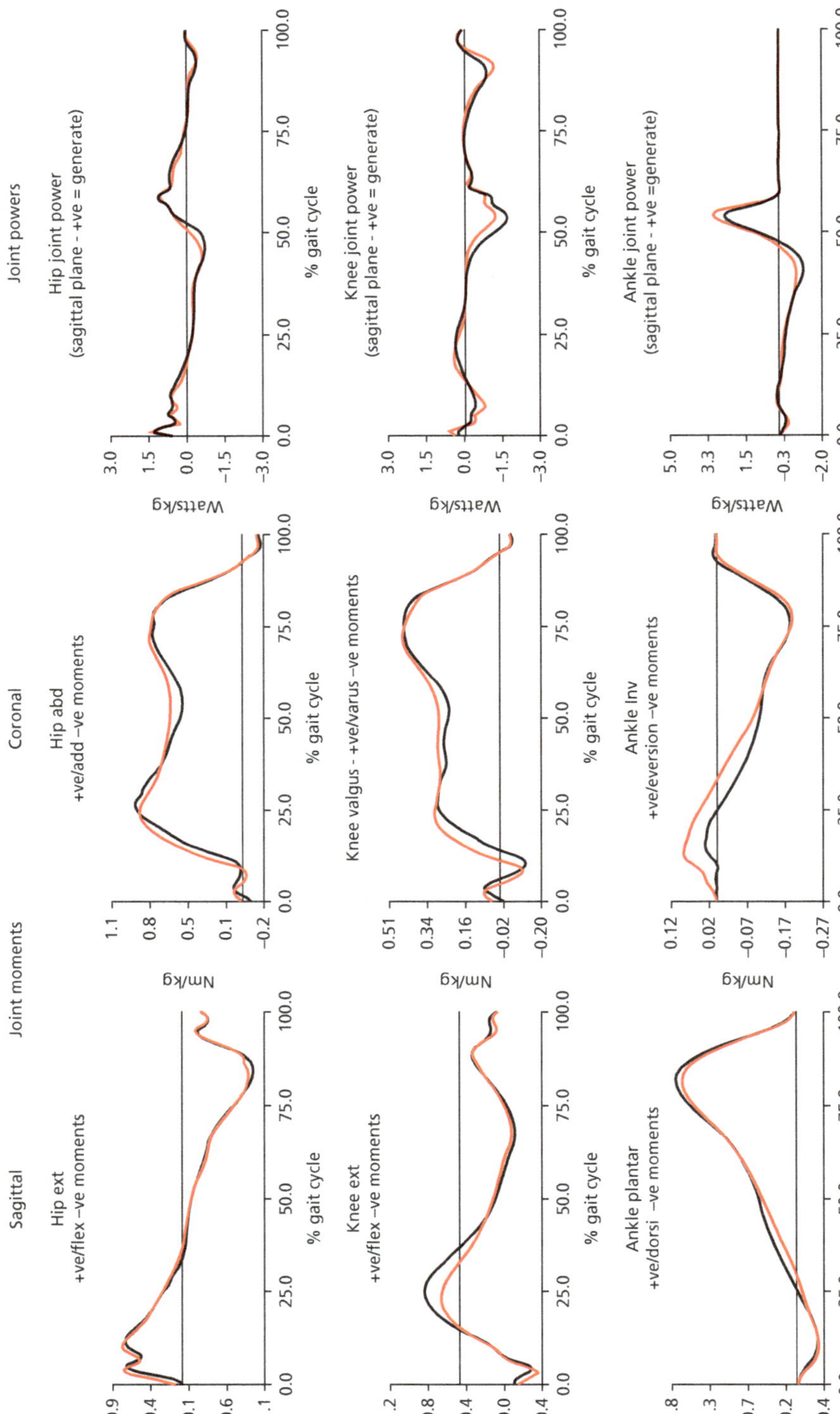

Figure 13.15 An example of hip, knee, and ankle moments (top to bottom) and for sagittal (left column) and coronal (right column) and hip, knee, and ankle powers. Red and black lines correspond to right and left foot, respectively.

Modelling

As technology and software have improved so have the capabilities of multi-body modelling, which allows for the calculations and predictions of internal forces on any given joint. Understanding how forces act within the joint is essential to be able to improve treatment and/or prescribe the correct treatment for a patient. Multi-body modelling can be computed in two separate methods, either forward dynamics or inverse dynamics. Forward dynamics uses known muscle forces to predict joint forces and moments, whereas inverse dynamics uses measured forces and moments to calculate muscle forces. Two commercially available multi-body modelling software packages, AnyBody Technologies (Aalborg, Denmark) and Open SIMM (21), are commonly used within musculoskeletal research settings.

In this chapter so far, we have discussed how to measure movement (i.e., kinematics), forces (i.e., kinetics), and, as a result, we can calculate internal moments. The main limitations of current gait analysis techniques are their inability to measure joint contact forces or muscle forces accurately owing to the invasive nature of collecting such data. With respect to the foot/ankle, we are unable to measure/analyse how all the bones/joints move and therefore how the forces act on these many joints. As a result, researchers and some clinicians are using multi-body modelling to compute internal forces and joint movement during walking and other activities of daily living and/or to understand how pathologies affect foot/ankle function.

Previously, detailed modelling of the complex ankle/foot movements required insertion of invasive intracortical bone pins directly into the bones of the foot (22) or simplified models that allow only for approximations of function (16, 19, 23). One example of multi-body modelling that has been applied to the foot and ankle is work by Oosterwaal et al. (24), who recently used a combination of very detailed foot/ankle kinematics (Figure 13.16), kinetics, and plantar pressures as well as computed tomography to develop the Glasgow–Maastricht subject-specific ankle/foot model. This model can measure kinematics and kinetics of all 26 joints in healthy control participants, demonstrating accurate and detailed modelling of ankle/foot function, and thus allows researchers and clinicians a greater insight into how pathology affects foot/ankle function.

Although multi-body modelling is unlikely to be used routinely in the clinical setting, it is hoped that findings from pathological musculoskeletal modelling will lead to a greater understanding of

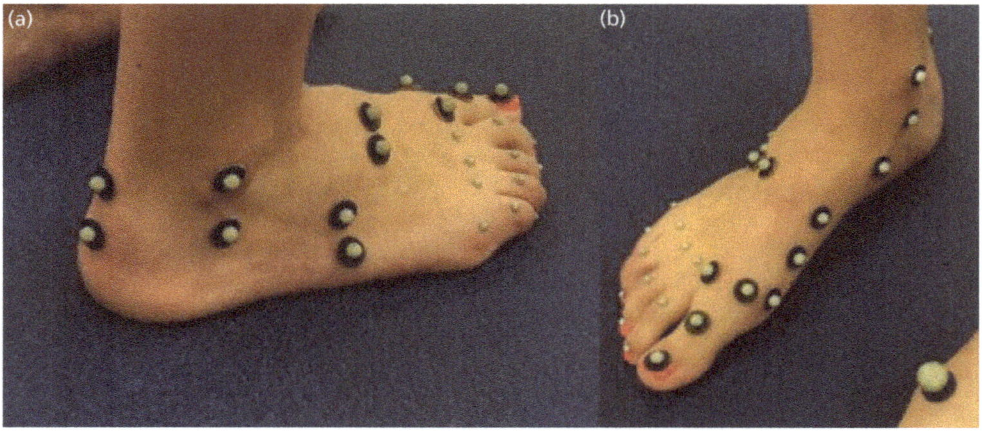

Figure 13.16 (a) Posterior-lateral and (b) anterior-medial view of the Glasgow–Maastricht Foot Model.

the pathological processes involved in musculoskeletal conditions and result in novel, evidence-based treatments for musculoskeletal conditions.

Electromyography

Electromyography (EMG) is a technique that can be used in isolation or in conjunction with 3D motion capture and subsequent modelling. EMG records the electrical signal associated with contracting muscles and can detect the onset of muscle contractions or abnormal muscle contractions that may occur in different musculoskeletal diseases. The most common method for collecting EMG is through attaching surface electrodes to the skin overlying the muscle(s) of choice. A good sensor-to-skin contact is essential to obtain a clean EMG signal with minimal noise. Recommendations are to shave the site where the electrode will be placed, if being placed on hair, and also to wipe the skin site with an alcohol swab. Similar to marker placement for 3D kinematics, a good knowledge of (lower limb) muscles and the direction in which the muscle fibres run are important factors for a good signal. Typically, the sensor location for the sensor is the midline of the belly of the muscle between the nearest innervation zone and the myotendinous junction. If the sensor is not placed accurately there is potential for cross-talk from other neighbouring muscles, thus giving an unrealistic signal of the muscle of choice. Skin-mounted EMG is ideal for those clinicians/researchers interested in muscle activation of superficial muscles, but will not capture muscle contractions of deeper muscles. For further guidelines on skin-mounted EMG, see www.SENIAM.org

The other method for collecting EMG data is intramuscular, fine-wire EMG. This allows the user to collect EMG signals on much deeper muscles than skin-mounted electrodes can achieve and targeting leads to greater muscle specificity. This technique requires the user to insert a needle electrode into the muscle with the aid of a hypodermic needle, often using ultrasound guidance. In the research setting fine-wire EMG has been used to confirm that altered activation of the posterior tibialis is associated with abnormal foot mechanics in RA patients with pes planovalgus foot deformity (25, 26). Recently, Barn et al. (27) used the combination of fine-wire EMG with gait analysis to determine the effect of customized foot orthoses on tibialis posterior muscle activation and foot kinematics in RA patients with pes planovalgus foot deformity. The results demonstrated that wearing an FFO compared to the barefoot condition demonstrated altered foot/ankle kinematics and surface EMG activation of the soleus and gastrocnemius closer to those of a healthy population. Fine-wire EMG of the tibialis posterior demonstrated a trend in the reduction of magnitude of contraction in the FFO condition compared to barefoot.

Clinical implications of laboratory gait analysis

As clinicians we all use qualitative gait analysis when assessing our patients. From the moment they enter the clinic through to a more perceptive assessment, both with and without clothes/shoes, we are appraising their gait. The more experienced the observer the more information will be obtained. How much more information could be obtained by formalizing this process and obtaining quantitative gait data—would it change the way we treat our patients? This remains a contentious area. The cost and therefore availability of a gait analysis laboratory is prohibitive for most units, but are they offering substandard care as a result of this? When might a clinician request detailed gait analysis were it available? In Leeds, gait analysis is carried out following referral from the multidisciplinary team:

- The podiatrist requesting plantar pressure measurement to assist the design of a custom off-loading foot orthosis.

- Physicians may request gait analysis to help explain foot mechanics for a patient with persistent unresolved tibialis posterior tenosynovitis after recognizing the foot was pronated.
- The surgeon wanting to understand the peak forefoot pressures when planning forefoot surgery, particularly in RA.
- The surgeon planning a total ankle replacement may request an analysis of the ankle 3D kinematics and kinetics as a baseline to evaluate prospectively any restoration of ankle function.
- Finally, the orthotist may request simple spatial and temporal measurements to check the gait symmetry when prescribing orthopaedic footwear and orthoses.

The laboratory strategy uses gait analysis to understand more fully the relationship between joint disease, impairment, foot structure and function, and the compensatory gait strategies adopted to overcome painful and disabling deformity. Gait analysis is better interpreted with prior knowledge of the nature and severity of impairments and the general and localized inflammatory status. It adds to the patient history and extends the clinical examination. It complements other investigations, particularly imaging, which aim to localize and quantify joint pathology and impairment.

There is still a lot of work to be done. The extent of 'normality' remains a problem, for how can we tell what is abnormal if we cannot define normal, especially in early disease? The real benefits for gait analysis will emerge if we can identify abnormal function in early disease. More data is required and agreement on what is to be measured, its reliability, and responsiveness. These are real issues that need to be tackled if gait analysis is to become a necessary laboratory investigation (28). At the moment it cannot work as a diagnostic test—there are far more powerful laboratory and imaging tests for that purpose. Gait analysis is used to help plan surgical interventions and to aid the prescription of orthoses. However, it is as a research tool that gait analysis has been most prominent and has led to insights into pathomechanics, particularly in RA.

References

1. **Helliwell P, Woodburn J, Redmond A, Turner D, Davys HJ.** *The Foot and Ankle in Rheumatoid Arthritis: A Comprehensive Guide.* London: Churchill Livingstone: Elsevier; 2007.
2. **Woodburn J, Barker S, Helliwell PS.** A randomised controlled trial of foot orthoses in rheumatoid arthritis. *J Rheumatol.* 2002;**29**:1377–83.
3. **Turner DE, Woodburn J, Helliwell PS, Cornwall ME, Emery P.** Pes planovalgus in rheumatoid arthritis: a descriptive and analytical study of foot function determined to gait analysis. *Musculoskel Care.* 2003;**1**:21–33.
4. **Lundberg A, Svensson O, Bylund C, Goldie I.** Kinematics of the ankle/foot complex—Part 2. Pronation & supination. *Foot Ankle.* 1989;**9**:248–53.
5. **Menz HB, Latt MD, Tiedemann A, Mun San Kwan M, Lord SR.** Reliability of the GAITRite walkway system for the quantification of temporo-spatial parameters of gait in young and older people. *Gait Posture.* 2004;**20**:20–5.
6. **Rome K, Hanchard NC.** Within-day reliability of temporal-spatial gait parameters associated with rheumatoid arthritic feet. *Musculoskel Care.* 2005;**3**:17–23.
7. **Debi R, Mor A, Segal O, et al.** Differences in gait patterns, pain, function and quality of life between males and females with knee osteoarthritis: a clinical trial. *BMC Musculoskel Dis.* 2009;**10**:127.
8. **Carroll M, Parmar P, Dalbeth N, Boocock M, Rome K.** Gait characteristics associated with the foot and ankle in inflammatory arthritis: a systematic review and meta-analysis. *BMC Musculoskel Dis.* 2015;**16**:134.
9. **Backhouse MR, Pickles DA, Mathieson HR, et al.** Diurnal variation of gait in patients with rheumatoid arthritis: the DIVIGN study. *Clin Biomech (Bristol, Avon).* 2014;**29**:811–14.

10. **Halstead J, Chapman GJ, Gray JC, et al.** Foot orthoses in the treatment of symptomatic midfoot osteoarthritis using clinical and biomechanical outcomes: a randomised feasibility study. *Clin Rheumatol.* 2016;**35**:987–96.
11. **Chapman GJ, Halstead J, Redmond AC.** Comparability of off the shelf foot orthoses in the redistribution of forces in midfoot osteoarthritis patients. *Gait Posture.* 2016;**49**:235–40.
12. **Wilkins RA, Siddle H, Redmond A, Helliwell P.** Plantar forefoot pressures in psoriatic arthritis-related dactylitis: an exploratory study. *Clin Rheumatol.* 2016;**35**(9):2333–8.
13. **Carson MC, Harrington ME, Thompson N, O'Connor JJ, Theologis TN.** Kinematic analysis of a multi-segment foot model for research and clinical applications: a repeatability analysis. *J Biomech.* 2001;**34**:1299–307.
14. **Leardini A, Benedetti MG, Berti L, Bettinelli D, Nativo R, Giannini S.** Rear-foot, mid-foot and fore-foot motion during the stance phase of gait. *Gait Posture.* 2007;**25**:453–62.
15. **Portinaro N, Leardini A, Panou A, Monzani V, Caravaggi P.** Modifying the Rizzoli foot model to improve the diagnosis of pes-planus: application to kinematics of feet in teenagers. *J Foot Anke Res.* 2014;**7**:754.
16. **Levinger P, Menz HB, Morrow AD, Feller JA, Bartlett JR, Bergman NR.** Foot kinematics in people with medial compartment knee osteoarthritis. *Rheumatology (Oxford, England).* 2012;**51**:2191–8.
17. **Levinger P, Murley GS, Barton CJ, Cotchett MP, McSweeney SR, Menz HB.** A comparison of foot kinematics in people with normal- and flat-arched feet using the Oxford Foot Model. *Gait Posture.* 2010;**32**:519–23.
18. **Turner DE, Helliwell PS, Emery P, Woodburn J.** The impact of rheumatoid arthritis on foot function in the early stages of disease: a clinical case series. *BMC Musculoskel Dis.* 2006;**7**:102.
19. **Woodburn J, Nelson KM, Siegel KL, Kepple TM, Gerber LH.** Multisegment foot motion during gait: proof of concept in rheumatoid arthritis. *J Rheumatol.* 2004;**31**:1918–27.
20. **Turner DE, Woodburn J.** Characterising the clinical and biomechanical features of severely deformed feet in rheumatoid arthritis. *Gait Posture.* 2008;**28**:574–80.
21. **Delp SL, Anderson FC, Arnold AS, et al.** OpenSim: open-source software to create and analyze dynamic simulations of movement. *IEEE T Bio-Med Eng.* 2007;**54**:1940–50.
22. **Lundgren P, Nester C, Liu A, et al.** Invasive in vivo measurement of rear-, mid- and forefoot motion during walking. *Gait Posture.* 2008;**28**:93–100.
23. **Stebbins J, Harrington M, Thompson N, Zavatsky A, Theologis T.** Repeatability of a model for measuring multi-segment foot kinematics in children. *Gait Posture.* 2006;**23**:401–10.
24. **Oosterwaal M, Carbes S, Telfer S, et al.** The Glasgow-Maastricht foot model, evaluation of a 26 segment kinematic model of the foot. *J Foot Ankle Res.* 2016;**9**:19.
25. **Barn R, Turner DE, Rafferty D, Sturrock RD, Woodburn J.** Tibialis posterior tenosynovitis and associated pes plano valgus in rheumatoid arthritis: electromyography, multisegment foot kinematics, and ultrasound features. *Arthritis Care Res.* 2013;**65**:495–502.
26. **Keenan MA, Peabody TD, Gronley JK, Perry J.** Valgus deformities of the feet and characteristics of gait in patients who have rheumatoid arthritis. *J Bone Joint Surg—Am.* 1991;**73-A**:237–47.
27. **Barn R, Brandon M, Rafferty D, et al.** Kinematic, kinetic and electromyographic response to customized foot orthoses in patients with tibialis posterior tenosynovitis, pes plano valgus and rheumatoid arthritis. *Rheumatology (Oxford, England).* 2014;**53**:123–30.
28. **Baan H, Dubbeldam R, Nene A, van der Laar M.** Gait analysis of the lower limb in patients with rheumatoid arthritis: a systematic literature review. *Semin Arthritis Rheum.* 2012;**41**:768–8.

Chapter 14

Foot health management

Heidi Siddle and Gordon Hendry

Introduction

The impact of foot problems in patients with rheumatic and musculoskeletal diseases has been detailed in Chapters 4–10, and frequently results in deformity, loss of function, and considerable pain, which impacts on the ability to enjoy simple activities with friends and family. Despite advances in the management of systemic diseases, persistent foot and ankle problems are associated with pain, physical disability, and cumulative joint damage, ultimately reducing mobility and functional capacity. During our experience of working with this group of patients we often hear that their feet are 'the first to be affected and last to be treated'.

Although in recent years National Institute for Health and Care Excellence (NICE) guidelines have included recommendations for managing foot and ankle problems in diseases such as rheumatoid arthritis (RA) (1) and osteoarthritis (OA) (2), the recommendations focus on treating the systemic disease and, together with the lack of evidence to support individual interventions, are therefore not specific enough for the treating clinician.

The current 'tight control' approach to managing RA, which is now being adopted for other inflammatory diseases, aims to achieve clinical remission and target treatment strategies at individual patients' disease activity (3–5). Various criteria have been proposed and subsequently validated for measuring remission in RA. These include the 28-joint disease activity score (DAS28), simplified disease activity index (SDAI), and clinical disease activity index (CDAI), which have all been developed to reduce time and complexity in clinic but do not include the feet and ankles. Recent evidence has demonstrated that patients in disease remission based on the DAS28, SDAI, and CDAI classification criteria foot synovitis is found in a substantial proportion (25–36%) of patients with RA (6). In a cohort study of 848 patients with recent-onset RA, of those reaching the DAS28 <2.6 remission criteria (7), 29% of cases had at least one painful metatarsophalangeal (MTP) joint and 31% had at least one swollen MTP during an 8-year follow-up (8). Conversely, a study comparing the 28-joint count with the 32-joint count, which includes the MTP joints and ankles, showed that the additional joint activity assessment does not convey significant added value to the evaluation of disease activity (9). However, recent evidence from patients in remission has identified that foot synovitis increased likelihood of relapse by up to twofold and also predicted worse long-term radiographic and functional outcomes (6). Hence, clinical examination of the foot and ankle joints in the presence of local symptoms has been recommended, along with, in some instances, therapy escalation to improve long-term outcomes irrespective of the patient's state of disease activity and/or remission status (6, 8, 9).

Since the introduction of the 2011 American College of Rheumatology/The European League Against Rheumatism (ACR/EULAR) remission criteria, which utilizes full joint counts (10) (as did the original 1981 ACR remission criteria [11]), it has been recognized that residual disease can be present in the feet of patients deemed to be in remission, putting patients at risk of ongoing damage if the criteria omit foot joint assessment (12). Interestingly, evidence from a cohort study identifying the use of foot care during the first 9 years following disease onset indicates that patients with higher disease activity at onset were more likely to receive foot care, whether it be surgical or conservative therapy (13).

The current evidence advocates including the feet in disease and remission assessment, and, as such, a paradigm of podiatry foot healthcare has been proposed in early RA (14). The paradigm promotes the early detection of joint disease utilizing the MTP joint squeeze test (15), a combination of targeted therapy at inflammatory lesions, and associated mechanically based impairments using ultrasound-guided corticosteroid injections and custom orthoses, 'tight control' of foot arthritis, and disease monitoring using disease measures (DAS), imaging methods, and foot-related outcome measures (14). Although this paradigm of care has been identified for patients with RA, we advocate using this treatment approach for all of our rheumatology patients who present with foot and ankle symptoms. As well as being able to recognize when there is disease activity in the foot or the patient is experiencing a flare of their systemic disease, it is important to liaise with the patient's rheumatology multidisciplinary team to review systemic therapy as appropriate. Hence, it is essential to get to know the local team to improve the efficiency of care.

Patient education and self-management

Education and self-management recommendations

Over the past decade there has been an increasing emphasis placed upon the importance of the promotion of patient education and self-management initiatives for people who suffer from long-term conditions (16, 17). These initiatives are designed to build upon the public's desire for better health by allowing them to develop the knowledge, skills, and confidence to care for themselves effectively with support from health professionals (16). Supported self-management is now considered to be one of the key components of the National Health Service (NHS) long-term conditions care model following the implementation of policies promoting patient-centred care (17, 18). The two main factors that are integral to this paradigm shift are: 1) the potential for empowerment of patients and improved self-efficacy leading to better outcomes; and 2) the potential for less healthcare utilization by reducing demand on limited resources (19). One of the recommendations from the State of Play in UK Rheumatology report was that commissioners and health boards should give greater priority to education and self-management programmes for managing long-term conditions (20).

Simple patient education can be defined as the process by which healthcare information from health professionals is delivered to patients with the expectation that this information will alter behaviours and improve health outcomes. In contrast, self-management educational interventions are more complex psychosocial and cognitive-behavioural interventions that are designed to allow patients to take an active part in the management of their own condition by improving their self-efficacy (21, 22). As a minimum, the following core components are considered essential for behaviour change via self-management programmes: 1) engaging in activities that promote health and prevent adverse sequelae; 2) interaction between patients and healthcare providers; 3) improved self-monitoring of physical and/or emotional status; 4) managing the effects of illness on functional ability and other aspects of general health and wellbeing (23–25).

General disease education

General disease education provision for conditions such as RA and OA is advised early (usually within 1 month of diagnosis) and should be ongoing (1, 2). The goal of early delivery of education is to improve patients' understanding of important factors such as symptoms, disease course and progression, routine clinical examinations and tests, medication information, including side-effects, pain management, physical activity, and physical and relaxation therapies (26, 27). This also serves to manage expectations to make disease-related changes in outcomes less daunting for patients. Typically, this general disease education would be delivered by a rheumatology nurse specialist or another integrated member of the rheumatology multidisciplinary team in the rheumatology outpatients setting. Nevertheless, podiatrists and other professionals who contribute to managing foot health are often asked to provide general health and/or disease information and advice that does not directly relate to foot health (28). It is not unusual for patients to feel overwhelmed during the early disease stage and there is a risk that excessive provision of complex information could have a detrimental effect on patients' ability to retain that information, as well as their emotional wellbeing (26, 29). Mindfulness of the patient's disease stage and the educational programmes in which they may be enrolled can be useful to provide timely support for more profession-specific education.

Foot health education

Foot health education is recommended in foot health management guidelines for all patients with RA (30) and those with other musculoskeletal diseases, including OA, metabolic bone diseases (osteoporosis, Paget's disease, osteomalacia, and osteogenesis imperfecta), connective tissue diseases (systemic lupus erythematosus [SLE], systemic sclerosis [SSc], vasculitides), and inflammatory arthritis (inclusive of RA, psoriatic arthritis [PsA], and spondyloarthritis) (31). Historically, foot health advice and education in rheumatology has been centred on simple provision of information concerning the role of the podiatrist, the need for foot-specific interventions such as foot orthoses (FOs) and how they work, the impact of disease on the foot and lower limb, and how to look after the feet in terms of joint protection, identifying red flags that require urgent attention, good foot hygiene, and what constitutes good and poor footwear habits (28, 31–33). Much of this information would normally be imparted verbally during outpatient podiatry appointments and supplemented with written material and signposting to other sources of information (such as the Versus Arthritis website), where the patient can find out more (Figure 14.1). However, at present very little is known about the impact of routine foot health education on patient behaviours and foot-specific outcomes. Nevertheless, to maximize the potential for success of educational interventions, clinicians should be aware of the potential barriers to behavioural change.

When providing foot health education, it is important to consider the degree of health literacy the patient has so that he or she can process and understand the information that is being provided. Poor health literacy has been associated with poor functional outcomes, which have been largely attributed to non-adherence with educational advice (34, 35). This is a particularly challenging issue to overcome given the time pressures during podiatry appointments. As such, an important role of the podiatrist in providing education will be to evaluate the patient's individual needs concerning foot health and deliver tailored education to address these. For general disease education, the educational needs assessment tool (ENAT) was developed largely for use by rheumatology specialist nurses to help people with arthritis identify their educational needs, which can then be prioritized accordingly by the health professional (36, 37). Although no such tool exists to guide foot health education specifically, the same principle applies in that identification of patients' specific needs for foot health education provides a means for informing the content, method of delivery, and timing of specific aspects of foot health education. It is possible that identification of patients' foot health educational needs could be informed through simple extension of the patient history and physical examination of foot structure, function, and footwear.

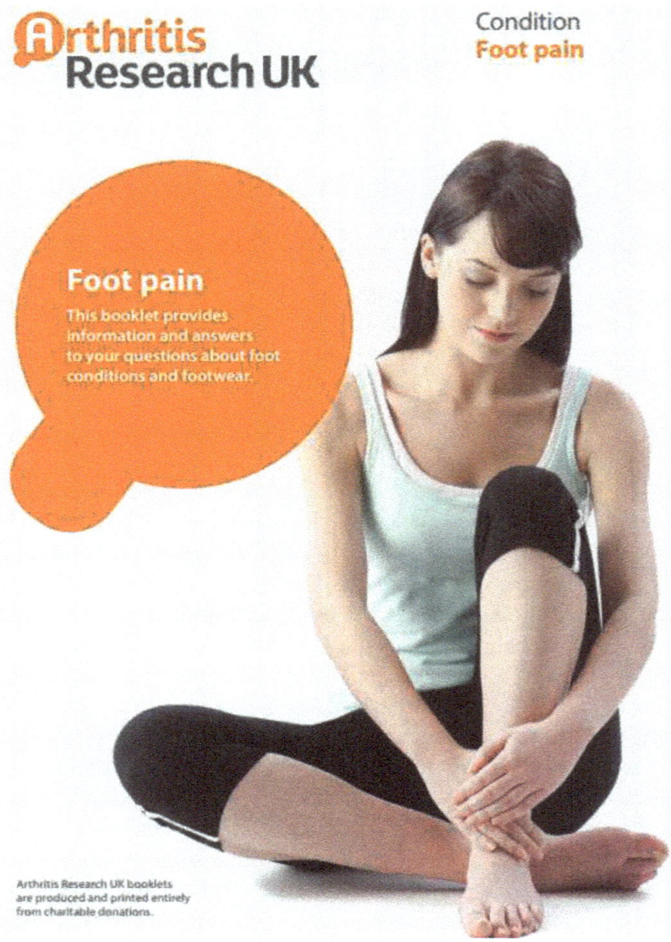

Figure 14.1 Arthritis Research UK (now Versus Arthritis) educational leaflet on foot pain.

There are several possible methods of delivery of foot health education, as well as educational aids, which provide new ways to support self-management for patients with a variety of health literacy levels. Qualitative research has highlighted that foot health education can be delivered by a practitioner on a one-to-one basis or to a group, verbally and/or with supplementary written information, or through signposting to internet resources (28, 32).

In recent years there has been an increase in the use of digital media technologies to deliver educational and self-management interventions. Armed with the knowledge that the vast majority of the adult population now own and use mobile smartphones with larger screen displays, tablets, and/or laptops to access the internet, many independent research groups and non-profit organizations have developed interactive educational programmes and applications using audiovisual animations (Figure 14.2) (38). One of the main advantages of these technological developments is that they provide patients with increased flexibility for accessing health information and resources at a convenient time and place that is suitable to the individual (38–41). Moreover, they are thought to be of benefit for those who have poor health literacy. Recent reviews of digital

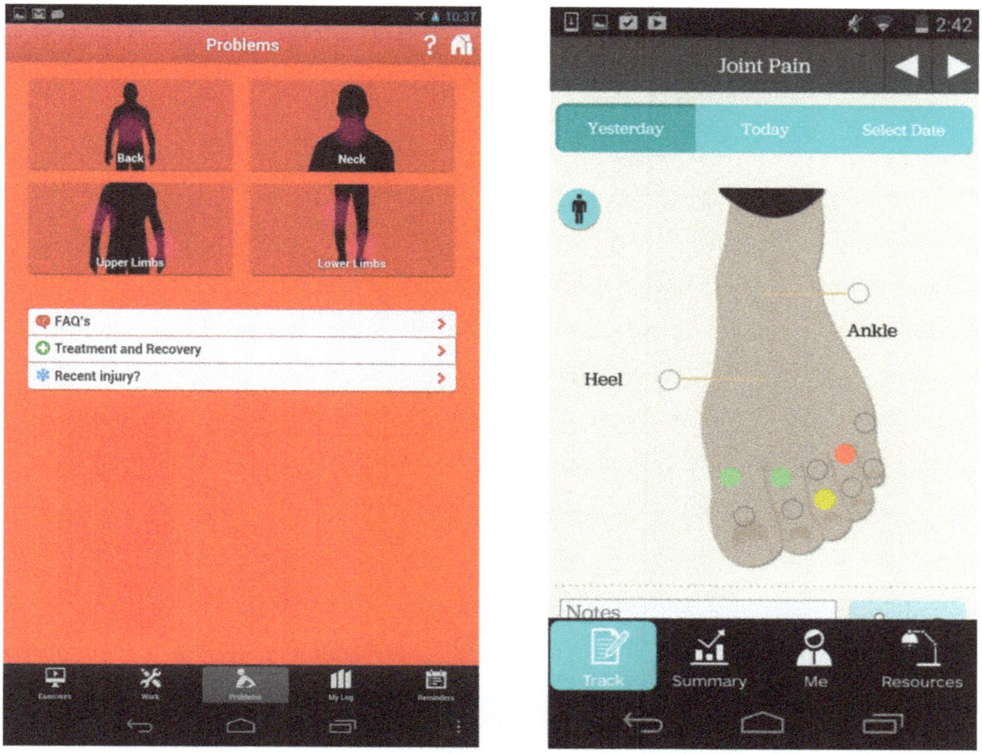

Figure 14.2 Screenshots from the National Health Service MSK and My RA smartphone self-management applications.

educational interventions for people with arthritis and/or long-term illnesses describe largely positive outcomes in terms of improved knowledge and self-efficacy, but urge caution owing to information gaps relating to long-term effects, acceptability (for those who are not computer-literate), costs (of maintenance and content updates), and risks of such interventions (38, 41, 42). As an alternative, there are several other educational tools that can be used alongside verbal and written information to aid patient education, such as physical examples of good footwear characteristics and anatomical models. In addition, a novel approach to improving patient education by utilizing musculoskeletal ultrasound to show patients their inflamed joints in real-time has recently been proposed (Figure 14.3) (43). Musculoskeletal ultrasound training is now available for podiatrists and other non-medical health professionals, and this novel method may provide an opportunity for increased patient understanding of the impact of the inflammatory disease process on the foot and ankle (43, 44).

In addition to poor health literacy, there are other important barriers to effective foot health education that require attention. Podiatrists and patients have identified that financial constraints in relation to costs of improving foot health behaviours, particularly in relation to seeking new and appropriate footwear, have been highlighted in several studies (28, 32, 45, 46). Unfortunately, when patients are unable to acquire appropriate shoes there are few alternative treatment options available to podiatrists beyond initiating access to surgical/accommodative footwear via an orthotist. Furthermore, patients are often dissatisfied with the prescribed footwear they receive (47). Development of a therapeutic relationship with patients built on empathy and compromise,

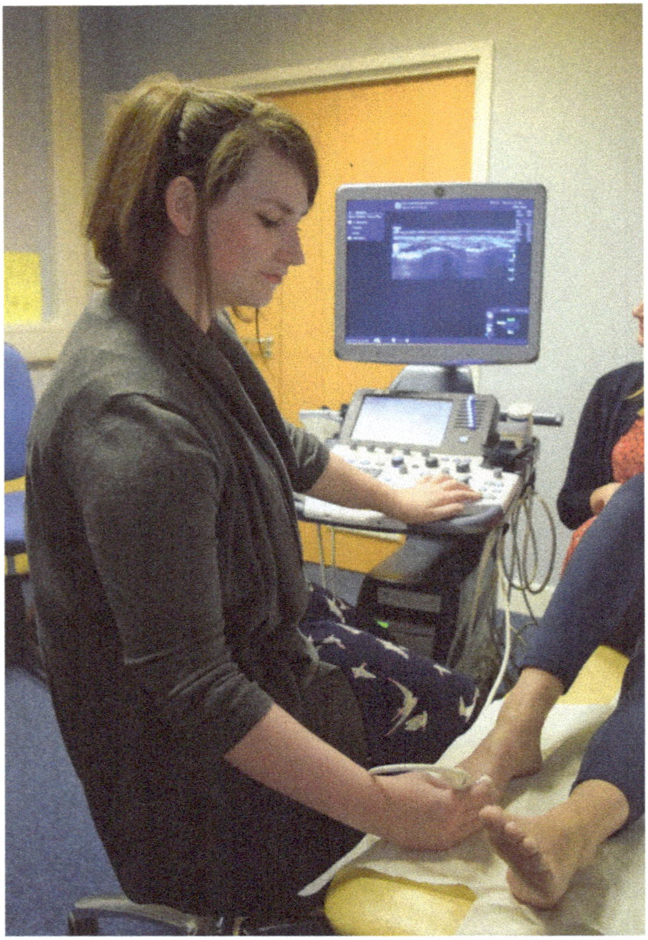

Figure 14.3 Musculoskeletal ultrasound real-time imaging capabilities being used as an educational tool to improve understanding of the inflammatory disease process in a patient with rheumatoid arthritis.

particularly where the goal is to influence footwear habits, has been highlighted as important for the success of education (28, 32). Clinicians should aim to consider patients' points of view regarding their foot health and should avoid being dismissive about seemingly unimportant issues as this may cause disillusionment and result in non-adherence.

Self-management programmes

A variety of self-management education programmes have been developed for use in rheumatology and in other chronic conditions (21, 22, 48–51), but only one has been developed specifically for the self-management of foot health that has been subsequently applied in a rheumatic disease population (52, 53). The FOOTSTEP self-management programme was developed to enable elderly adults who would normally seek foot care through podiatry services to undertake their own basic foot care (53). FOOTSTEP participants participated in hands-on workshops facilitated by podiatrists who delivered educational material with the aid of flashcards and who also performed demonstrations of skin and nail care (53). Encouragingly, there was no difference in outcomes between those who took part in the FOOTSTEP self-management programme versus those who accessed basic foot care via podiatry services (53). When this programme was applied in an established RA population, a large proportion of participants (43%) were found to be physically unable to undertake some aspects of the self-management programme adequately (52). Nevertheless, these studies have demonstrated that there may be scope for greater empowerment of patients with regard to managing their own foot health.

Skin and nail care

Nail care

Nail care alone provides challenges for patients who experience problems reaching their feet, as well as those who have lost strength or movement in their hands to be able to use nail-cutting equipment. Furthermore, it can be painful, particularly when the feet are swollen and tender. Inappropriate and inadequate nail care can result in spikes of nail being left in the nail sulci, which pose increased risks such as infection for those who are immunosuppressed and particularly those taking biologic therapies. Unfortunately, NHS podiatry services for routine treatments such as nail care are limited and there are often long periods between appointments. In such cases we would recommend that patients seek advice and treatment from a Health and Care Professions Council (HCPC)-registered chiropodist or podiatrist.

Hand nail care is often just as difficult, particularly when joints are swollen, deformity has occurred as a result of bony changes in arthritis, and in diseases such as scleroderma where the skin has tightened. Podiatrists are well placed to provide hand nail care, with the support of the rheumatology team.

Nail psoriasis and onychomycosis

The treatment of nail psoriasis is difficult and further details are provided in Chapter 7. Appropriate nail care, and in some situations nail avulsion, is important but there is little evidence to support the use of local therapy in this situation. Systemic medication has demonstrated efficacy in the treatment of nail disease in patients with psoriasis and psoriatic arthritis. It is, of course, important to rule out onychomycosis, known as a fungal infection of the toenails. Local nail-based treatments for onychomycosis can be beneficial but require persistent applications over an extended period of time. Short courses of oral antifungal treatments are available on prescription and appear to offer better efficacy and fewer side-effects than previously described. However, these may be contraindicated in patients taking disease-modifying antirheumatic drugs (DMARDs) and biologic therapies.

Onychocryptosis

Onychocryptosis is a condition in which a spike, shoulder, or serrated edge of the nail has pierced the epidermis of the sulcus and penetrated the dermal tissues (Figure 14.1). Since it is frequently accompanied by local sepsis it is a potentially serious complication in patients treated with biologic therapies. Infected onychocryptosis has been observed in patients with RA, all of whom were in receipt of biologic therapy. Suspension of biologic therapy following guidelines, along with antibiotics and podiatry treatment (largely nail avulsion [Figure 14.4]) results in a successful outcome for patients (54). These findings highlight the need to check the feet as a source of potential infection in patients commencing biologic therapies as well as the need to adhere to perioperative

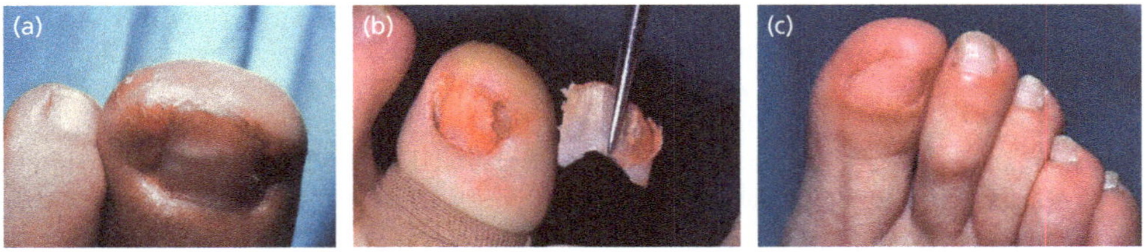

Figure 14.4 (a) Onychocryptosis of hallux nail. (b) Total nail avulsion of the hallux nail. (c) Healed nail bed following total nail avulsion of the hallux nail.

guidelines when undertaking a nail avulsion, ensuring foot health teams are working closely with the rheumatology team.

Callus debridement

Patients with RA frequently complain of 'walking on pebbles', usually the result of subluxed or dislocated MTP joints that are subject to excessive shear and compressive stresses during gait, frequently resulting in the buildup of painful plantar callosities over the metatarsal heads (55). The rationale and therapeutic benefit of callus reduction to reduce peak pressures, prevent ulceration, and facilitate wound healing is firmly established in patients with diabetes (56, 57). Anecdotal clinical evidence and a preliminary investigation in patients with RA showed a large but short-lived (7-day) reduction in pain following debridement (58). A pilot randomized controlled trial (RCT) investigated the effect of sharp scalpel debridement against a sham procedure. This RCT concluded that, although debridement reduced pain and focal pressures in patients with RA, these benefits were no greater in the treatment group than for the sham procedure group (59). The most recent findings from a full RCT have demonstrated that the long-term benefits of sharp scalpel debridement of painful forefoot plantar callosities in RA, when undertaken in conjunction with a combined therapeutic approach (prescription of orthoses and footwear), produced no additional benefit over the combined therapeutic approach alone. This RCT further questions the efficacy of callus removal in this group of patients and provides evidence to highlight that the causes of forefoot pain in RA are unlikely to be solely attributed to plantar callosities (60). However, it should be noted that patients with high-risk presentations such as extravasated blood in the callus and/or suspected ulceration underneath the callus were excluded from these studies. Hence, the authors recommend that sharp scalpel debridement should not be used routinely in the care of painful forefoot plantar callosities but should be confined to reduction of high-risk states or short-term alleviation of severe pain.

Ulceration/wound care

Although there are studies reporting the incidence of ulceration in the foot and ankle across the rheumatic diseases, little is known about the management strategies. Understanding the risk factors for ulceration will enable us to target our interventions appropriately and in a timelier manner. The risk factors for foot ulceration are described in previous disease-specific chapters (Chapters 5–8).

Recent epidemiological studies and case series have reported that ulceration in RA occurs at multiple sites and usually on the pressure-vulnerable bony sites in the forefoot; these include the dorsal aspect of hammer toes (48%), the plantar aspect of metatarsal heads (32%), and the medial aspect of the first MTP joint in patients with hallux valgus (20%) (60–64). Accommodation and off-loading of these bony sites are essential to aid healing and prevent ulceration. The provision of footwear and FOs will be discussed in further detail below (see Section on 'Foot orthoses').

Vasculitis has frequently been suggested as a primary cause of ulceration in patients with RA, and therefore treatment of the underlying systemic disease is key to managing foot ulceration. However, it has consistently been shown that this is unlikely to be true. The first study of patients with RA and foot problems reported that only two patients out of the 204 studied showed evidence of vasculitis in their feet (65) and stated that ulceration on the dorsum of the foot and lower leg are more likely to be of predominantly vasculitic origin (66). However, recent evidence has not identified vasculitis in RA patients with ulceration only affecting the feet (64, 67).

Prevention of ulceration in any group of patients is essential foot health management. In a recent study undertaken by Firth and colleagues (68) to identify predictors of foot ulceration in patients with RA without diabetes, the findings indicate that foot ulceration occurring in patients with RA shares similarities with the causal pathway of diabetic foot ulceration. The analysis showed that risk of ulceration rose with increasing loss of sensation and foot deformity and with vascular insufficiency. Foot checks, which include vascular and sensation screening for patients with diabetes, are now firmly established; we encourage clinicians to include these screening methods in the management of their rheumatology patients, particularly those with RA and connective tissue diseases.

The management of foot infection in patients who are immunocompromised is essential to preventing further local and systemic deterioration. Identifying the presence of infection in wound sites can be difficult to ascertain by the clinician, and questions have been raised about the effectiveness of wound swabbing in identifying organisms responsible for infection in patients with RA as well as patients with diabetes (69, 70). The evidence supporting which organisms cause infection is limited; however, *Staphylococcus aureus* appears to be the most common microorganism, which is consistent with that found in the wounds of other patient groups (70). As with any infection, DMARDS and biologic therapies should be suspended until the infection has resolved and the course of antibiotics has been completed. However, suspending systemic treatment, which in turn potentially causes a flare of the inflammatory disease, may delay wound healing (67) and therefore we recommend re-starting patients' systemic medication as soon as the infection has resolved and the wound is improving.

Off-loading the site of ulceration is a key factor in healing wounds in patients with diabetes who have neuropathy (loss of sensation) and subsequent deformity (71) and therefore should form part of the management strategy for rheumatology patients who present with foot ulceration. Adequate or accommodative footwear and FOs are required, but in cases of acute and painful ulceration other methods need to be considered. Traditional methods of off-loading high-pressure sites can be used, and these include DH Pressure Relief Walkers and the Aircast Pneumatic Walkers. These are effective but may present some problems for patients with rheumatic diseases because, with hand impairments, they may be difficult to put on and take off, and, where muscle weakness is present in the lower limb, feel heavy and cumbersome to the patient. Alternatively, lightweight forefoot and rearfoot 'off-loader' boots are available, which rheumatology patients appear to use successfully. Healing is often accelerated in a pain-free or pain-reduced environment, which is significantly helped by off-loading a painful joint; however, pharmacological pain management strategies should also be considered for these patients.

Wound dressings are considered an essential therapy to managing ulceration in the foot but should not be used in isolation without addressing the need for off-loading or accommodating deformity and managing vascular complications, when indicated. There are multiple dressings available, but none that have been evaluated for wounds in rheumatology patients. Those that cushion the often-painful ulcer site and provide an optimal healing environment by absorbing exudate and de-sloughing the wound are recommended. Bulky dressings, particularly for interdigital ulcers, should be avoided as they may serve to increase local pressures further. Adherent dressings are not recommended as they usually cause a deterioration of both the wound bed and the surrounding fragile tissues.

Footwear

Poor footwear characteristics

Broadly speaking, the physical characteristics of modern-day footwear have been designed to provide protection from the environment, facilitate foot function, and treat musculoskeletal injury (72, 73). However, it is well recognized that certain footwear characteristics have been implicated as contributors to foot and ankle impairments. There are several negative physical characteristics of footwear, which, as a general rule, should be avoided by the general adult population. Excessive heel height has been associated with forefoot deformities, development of soft-tissue lesions such as corns and calluses, forefoot deformities, foot pain, impaired balance, and ankle sprain risk (74–79). Characteristics such as a lack of, or an inadequate fixation/retaining medium, excessive heel counter flexibility, and excessive longitudinal sole flexibility have been associated with the onset of foot pain, discomfort, and localized fatigue owing to insufficient motion control (72, 80–82). In addition, shoes with outer-sole materials that do not have slip resistance properties may be a risk factor for falls and subsequent injury (83). However, perhaps a more concerning issue is that studies have demonstrated that a high proportion of the adult population (26–50%) wear ill-fitting shoes (84–88). Research evidence from large-sample epidemiological studies of the general adult population have demonstrated that ill-fitting footwear is associated with foot pain, deformities, and soft-tissue lesions (74, 89–92). Given that foot and ankle joint pain, impairments, and deformities are frequently reported in chronic rheumatological conditions, it is clear that good footwear habits in terms of both physical characteristics and adequate fitting are important for maintaining foot health.

Footwear provision and advice/education

For adequate management of foot problems associated with rheumatological conditions, there are two main approaches relating to footwear: 1) provision of footwear education/advice; and 2) provision of therapeutic/bespoke/customized footwear. Several studies have highlighted that many people with rheumatic diseases do not wear suitable footwear and that poor footwear can exacerbate symptoms (93–95). As a result, footwear education is now considered to be a core component of podiatry care for people with rheumatological conditions (28, 32). However, there are important considerations for health professionals who are tasked with delivering footwear education, such as individual patient footwear needs, personal tastes, seasonal footwear trends (Figure 14.5), timing of education delivery, and the ability of the patient to assume the high costs associated with acquiring new shoes (28, 32, 45, 96). Consideration of these factors is important to ensure that the patient is at least partially compliant in altering their footwear habits. For women in particular, footwear is considered to be an important element of desirable self-image of being/appearing able-bodied (93, 97). Therefore, the restrictions in available choices of suitable retail footwear as a result of foot joint arthritis can be a source of considerable distress (93, 97, 98). Recent research has highlighted that people with chronic rheumatological conditions such as RA, OA, gout, PsA, spondyloarthritis, SLE, and SSc may experience difficulties in finding appropriate footwear as a result of their disease-specific foot problems, the lack of desirable footwear design features and styles, and/or the burden of seeking appropriate footwear (45). The main driver of

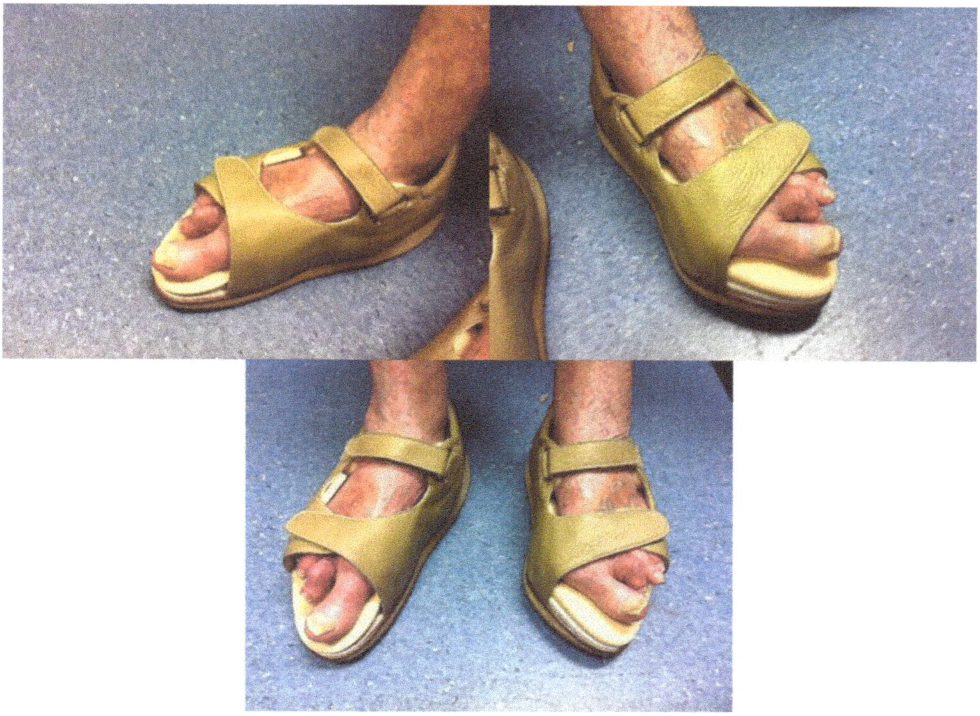

Figure 14.5 Therapeutic footwear designed specifically for a patient with established rheumatoid arthritis for wear during warmer weather/seasons/climates.

footwear difficulties in this population is the development of disease-related foot deformities, resulting in problems with finding a suitable shoe that both fits the foot and accommodates the deformity (45, 99).

Patients with severe RA and foot deformities may require specialist therapeutic footwear over the course of their disease, especially in the presence of rigid deformity, high focal pressures and pain, and/or ulceration (Figure 14.6).

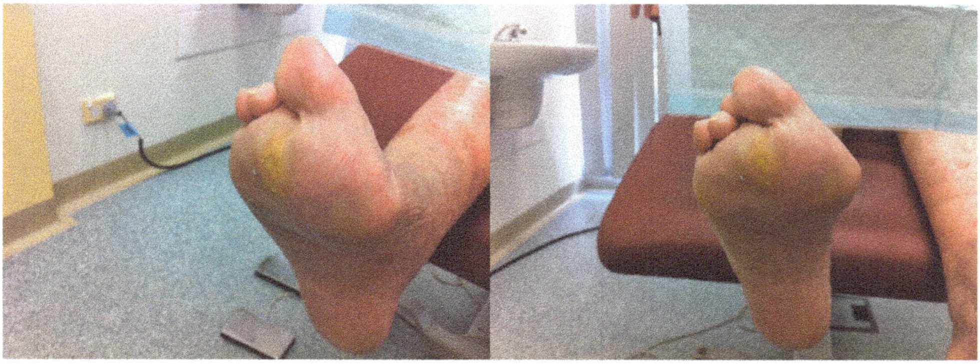

Figure 14.6 Rheumatoid arthritis patient at risk of ulceration presenting with severe forefoot deformity, raised focal forefoot pressures, and plantar heloma durum.

There is growing evidence that specialist accommodative footwear and rocker-shoes may be effective in reducing foot pain in RA (100–104). Recent research suggests that patients with first MTP OA may also benefit from rocker-sole shoes, which allow the body's centre of mass to progress over the base of support without recruiting first MTP joint dorsiflexion (105). However, there are major unresolved issues concerning patient adherence to accommodative footwear interventions (47), and care should be taken to ensure that patients are aware of the proposed designs at an early stage to avoid wasted healthcare resources through non-adherence.

Foot orthoses

Foot orthoses: current evidence and recommendations

FOs are a recognized non-pharmacological adjunct therapy to standard medical care for people who present with foot and ankle problems. FOs are designed to redistribute load from weightbearing sites such as painful MTP joints and to correct medial longitudinal arch shape through control of subtalar and midtarsal joint forces (Figure 14.7) (106–109). The best available research evidence from systematic reviews with meta-analyses indicate that FOs may be beneficial in reducing pain and elevated forefoot pressures in RA (110, 111). As a result, clinical management guidelines for foot care for people with RA typically recommend the use of FOs in the management of those with relevant foot problems (1, 30, 112–115). At present, there is little evidence-based guidance available to inform FO prescriptions for people with RA. The preliminary evidence suggests that FO design rules based on biomechanistic target variables (peak rearfoot eversion to guide rearfoot posting, minimum navicular height to guide FO medial arch height, and plantar pressure thresholds for individual metatarsal heads to guide presence/absence of forefoot cushioning) may result in greater mode-of-action responses and more positive patient experiences (such as improved perceptions of comfort) relative to FOs manufactured using standard clinical protocols (116). Research on FO efficacy in other rheumatic conditions is in its infancy. However, there is some emerging evidence to suggest that FOs may result in improvements in pain and function in people with OA of the midfoot (117–119) and the first MTP joint (105).

Timing of intervention with foot orthoses

A key issue concerning FO prescription in RA that is yet to be explored in detail is when to intervene through orthotic therapy. Evidence from cohort studies suggests that there is a high prevalence

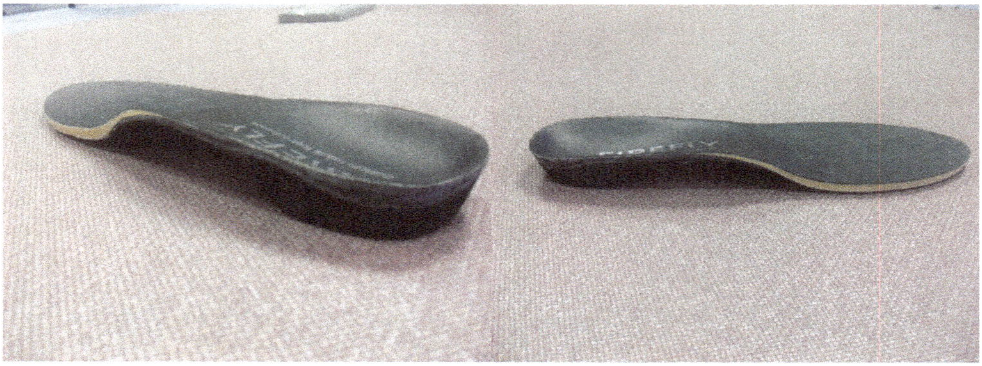

Figure 14.7 Customized rigid (carbon fibre) foot orthoses with rearfoot posting and cushioned forefoot extension.

of foot joint arthritis and pain in patients with early RA (within 2 years of diagnosis) (120–122). Significant advancements in the medical management of RA have recently been achieved with the focus on the treat-to-target approach, where low disease activity or remission states are targeted through early detection, disease monitoring, and tight control strategies (123–125). Several RCTs of relatively new biologic drugs have demonstrated marked reductions in overall pain and disease activity scores, but there is often persistence of foot pain and disability (122, 126). Indeed, several functionally important kinematic alterations in foot function have been detected early in the disease process (127). A recent prospective cohort has demonstrated that earlier intervention with FOs for patients with RA predicts more favourable foot pain and disability outcomes (128). As a result, it is probable that prescription of FOs should be targeted earlier in the course of the disease to provide the best opportunity for achieving desirable outcomes (14).

Injection techniques

Injections into the foot and ankle are generally used as therapy (corticosteroid) but may be used as a diagnostic aid (local anaesthetic) to determine which structure is the most troublesome. NICE recommends intra-articular steroids to improve symptoms rapidly in people with newly diagnosed RA (1) if they are not already receiving glucocorticoids as part of their systemic disease management. For people with OA, NICE recommends that intra-articular corticosteroid injection should be considered as an adjunct to core treatments for the relief of moderate to severe pain (2).

Administering local intra-articular or soft-tissue steroid injections means that the patient is not exposed to the usual systemic side-effects of these drugs and typically there is a low incidence of side-effects. Local injection therapy of the foot and ankle is indicated for acute inflammation, tendinopathy, and fasciopathy at specific sites. Corticosteroid injections are typically given for inflamed and swollen joints and therefore the aim is not to place the needle tip within the joint cavity but to place it within the joint capsule. The close proximity of joints in the foot may make accurate clinical localization of the pain difficult (129) and hence lead to wrong placement of the injection, often leading to poor clinical outcome. In recent years there have been multiple evaluations of the use of image-guided injections in the foot and ankle. However, although these have been specific to conditions such as plantar fasciitis and Achilles tendon disease, which affect rheumatology patients, the majority of studies have not been in patients specifically with inflammatory arthritis. D'Agostino and colleagues (130) evaluated the impact of ultrasound on therapeutic decision-making and clinical outcome of local corticosteroid injection performed as a treatment of painful ankle, hindfoot, and midfoot in chronic inflammatory diseases. The use of ultrasound led the physician to change the diagnosis in 32.4% of sites imaged and subsequently alter the planning of corticosteroid injections into the foot and ankle in 82.5% of patients. The authors also reported a trend toward improved short-term symptomatic treatment effect.

In a more recent study, Cunnington et al. (131) investigated whether ultrasound guidance improves the accuracy and clinical outcome of joint injections, including those into the ankle, compared with injections guided by clinical examination alone in patients with inflammatory arthritis (131). They reported that ultrasound guidance significantly improved the accuracy of joint injections; however, in this study it did not improve the short-term outcome of the joint injection. Accuracy is considered important, particularly in patients with tenosynovitis to ensure that the clinician avoids injecting directly into the tendon, which has the potential to cause a tear or rupture. Although this evidence supports the use of ultrasound-guided injection, access to ultrasound machines and clinicians who are appropriately trained is still limited and therefore this chapter will provide advice on so-called blind injections for the foot and ankle.

Before considering a steroid injection, it is also important to assess for functional and biomechanical causes that might be contributing to the problem. We advocate correcting or improving any structural deformity or biomechanical problem using orthoses and/or footwear prior to injecting foot and ankle sites to reduce the risk of the problem recurring. It is also important to consider the level of disease activity/inflammation in the feet as well the patient's systemic disease. It would be inappropriate to inject multiple foot sites in the presence of persistent disease that would benefit in the first instance from a review of systemic therapy.

Prior to injecting the foot and ankle with steroid it is essential, as with any injection, to check for any contraindications. Absolute contraindications include the presence of local or systemic infection, any allergies or hypersensitivities to the drugs being used, i.e., steroid and/or local anaesthetic, injections into a prosthetic joint or at the site of a recent fracture, and without informed consent by the patient. Relative contraindications include those at risk of increased bleeding, people with diabetes, pregnancy, and large tendinopathies such as the Achilles tendon. If patients with inherited bleeding disorders (haemophilia) or acquired bleeding disorder (such as those taking warfarin) require a steroid injection, it is important to reduce the risk of bleeding into the injected joint by correcting the coagulation therapy or omitting it for a few days prior to the procedure.

It is important to consider your choice of steroid: methylprednisolone (Depo-Medrone) and triamcinolone acetonide (Kenalog) are long-acting steroids, with Depo-Medrone available in premixed vials with lidocaine. Hydrocortisone is a shorter-acting, less potent steroid and is often considered more appropriate for soft-tissue injections, particularly in the proximity and within tendons around the ankle, as rupture may follow. It is up to individual clinicians to decide if they want to include local anaesthetic with their steroid injection. Generally, patients would prefer not to have two injections and, as allied health professionals in the UK without the appropriate qualifications are not allowed to mix medicines, then a pre-mixed solution should be considered.

Patients should be positioned in a comfortable position to reduce the risk of unwanted movement and so that the injection site is easily accessible for the clinician. Injections should be administered using an aseptic technique, having identified and marked your injection site. Use disposable needles and syringes and change the needle after drawing up the solution. The area should then be thoroughly cleansed and your hands washed before applying gloves. It is important not to touch the injection site once it has been cleaned; an ethyl chloride spray can be used to numb the skin before the needle is inserted. Having inserted your needle, aspirate to check that you have not inserted it into a vessel or there are any signs of infected fluid in the area. The injection site should be covered afterwards for 24 hours.

It is important to inform patients of the symptoms they will experience post injection—the likely immediate improvement owing to local anaesthetic (if used), that the site may be more painful for the first 24 hours because of a flare effect of the steroid, and then they should notice an improvement, which will hopefully last up to 3 months, depending on the steroid and dose given. Patients may also experience a systemic effect depending on the dose; flushing is a common symptom and the menstrual cycle may be affected in women. Patients should be warned of the signs and symptoms of infection and the action to take. If patients are diabetic, they should be advised that their normal control may fluctuate in the days following the steroid injection. There is also the risk of subcutaneous tissue atrophy, particularly if the steroid is not placed accurately in the joint. Patients should be advised that the tissue should return to normal, but it may take several months. Following a steroid injection into a weightbearing joint it is advisable to rest the joint for 24–48 hours (132). The reason for rest is to ensure the steroid preparation stays in the joint to achieve maximum benefit.

Intra-articular injections

Tibiotalar joint

The patient should be sat on the treatment couch with the knee bent to 90° and the foot slightly plantar flexed. Approach the joint anteriorly, inserting the needle into the joint space between the tibia and the talus, medial to the tibialis anterior tendon (Figure 14.8). It is important to avoid the dorsalis pedis artery, which is lateral to the tendon of extensor hallucis longus. We recommend using a 23-gauge (g) (blue) needle or a 21-g (green) needle injecting 40 mg of methylprednisolone.

Subtalar joint

The subtalar joint is a complex synovial joint with anterior and posterior 'facets', and appreciation of the anatomy (see Chapter 2) is recommended before injecting it. The joint is generally felt to be relatively difficult to enter without some form of imaging. The traditional approach to the subtalar joint is either medially using the sustentaculum tali as a bony landmark, where the needle can be directed anteriorly or posteriorly to enter the respective parts of the joint, or posteriorly, approaching just lateral to the Achilles tendon and entering the posterior part of the joint (133). An alternative approach laterally, via the sinus tarsi, provides a simpler approach through which aspiration and injection can be performed without imaging (134) (Figure 14.9). The patient should be sat on the treatment coach with the knee bent (approximately 45°) and the foot inverted. The sinus tarsi is located by palpation just anterior to the lateral malleolus. If the location is tender, local anaesthetic can be used. The needle (either a 21- or 23-g) is directed toward the tip of the medial malleolus. The joint space is entered at a depth of 1–2 cm. The approach should encounter no bony obstruction and the injection of 40 mg of methylprednisolone is performed without resistance.

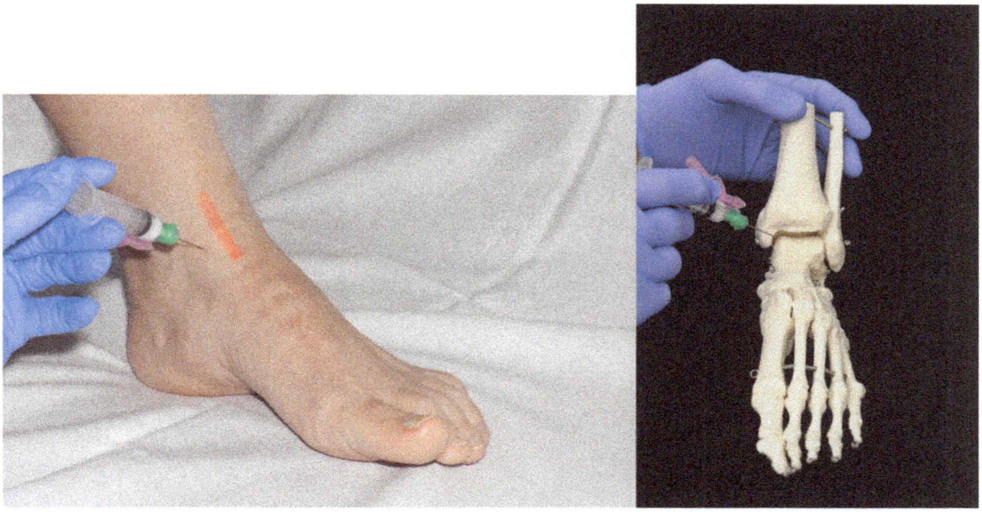

Figure 14.8 Corticosteroid injection into the tibiotalar joint (extensor hallucis longus tendon marked in red).

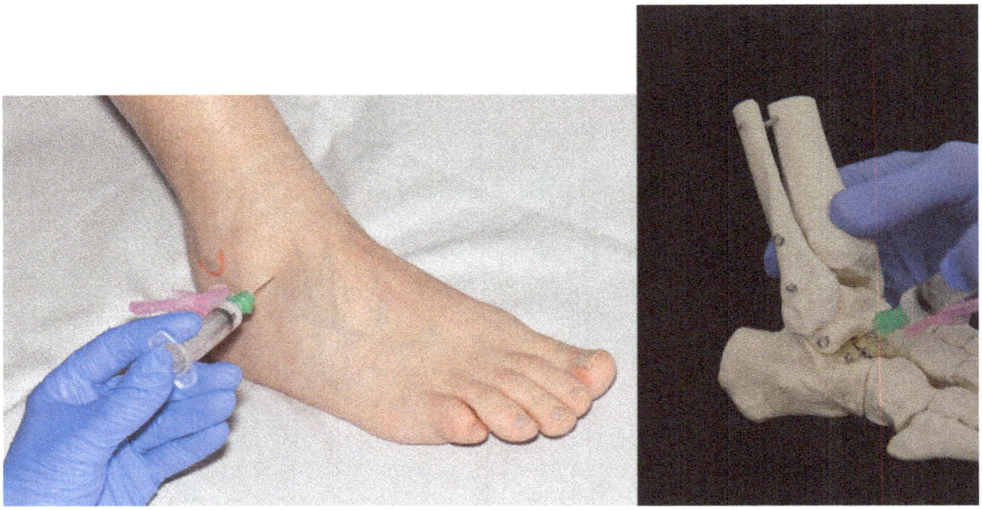

Figure 14.9 Injection of corticosteroid injection into the subtalar joint via the sinus tarsi (lateral malleolus outlined in red).

Talonavicular joint

This joint is a common source of symptoms in RA but is not always easy to inject. The patient should be sat on the treatment coach with the knee bent (approximately 45°) and the foot everted. Identify the tuberosity of the navicular and the joint line of the talonavicular joint just proximal to this landmark. The joint is situated near the surface of the skin so a 25-g 'orange' needle is used to inject perpendicular to the skin (Figure 14.10). This is not a very capacious joint and 20 mg of methylprednisolone or equivalent is recommended.

First metatarsal joint

Palpate the joint space whilst passively flexing and extending the toe. Using an oblique dorsal approach, the needle tip is placed under the extensor tendon, which is contiguous with the dorsal 'hood' of the capsule (Figure 14.11) inserting into the joint capsule. The approach to the joint may

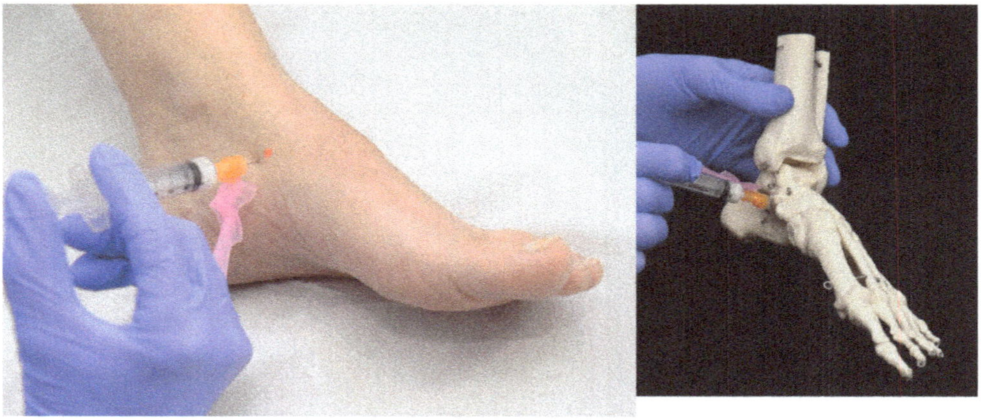

Figure 14.10 Injection of the talonavicular joint just proximal to the tuberosity of the navicular.

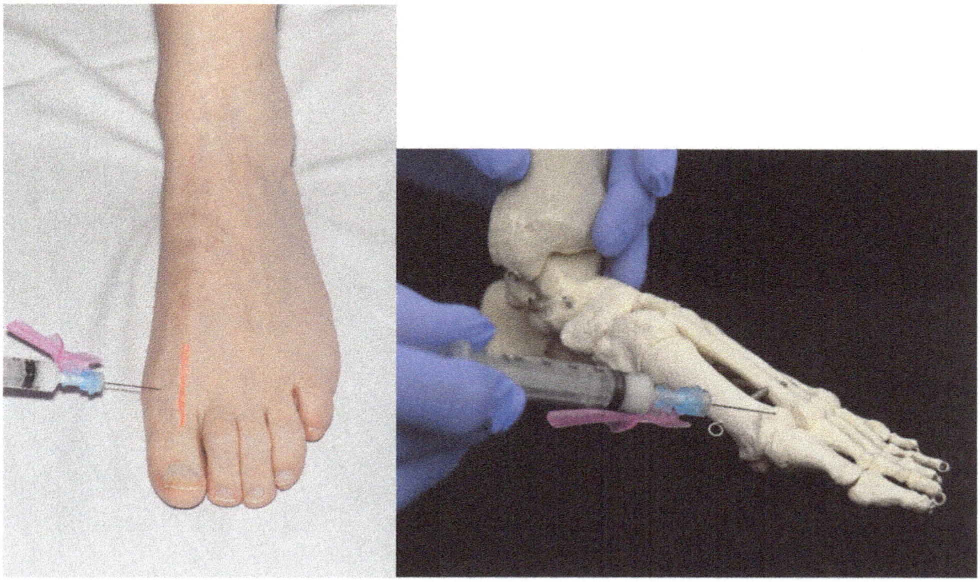

Figure 14.11 Injection of the first metatarsophalangeal joint using a dorsal approach guiding the needle beneath the extensor hallucis longus tendon, marked in red, to within the capsule of the joint.

be obstructed by large amounts of new bone if severe hallux abducto valgus or first MTP joint OA is present, and the use of imaging and guided techniques has obvious advantages in such cases. A fine 25-g needle should be used, injecting approximately 20 mg of methylprednisolone.

Lesser metatarsal joints

By analogy to the technique for injecting the first MTP joint the aim is not to enter the joint cavity but to place the needle within the capsule using the dorsal approach, injecting beneath the extensor tendon (Figure 14.12). A fine needle, such as a 25-g needle, is used to inject 10 mg of methylprednisolone into the joint.

Interphalangeal joints

Injection into the interphalangeal joints is required more often in patients with PsA where one or two proximal and distal interphalangeal joints are typically affected. A fine 25-g 'orange' needle is required. The approach is similar to the MTP joints: the joint is approached dorsally from either side and the needle slipped under the extensor tendon to rest within the joint capsule (Figure 14.13). When the injection is made a bulge is felt on the opposite side of the joint. If the needle is placed dorsal to the extensor tendon the bulge appears at the tip of the needle and the needle should be repositioned. The joint, like those of the lesser MTP joints, will only accept a small volume of fluid (approximately 10 mg of methylprednisolone).

Soft-tissue injections

Retrocalcaneal bursae

The retrocalcaneal bursa is situated in a triangle anterior to the Achilles tendon and posterior to the base of the talus and the posterior-superior aspect of the calcaneum. It can become inflamed in patients with inflammatory arthritis, particularly those with spondyloarthropathies, and may

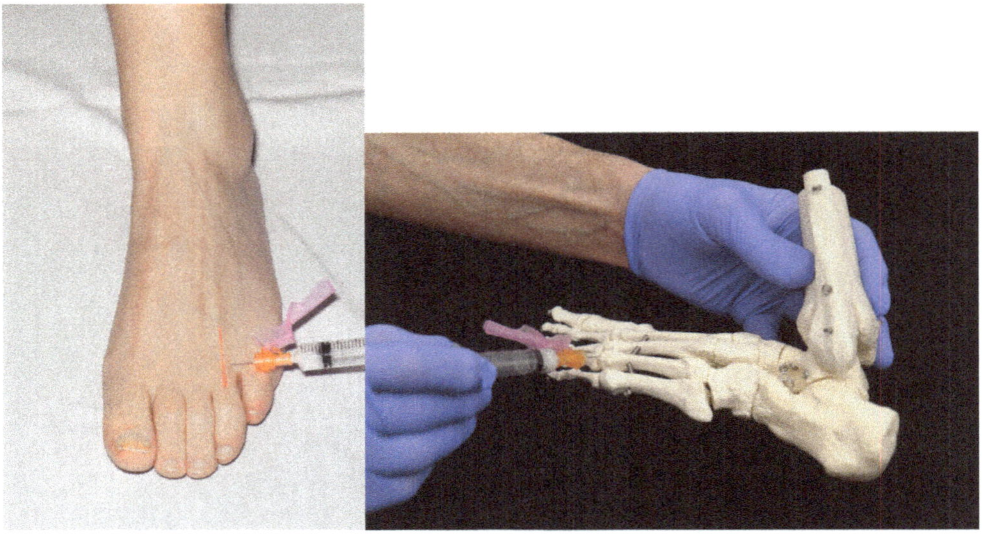

Figure 14.12 Injection into the capsule of the fourth metatarsophalangeal joint lateral to the extensor digitorum longus tendon (marked in red).

occasionally require injection with steroids. The patient lies prone with the foot hanging over the edge of the treatment couch and held in a dorsiflexed position. The bursa is approached at an angle to one side of the Achilles tendon close to its insertion into the calcaneum (Figure 14.14). There are no neurovascular tissues to be concerned about, although exact placement may be difficult because of the variable depth of the bursa. This injection is readily and probably best performed with ultrasound guidance. Use a 23-g (blue) needle and, once it is correctly positioned, you should be able to inject 20 mg of methylprednisolone into the area.

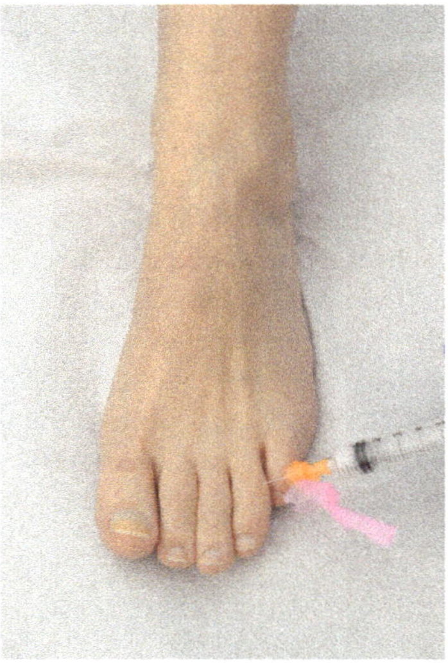

Figure 14.13 Dorsal injection of the fourth proximal interphalangeal joint, slipping the needle under the extensor tendon to rest within the joint capsule.

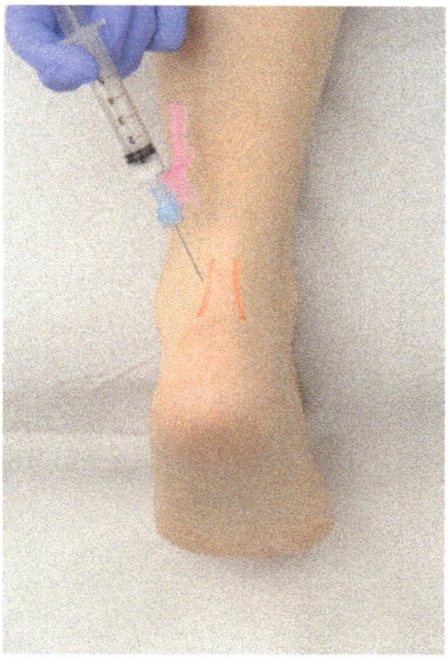

Figure 14.14 Injection into the retrocalcaneal bursa is approached at an angle to one side of the Achilles tendon (marked in red) close to its insertion into the calcaneum.

Tibialis posterior tendon sheath

The tibialis posterior tendon is frequently affected by florid tenosynovitis as it passes around the medial malleolus. Instability at the rearfoot with eversion of the calcaneum on weightbearing will exacerbate this. If the tenosynovitis is to be treated by local steroid injection it is imperative to address the foot biomechanics, in particular any subtalar joint instability, at the same time. The patient should be supine, with the knee bent and foot everted. The injection is performed using a 23-g needle along the axis of the tendon at the level of the medial malleolus, using a proximal approach (Figure 14.15). If the needle is correctly sited, the injected material can be seen and felt to pass up the tendon sheath. If the injection is difficult or there is an unusual amount of resistance, it is possible that the needle tip is within the substance of the tendon and the needle should be withdrawn slightly, owing to risk of rupture, before injecting 20 mg of methylprednisolone.

Peroneal tendon sheaths

A similar technique is used as for injection of the tibialis posterior tendon sheath, although with the foot placed in an inverted position. Typically, the peroneus longus and brevis tendons can be visualized as they pass around the lateral malleolus. In such circumstances the injection can be made using a proximal approach (Figure 14.16), injecting perpendicular to the skin, and turning and sliding horizontally under the skin toward the lateral malleolus using a 23-g needle and depositing 20 mg of methylprednisolone. With either of the approaches it should be possible to see and feel the injected material as it passes along the tendon sheath.

Morton's neuroma

The term 'Morton's neuroma' specifically refers to a neuroma in the third and fourth intermetatarsal space, and is often a misnomer in inflammatory arthritis as the condition and symptoms alike are reproduced by inflammatory tissue in the intermetatarsal space. For either of these conditions an injection of a long-acting steroid is efficacious. The patient sits on the treatment couch with the knee bent to 90° and the foot flat on the couch. The injection is made from the dorsal,

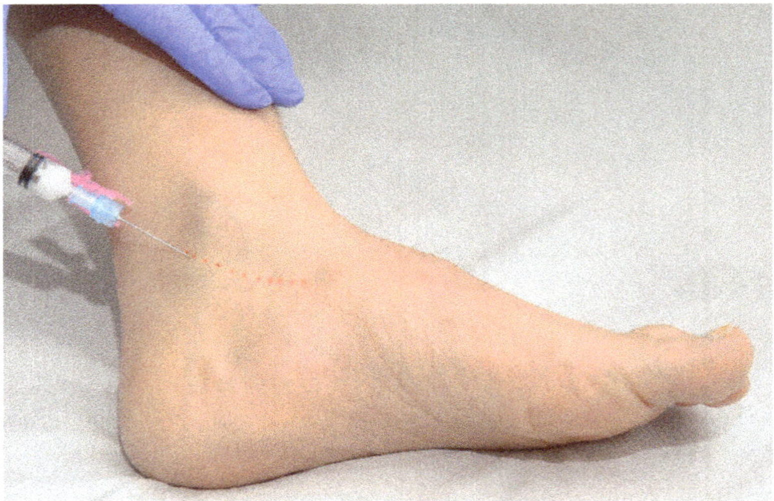

Figure 14.15 Injection of the tibialis posterior tendon sheath is made along the axis of the tendon at the level of the medial malleolus, using a proximal approach.

perpendicular approach directly into the space between the metatarsal heads, approximately 1 cm proximal to the web space (Figure 14.17) using a 23-g (blue) needle, depositing 20 mg of methylprednisolone.

Tarsal tunnel

The tarsal tunnel lies on the medial side of the ankle and is bounded by the calcaneus, the flexor retinaculum (ligamentum lacinatum), and the tendinous arch of abductor hallucis. Also found

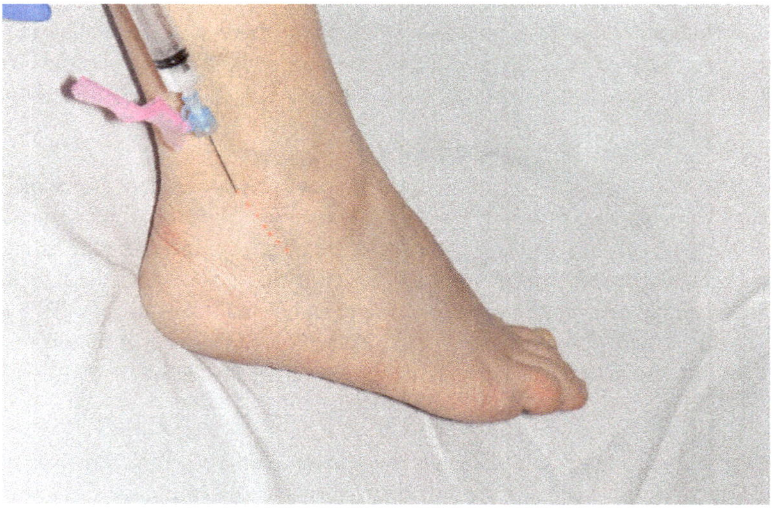

Figure 14.16 Injection of the peroneus longus and brevis tendons as they pass around the lateral malleolus using a proximal approach, injecting perpendicular to the skin, and turning and sliding the needle horizontally under the skin toward the lateral malleolus.

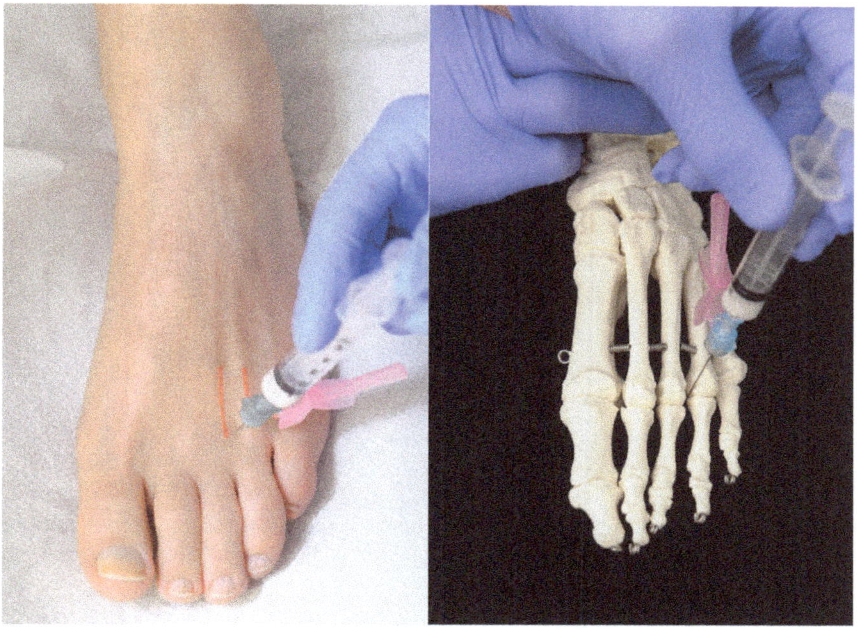

Figure 14.17 Injection of Morton's neuroma in the third and fourth intermetatarsal space from the dorsal aspect using a perpendicular approach directly into the space between the metatarsal heads, approximately 1 cm proximal to the web space.

passing through the 'tunnel' are the posterior tibial artery and the tendons of tibialis posterior and flexor hallucis longus. Tenosynovitis in the sheaths of the latter is the most likely cause of the tarsal tunnel syndrome in inflammatory arthritis, most notably RA. Neurophysiological testing will aid the diagnosis of tarsal tunnel syndrome as it is difficult to confirm in the clinic situation. The patient will be positioned as if the tibialis posterior tendon sheath is being injected. Mark the route of the posterior tibial artery. The injection is made from the proximal aspect of the site using a 23-g needle, attempting to avoid the neurovascular structures (Figure 14.18); placement of the needle at the inferior aspect of the ligament is the best way to do this 'blind' but, if in doubt, use an ultrasound-guided technique. If the condition persists despite injection, and the problem is confirmed by electrophysiology, surgery may be contemplated.

Plantar fascia

Thickening of the plantar fascia where it inserts into the medial tubercle of the calcaneum is more commonly seen in the seronegative spondyloarthropathies but has been shown to occur with a similar frequency in RA (135). The traditional approach to this injection has been directly onto the painful spot through the heel pad but this approach is painful, may result in excessive bleeding, and may also promote rupture of the plantar fascia. The alternative technique is to inject the attachment from the medial aspect of the ankle, aiming to target the 21-g (green) needle tip at the medial calcaneal tubercle, injecting 20 mg of methylprednisolone (Figure 14.19). This technique is slightly harder, as some degree of 'triangulation' is necessary. The patient should be supine, with the knee bent and foot everted. Either of the above injections may be made more comfortable by performing a tibial nerve block at the ankle; however, the nerve block may be considered more painful and the decision should be directed by the patient's preference for one

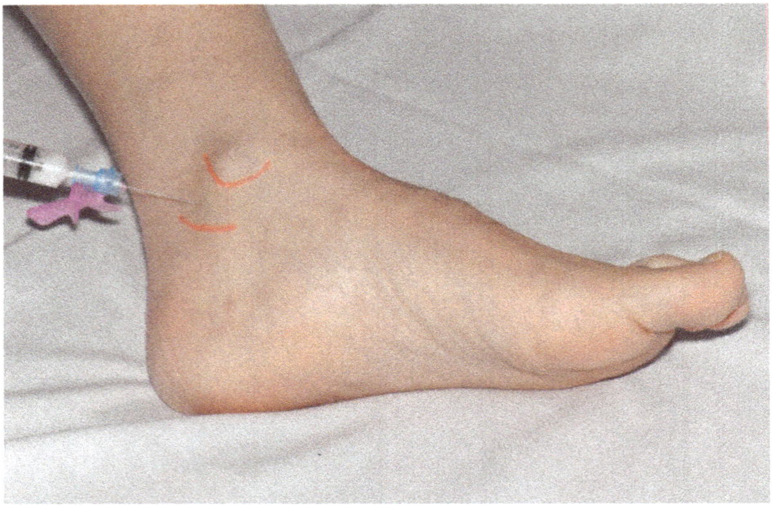

Figure 14.18 Injection of the tarsal tunnel is made from the proximal aspect of the site between the posterior tibial artery (red line) and the medial malleolus (red curve).

or two injections. Other options for the management of plantar fasciitis are discussed previously in Chapter 9.

Nerve blocks for the foot and ankle

There are several indications for nerve blockade in the foot and ankle, including those specific to patients with an inflammatory arthritis.

If the administration of steroid is contraindicated, then a nerve block can provide temporary relief of pain from synovitis or tendinitis. It has been noted that interrupting the chronic pain cycle even temporarily has some longer-term benefits for some patients (136). Nerve blocks are often used as a diagnostic aid to help identify painful structures or to estimate joint degeneration (129). This is particularly pertinent in the foot, where multiple joints and/or soft tissues are involved, but clinically it is difficult to differentiate the main cause of the symptoms.

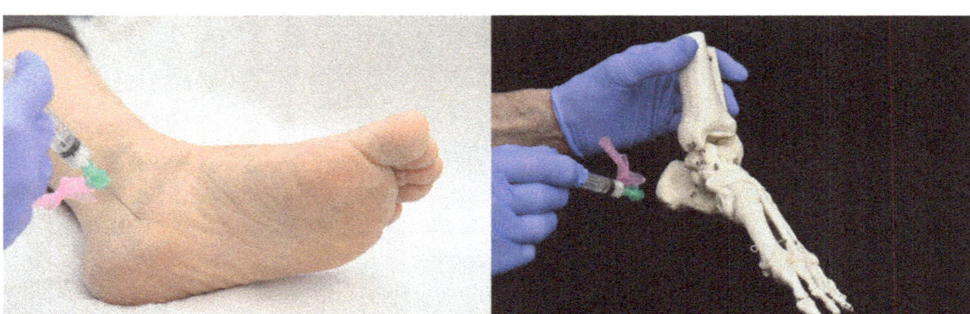

Figure 14.19 Injection of the plantar fascia attachment from the medial aspect of the ankle, targeting the needle tip at the medial calcaneal tubercle.

Prior to more invasive procedures or painful injections such as local corticosteroid infiltration or injection of the plantar fascia, nerve blocks can be helpful.

The most widely used local anaesthetic agents are lidocaine, mepivacaine, and bupivacaine. They are used without adrenaline in end structures such as the foot to avoid compromising the arterial supply.

Lidocaine is used at concentrations typically of 1% or 2% and may be used alone or mixed with other agents such as corticosteroids. The onset of analgesia is fairly rapid, usually within 1–2 minutes in a joint or soft tissue but relatively longer (20–30 minutes) for a nerve such as the tibial or peroneal. Hence nerve blocks require extra time in currently busy clinics and this should be factored in when considering the need. Lidocaine provides a relatively short duration of analgesia, typically of 2–3 hours. Mepivacaine, usually administered at a concentration of 1.5% or 3%, can have a slightly more rapid onset and has a similar duration of effect. For a longer lasting blockade, bupivacaine (typically 0.25% or 0.50%) will provide analgesia for up to 10 hours, although its onset of action is slow, at 20–40 minutes, and its toxicity is greater than lidocaine or mepivacaine.

Local analgesia is most often administered subcutaneously to desensitize the skin local to the site of a more painful procedure. Local anaesthetic may also be introduced directly into a painful structure such as a joint or soft-tissue lesion.

A clinician with good knowledge of anatomy can, however, use local anaesthetic to blockade individual nerves at the level of the ankle and so provide analgesia with a single injection to the moderately large areas of the foot associated with each dermatome.

There are as many as seven ankle nerve blocks that may be used, but most indications in rheumatology require only analgesia of the plantar foot (tibial nerve) or the dorsum of the forefoot (common peroneal nerve). All can be performed with the patient in a supine position, although the operator might find access better for the posterior approaches if the patient is put in a prone position.

Tibial nerve

The tibial nerve is a branch of the sciatic nerve. Its sensory dermatome includes the plantar surface of the foot (via the medial and lateral plantar nerves) and the lateral side of the foot (via the sural nerve). A single injection blockading the tibial nerve at ankle level gives satisfactory analgesia of the whole of the plantar surface of the foot, making this technique potentially suitable for painful plantar procedures such as for plantar fasciitis or ulcer debridement.

It is blocked at the level of the malleolus using a posterior or medial approach. If the patient is supine the foot should be abducted to expose the posteromedial aspect of the ankle. It may be possible to palpate or roll the nerve to identify its location precisely, although this is not common. The nerve lies medial to the rest of the neurovascular structures and so the approach should stay close to the medial side of the Achilles tendon. Palpation and subsequent marking of the tibialis posterior artery either by hand or using a hand-held Doppler is advised. The needle is introduced midway between the tip of the malleolus and the medial border of the Achilles tendon and advanced toward the posterior aspect of the tibia. The patient should be advised to warn the operator if paraesthesia is felt, as this indicates that the needle tip has touched the nerve itself. If this occurs, then the needle tip should be withdrawn a few millimetres prior to completing the injection. If the needle tip advances without encountering the nerve, then it will come to rest on the posterior aspect of the tibia. At this point the needle should again be withdrawn a few millimetres prior to completing the injection.

Once the desired spot is reached aspiration must be performed to ensure that the needle tip is not lying within any of the vascular structures closely associated with the tibial nerve in this region. If the aspirate is clear, the injection is completed by infiltrating 2–5 ml of solution around the nerve, the amount depending on concentration used. The diameter of the tibial nerve slows the rate of onset of analgesia slightly, and complete anaesthesia may take 20–30 minutes at this site.

Common/superficial peroneal nerve

The common peroneal nerve also derives from the sciatic nerve dividing into a superficial and deep branch at the level of the mid-tibia. The superficial branch passes anterior to the lateral malleolus to supply the majority of the dorsum of the foot, while the deep branch passes through the tibiofibular interosseous membrane along the dorsum of the foot to supply the first/second toe interspace. If the area of required anaesthesia includes the first/second toe interspace, then blockade is best achieved proximal to branching at the level of the fibular styloid process. If analgesia of the first/second toe interspace is not required, the common peroneal nerve can be blocked at the fibular styloid or the superficial branch alone can be blocked at the lateral malleolus.

To block the common peroneal nerve, it is usually directly palpable 1–2 cm distal to the styloid process of the fibula, and the nerve may be rolled under the finger tips. It is blocked with a straightforward subcutaneous injection close to the nerve. Onset of action is typically in the 15–20-minute range.

Blockade of the superficial branch is undertaken on the anterolateral aspect of the lateral malleolus. The nerve can be often be palpated directly or may even be seen and, if so, a direct subcutaneous deposition is made close to the nerve. If the nerve cannot be located precisely, then an alternative technique is used. The course of the nerve can be quite variable in this region, so a common technique is to pass the needle tip subcutaneously across the likely course of the nerve for 2–3 cm. The local analgesic is deposited as the needle is slowly withdrawing, leaving a 2–3-cm bleb of local anaesthetic subcutaneously. Blocking the nerve directly at the ankle can give rapid onset of action.

Exercise therapy

Muscle weakness, restricted range of motion of joints, and reduced physical function are commonly seen in rheumatology patients. Significant muscle loss (~67%) and obesity (~80%) are regularly observed in patients with arthritis and in RA is termed 'rheumatoid cachexia'. In a recent editorial, Lemmey and colleagues highlighted the contribution of rheumatoid cachexia to the disability and exacerbated comorbidity risk in this patient group (137).

Although current guidelines identify the need to encourage patients to undertake exercise, these are not specific to the foot and ankle. However, patients may require other foot health management strategies first to ensure they are able to take part in exercise therapy; for example, that they are wearing the most effective footwear and are provided with orthoses, if required, to prevent any additional complications. The NICE guidelines (1) recommend that people with RA should have access to specialist physiotherapy, with periodic review to:

- Improve general fitness and encourage regular exercise.
- Learn exercises for enhancing joint flexibility, muscle strength, and managing other functional impairments.

Further recommendations from the NICE guidelines for OA state that clinicians should offer advice on core treatments to all people with clinical OA, which should include activity and exercise, as well as interventions to achieve weight loss if the person is overweight or obese (2). Our exercise advice to people with OA should be irrespective of age, comorbidity, pain severity, or disability. Exercise should include both local muscle strengthening and general aerobic fitness.

Historically, patients with arthritis, particularly those with RA, were recommended to avoid weightbearing exercise and concentrate on isometric non-weightbearing exercises and range-of-motion exercises to avoid aggravating joint inflammation and accelerating joint damage. In 1996 Rall and colleagues examined the feasibility of high-intensity progressive resistance training in patients with RA compared with healthy young and old patients (138). Patients with RA had no change in the number of painful or swollen joints but had significant reductions in self-reported pain score and fatigue score, as well as improved 50-foot walking times and improved balance and gait scores. They concluded that high-intensity strength training is feasible and safe in selected patients with well-controlled RA and leads to significant improvements in strength, pain, and fatigue without exacerbating disease activity or joint pain (138). As well as improving symptoms reported by patients, long-term high-intensity weightbearing exercise programmes, compared with usual care physical therapy, have been shown to be effective in increasing the physical capacity and functional ability of patients with RA without causing additional damage to the weightbearing joints (139, 140). A further advantage is that such programmes help to prevent systemic bone loss.

More recently, Lemmey and colleagues conducted an RCT and confirmed that high-intensity progressive resistance training is a safe and effective means of restoring muscle mass and functional capacity in patients with established, stable RA, advocating that such training should be included in disease management (141).

Enabling Self-management and Coping with Arthritic Pain using Exercise (ESCAPE-pain) is a rehabilitation programme for people with chronic joint pain that integrates educational self-management and coping strategies with an exercise regimen individualized for each participant. ESCAPE-pain appears to achieve improvements by increasing people's treatment belief in the safety and utility of exercise to control symptoms, rather than alteration in their beliefs about causation or prognosis. Although this programme has only been evaluated for people with knee pain (142–144), clinicians have already suggested that it offers a mechanism to improve musculoskeletal symptoms in all rheumatology patients.

In patients with RA and OA proprioceptive deficits, as well as loss of muscle strength and functional ability, have been shown (145, 146). Quadriceps sensorimotor deficits are associated with lower limb disability and have been shown to improve with a rehabilitation programme that incorporates both physical activity and strength training without exacerbating pain and disease activity. Furthermore, it has been suggested that improvements in proprioceptive acuity may reduce harmful impact forces during gait, resulting in better timing of placement of the foot.

Gait training and re-education for patients is not routinely carried out in rheumatology clinics. However, gait training has been shown to be beneficial in the rehabilitation of patients who have had strokes, patients with Parkinson's disease, amputee patients using artificial limbs, and in reducing falls in the elderly population. Gait training using the rhythmic auditory stimulation method consists of audiotapes with metronome-pulse patterns embedded into the on/off beat structure of rhythmically accentuated instrumental music has been shown to increase gait velocity, stride length, and step cadence. Further work is needed to determine the effectiveness of gait training for patients with rheumatic and musculoskeletal diseases.

Conclusion

Rheumatic and musculoskeletal diseases are complex multisystem diseases that affect the feet and therefore usually require a multidisciplinary approach to their management. The challenge often faced is in coordinating the care of patients and ensuring that all those involved, including the patient, are aware of each other's roles; organizing care for patients will be discussed in further detail in Chapter 16. This chapter has discussed and highlighted the relevant non-surgical foot health management strategies for rheumatology patients, who frequently present with both inflammatory and mechanical disease in their feet, with the aim of minimizing the impact on the foot and ankle.

References

1. **National Institute for Health and Care Excellence**. *Clinical Guideline 79: Rheumatoid Arthritis. The Management of Rheumatoid Arthritis in Adults*. London: NICE; 2009.
2. **National Institute for Health and Care Excellence**. *Clinical Guideline 177: Osteoarthritis: Care and Management*. London: NICE; 2014.
3. **Grigor C, Capell H, Stirling A, et al.** Effect of a treatment strategy of tight control for rheumatoid arthritis (the TICORA study): a single-blind randomised controlled trial. *Lancet*. 2004;**364**(9430):263–9.
4. **Kiely PD, Brown AK, Edwards CJ, et al.** Contemporary treatment principles for early rheumatoid arthritis: a consensus statement. *Rheumatology (Oxford)*. 2009;**48**(7):765–72.
5. **Ostor AJ, Conaghan PG.** Tight control in rheumatoid arthritis improves outcomes. *Practitioner*. 2009;**253**(1716):29–32.
6. **Wechalekar MD, Lester S, Hill CL, et al.** Active foot synovitis in patients with rheumatoid arthritis: unstable remission status, radiographic progression, and worse functional outcomes in patients with foot synovitis in apparent remission. *Arthritis Care Res (Hoboken)*. 2016;**68**(11):1616–23.
7. **Fransen J, Creemers MC, Van Riel PL.** Remission in rheumatoid arthritis: agreement of the disease activity score (DAS28) with the ARA preliminary remission criteria. *Rheumatology (Oxford)*. 2004;**43**(10):1252–5.
8. **van der Leeden M, Steultjens MP, van Schaardenburg D, Dekker J.** Forefoot disease activity in rheumatoid arthritis patients in remission: results of a cohort study. *Arthritis Res Ther*. 2010;**12**(1):R3.
9. **Kapral T, Dernoschnig F, Machold KP, et al.** Remission by composite scores in rheumatoid arthritis: are ankles and feet important? *Arthritis Res Ther*. 2007;**9**(4):R72.
10. **Felson DT, Smolen JS, Wells G, et al.** American College of Rheumatology/European League Against Rheumatism provisional definition of remission in rheumatoid arthritis for clinical trials. *Arthritis Rheum*. 2011;**63**(3):573–86.
11. **Pinals RS, Masi AT, Larsen RA.** Preliminary criteria for clinical remission in rheumatoid arthritis. *Arthritis Rheum*. 1981;**24**(10):1308–15.
12. **Wechalekar MD, Lester S, Proudman SM, et al.** Active foot synovitis in patients with rheumatoid arthritis: applying clinical criteria for disease activity and remission may result in underestimation of foot joint involvement. *Arthritis Rheum*. 2012;**64**(5):1316–22.
13. **Backhouse MR, Keenan AM, Hensor EM, et al.** Use of conservative and surgical foot care in an inception cohort of patients with rheumatoid arthritis. *Rheumatology (Oxford)*. 2011;**50**(9):1586–95.
14. **Woodburn J, Hennessy K, Steultjens MP, McInnes IB, Turner DE.** Looking through the 'window of opportunity': is there a new paradigm of podiatry care on the horizon in early rheumatoid arthritis? *J Foot Ankle Res*. 2010;**3**:8.
15. **Emery P, Breedveld FC, Dougados M, Kalden JR, Schiff MH, Smolen JS.** Early referral recommendation for newly diagnosed rheumatoid arthritis: evidence based development of a clinical guide. *Ann Rheum Dis*. 2002;**61**(4):290–7.
16. **Department of Health**. *Supporting People with Long Term Conditions. An NHS and Social Care Model to Support Local Innovation and Integration*. London: Department of Health; 2005.
17. **Department of Health**. *Long Term Conditions Compendium of Information*, 3rd edition. London: Department of Health; 2012.
18. **The Scottish Government**. *Long Term Conditions Collaborative: Improving Care Pathways*. Edinburgh: The Scottish Government; 2010.

19. **Panagioti M, Richardson G, Small N, et al.** Self-management support interventions to reduce health care utilisation without compromising outcomes: a systematic review and meta-analysis. *BMC Health Services Research.* 2014;**14**:356.
20. **The British Society for Rheumatology.** *The State of Play in UK Rheumatology: Insights into Service Pressures and Solutions.* UK: The British Society for Rheumatology; 2015.
21. **Kroon FPB, van der Burg LRA, Buchbinder R, Osborne RH, Johnston RV, Pitt V.** Self-management education programmes for osteoarthritis. *Cochrane Database of Systematic Reviews.* 2014;CD008963. DOI: 10.1002/14651858.CD008963.pub2.
22. **Lefevre-Colau MM, Buchbinder R, Regnaux JP, Roren A, Poiraudeau S, Boutron I.** Self-management education programmes for rheumatoid arthritis. *Cochrane Database of Systematic Reviews.* 2014;CD011338. DOI: 10.1002/14651858.CD011338.
23. **Osborne RH, Spinks JM, Wicks IP.** Patient education and self-management programs in arthritis. *Med J Aust.* 2004;**180**(5 Suppl):23–6.
24. **Lorig KR, Holman H.** Self-management education: history, definition, outcomes, and mechanisms. *Ann Behav Med.* 2003;**26**(1):1–7.
25. **Von Korff M, Gruman J, Schaefer J, Curry SJ, Wagner EH.** Collaborative management of chronic illness. *Ann Int Med.* 1997;**127**(12):1097–102.
26. **Haywood H, Adams J.** Patients' experiences of rheumatoid arthritis education: a short report. *Musculoskelet Care.* 2011;**9**:113–19.
27. **Makelainen P, Vahvilainen-Julkunen K, Pietila A-M.** Rheumatoid arthritis patients' education—context and methods. *J Clin Nurs.* 2007;**16**:258–67.
28. **Graham AS, Hammond A, Williams AE.** Foot health education for people with rheumatoid arthritis: the practitioner's perspective. *J Foot Ankle Res.* 2012;**5**:2.
29. **Makelainen P, Vahvilainen-Julkunen K, Pietila A-M.** Rheumatoid arthritis patient education: RA patients' experience. *J Clin Nurs.* 2009;**18**:2058–65.
30. **Williams AE, Davies S, Graham A, et al.** Guidelines for the management of foot health problems associated with rheumatoid arthritis. *Musculoskelet Care.* 2011;**9**:86–92.
31. **PRCA** (2010). PRCA Standards of Care for People with Musculoskeletal Foot Health Problems. Available at http://www.prcassoc.org.uk/standards-project.
32. **Graham AS, Hammond A, Walmsley S, Williams AE.** Foot health education for people with rheumatoid arthritis—some patient perspectives. *J Foot Ankle Res.* 2012;**5**:23.
33. **Graham AS, Hammond A, Williams AE.** Therapeutic foot health education for patients with rheumatoid arthritis: a narrative review. *Musculoskelet Care.* 2011;**9**:141–51.
34. **Caplan L, Wolfe F, Michaud K, Quinzanos I, Hirsh JM.** Strong association of health literacy with functional status among rheumatoid arthritis patients: a cross-sectional study. *Arthritis Care Res.* 2014;**66**:508–14.
35. **van Onna M, Hinsenveld E, de Vries H, Boonen A.** Health literacy in patients dealing with gout: a qualitative study. *Clin Rheumatol.* 2015;**34**:1599–603.
36. **Hardware B, Johnson D, Hale C, Ndosi M, Adebajo A.** Patients and nursing staff views of using the education needs assessment tool in rheumatology clinics: a qualitative study. *J Clin Nurs.* 2015;**24**:1048–58.
37. **Hardware B, Lacey AE, Shewan J.** Towards the development of a tool to assess educational needs in patients with arthritis. *Clin Effect Nurs.* 2004;**8**:111–17.
38. **Li LC, Townsend AF, Badley EM.** Self-management interventions in the digital age: new approaches to support people with rheumatologic conditions. *Best Pract Res Clin Rheumatol.* 2012;**26**:321–33.
39. **Azevedo ARP, de Sousa HML, Monteiro JAF, Lima ARNP.** Future perspectives of smartphone applications for rheumatic disease self-management. *Rheumatol Int.* 2015;**35**:419–31.
40. **Poole JL, Mendelson C, Skipper B, Khanna D.** Taking charge of systemic sclerosis: a pilot study to assess the effectiveness of an internet self-management program. *Arthritis Care Res.* 2014;**66**:778–82.

41. **de Jongh T, Gurol-Urganci I, Vodopivec-Jamsek V, Car J, Atun R.** Mobile phone messaging for facilitating self-management of long-term illnesses. *Cochrane Database of Systematic Reviews.* 2012;CD007459.
42. **Shigaki CL, Smarr KL, Siva C, Ge B, Musser D, Johnson R.** RAHelp: an online intervention for individuals with rheumatoid arthritis. *Arthritis Care Res.* 2013;**65**:1573–81.
43. **Joplin S, van der Zwan R, Joshua F, Wong PKK.** Medication adherence in patients with rheumatoid arthritis: the effect of patient education, health literacy and musculoskeletal ultrasound. *Biomed Res Int.* 2015;150658.
44. **Joplin SK, van der Zwan R, Bagga H, Joshua F, Wong PKK.** Pilot study assessing the novel use of musculoskeletal ultrasound in patients with rheumatoid arthritis to improve patient attitudes and adherence to medication. *Int J Rheum Dis.* 2014;**19**:658–64.
45. **Hendry GJ, Brenton-Rule A, Barr G, Rome K.** Footwear experiences of people with chronic musculoskeletal diseases. *Arthritis Care Res.* 2015;**67**:1164–72.
46. **Hendry GJ, Gibson KA, Pile K, et al.** 'They just scraped off the calluses': a mixed methods exploration of foot care access and provision for people with rheumatoid arthritis in south-western Sydney, Australia. *J Foot Ankle Res.* 2013;**6**:34.
47. **Williams AE, Nester CJ, Ravey MI.** Rheumatoid arthritis patients' experiences of wearing therapeutic footwear—a qualitative investigation. *BMC Musculoskelet Disord.* 2007;**8**:104.
48. **Gronning K, Rannestad T, Skomsvoll JF, Rygg LO, Steinsbekk A.** Long-term effects of a nurse-led group and individual patient education programme for patients with chronic inflammatory polyarthritis—a randomised controlled trial. *J Clin Nurs.* 2013;**23**:1005–17.
49. **Iversen MD, Hammond A, Betteridge N.** Self-management of rheumatic diseases: state of the art and future perspectives. *Ann Rheum Dis.* 2010;**69**:955–63.
50. **Barlow J, Turner A, Swaby L, Gilchrist M, Wright C, Doherty M.** An 8-year follow-up of arthritis self-management programme participants. *Rheumatology.* 2009;**48**:128–33.
51. **Hammond A, Freeman K.** One-year outcomes of a randomized controlled trial on an educational-behavioural joint protection programme for people with rheumatoid arthritis. *Rheumatology.* 2001;**40**:1044–51.
52. **Semple R, Newcombe LW, Finlayson GL, Hutchison CR, Forlow JH, Woodburn J.** The FOOTSTEP self-management foot care programme: are rheumatoid arthritis patients physically able to participate? *Musculoskelet Care.* 2009;**7**:57–65.
53. **Waxman R, Woodburn H, Powell M, Woodburn J, Blackburn S, Helliwell P.** FOOTSTEP: a randomized controlled trial investigating the clinical and cost effectiveness of a patient self-management program for basic foot care in the elderly. *J Clin Epidemiol.* 2003;**56**:1092–9.
54. **Davys HJ, Woodburn J, Bingham SJ, Emery P.** Onychocryptosis (ingrowing toe nail) in patients with rheumatoid arthritis on biologic therapies. *Rheumatology (Oxford).* 2006;**45**(Suppl. 1):i171.
55. **Woodburn J, Helliwell PS.** Relation between heel position and the distribution of forefoot plantar pressures and skin callosities in rheumatoid arthritis. *Ann Rheum Dis.* 1996;**55**(11):806–10.
56. **Young MJ, Cavanagh PR, Thomas G, Johnson MM, Murray H, Boulton AJ.** The effect of callus removal on dynamic plantar foot pressures in diabetic patients. *Diabet Med.* 1992;**9**(1):55–7.
57. **Murray HJ, Young MJ, Hollis S, Boulton AJ.** The association between callus formation, high pressures and neuropathy in diabetic foot ulceration. *Diabet Med.* 1996;**13**(11):979–82.
58. **Woodburn J, Stableford Z, Helliwell PS.** Preliminary investigation of debridement of plantar callosities in rheumatoid arthritis. *Rheumatology (Oxford).* 2000;**39**(6):652–4.
59. **Davys HJ, Turner DE, Helliwell PS, Conaghan PG, Emery P, Woodburn J.** Debridement of plantar callosities in rheumatoid arthritis: a randomized controlled trial. *Rheumatology (Oxford).* 2005;**44**(2):207–10.
60. **Siddle HJ, Redmond AC, Waxman R, et al.** Debridement of painful forefoot plantar callosities in rheumatoid arthritis: the CARROT randomised controlled trial. *Clin Rheumatol.* 2013; **32**(5):567–74.

61. **Davys HJ, Turner DE, Helliwell PS, Emery P.** Foot ulceration in patients with rheumatic diseases. *Ann Rheum Dis.* 2006;**65**(Abstract Suppl. 2):ii241.
62. **Firth J, Hale C, Helliwell P, Hill J, Nelson EA.** The prevalence of foot ulceration in patients with rheumatoid arthritis. *Arthritis Rheum.* 2008;**59**(2):200–5.
63. **Firth J, Helliwell P, Hale C, Hill J, Nelson EA.** The predictors of foot ulceration in patients with rheumatoid arthritis: a preliminary investigation. *Clin Rheumatol.* 2008;**27**(11):1423–8.
64. **Siddle HJ, Firth J, Waxman R, Nelson EA, Helliwell PS.** A case series to describe the clinical characteristics of foot ulceration in patients with rheumatoid arthritis. *Clin Rheumatol.* 2012;**31**(3):541–5.
65. **Vidigal E, Jacoby RK, Dixon AS, Ratliff AH, Kirkup J.** The foot in chronic rheumatoid arthritis. *Ann Rheum Dis.* 1975;**34**(4):292–7.
66. **Cawley MI.** Vasculitis and ulceration in rheumatic diseases of the foot. *Bailliere's Clin Rheumatol.* 1987;**1**(2):315–33.
67. **Shanmugam VK, Demaria DM, Attinger CE.** Lower extremity ulcers in rheumatoid arthritis: features and response to immunosuppression. *Clin Rheumatol.* 2011;**30**(6):849–53.
68. **Firth J, Waxman R, Law G, et al.** The predictors of foot ulceration in patients with rheumatoid arthritis. *Clin Rheumatol.* 2014;**33**(5):615–21.
69. **Fitzgerald P, Siddle HJ, Backhouse MR, Nelson EA.** Prevalence and microbiological characteristics of clinically infected foot-ulcers in patients with rheumatoid arthritis: a retrospective exploratory study. *J Foot Ankle Res.* 2015;**8**:38.
70. **Backhouse M, Nelson A, Wright-Hughes A, et al.** CODIFI (Concordance in Diabetic Foot Infection): agreement in reported presence of likely pathogens in swabs and tissue samples from infected diabetic foot ulcers. *J Foot Ankle Res.* 2015;**8**(Suppl. 1):A2.
71. **National Institute for Health and Care Excellence.** *Clinical Guideline 15: Diabetic Foot Problems: Prevention and Management.* London: NICE; 2015.
72. **Barton CJ, Bonanno D, Menz HB.** Development and evaluation of a tool for the assessment of footwear characteristics. *J Foot Ankle Res.* 2009;**2**:10.
73. **McPoil T.** Footwear. *Phys Ther.* 1988;**68**:1857–65.
74. **Dufour AB, Casey VA, Gologhtly YM, Hannan MT.** Characteristics associated with hallux valgus in a population-based foot study of older adults. *Arthritis Care Res.* 2014;**66**:1880–6.
75. **Foster A, Blanchette MG, Chou Y-C, Powers CM.** The influence of heel height on frontal plane ankle biomechanics: implications for lateral ankle sprains. *Foot Ankle Int.* 2012;**33**:64–9.
76. **Menant J, Perry S, Steele J, Menz H, Munro B, Lord S.** Effects of shoe characteristics on dynamic stability when walking on even and uneven surfaces in young and older people. *Arch Phys Med Rehabil.* 2008;**89**:1970–6.
77. **Menant JC, Steele JR, Menz HB, Munro BJ, Lord SR.** Effects of walking surfaces and footwear on temporo-spatial gait parameters in young and older people. *Gait Posture.* 2009;**29**(3):392–7.
78. **Menz HB, Morris ME.** Determinants of disabling foot pain in retirement village residents. *J Am Podiatr Med Assoc.* 2005;**95**:573–9.
79. **Lord S, Bashford G.** Shoe characteristics and balance in older women. *J Am Geriatr Soc.* 1996;**44**:429–33.
80. **van der Zwaard BC, van der Horst HE, Knol DL, Vanwanseele B, Elders PJM.** Treatment of forefoot problems in older people: a randomized clinical trial comparing podiatric treatment with standardised shoe advice. *Ann Fam Med.* 2014;**12**:432–40.
81. **Menz HB, Sherrington C.** The footwear assessment form: a reliable clinical tool to assess footwear characteristics of relevance to postural stability in older adults. *Clin Rehabil.* 2000;**14**:657–64.
82. **Frey C.** Foot health and shoewear for women. *Clin Orthop Rel Res.* 2000;**372**:32–44.
83. **Menz HB, Lord SR, McIntosh AS.** Slip resistance of casual footwear: implications for falls in older adults. *Gerontology.* 2001;**47**:145–9.

84. **Menz HB, Auhl M, Ristevski S, Frescos N, Munteanu SE.** Evaluation of the accuracy of shoe fitting in older people using three-dimensional foot scanning. *J Foot Ankle Res.* 2014;**7**:3.
85. **McInnes AD, Hashmi F, Farndon LJ, et al.** Comparison of shoe-length fit between people with and without diabetic peripheral neuropathy: a case–control study. *J Foot Ankle Res.* 2012;**5**:9.
86. **Schwartzkopf R, Perretta DJ, Russell TA, Sheskier SC.** Foot and shoe size mismatch in three different New York City populations. *J Foot Ankle Surg.* 2011;**50**:391–4.
87. **Chaiwanichsiri D, Tantisiriwat N, Janchai S.** Proper shoe sizes for Thai elderly. *Foot.* 2008;**18**:186–91.
88. **Nixon BP, Armstrong DG, Wendell C, Vazquez JR, Rabinovich Z.** Do US veterans wear appropriately sized shoes? The Veteran Affairs Shoe Size Selection Study. *J Am Podiatr Med Assoc.* 2006;**96**:290–2.
89. **Nguyen US, Hillstrom HJ, Li W, et al.** Factors associated with hallux valgus in a population-based study of older women and men: the MOBILIZE Boston Study. *Osteoarthritis Cartilage.* 2010;**18**:41–6.
90. **Dufour AB, Broe KE, Nguyen UDT, et al.** Foot pain: is current or past footwear a factor? *Arthritis Rheum.* 2009;**61**:1352–8.
91. **Menz HB, Morris ME.** Determinants of disabling foot pain in retirement village residents. *J Am Podiatr Med Assoc.* 2005;**95**:573–9.
92. **Burns SL, Leese GP, McMurdo MET.** Older people and ill fitting shoes. *Postgrad Med J.* 2002;**78**:344–6.
93. **Naidoo S, Anderson S, Mills J, et al.** 'I could cry, the amount of shoes I can't get into': a qualitative exploration of the factors that influence retail footwear selection in women with rheumatoid arthritis. *J Foot Ankle Res.* 2011;**4**:21.
94. **Rome K, Frecklington M, McNair P, Gow P, Dalbeth N.** Footwear characteristics and factors influencing footwear choice in patients with gout. *Arthritis Care Res.* 2011;**63**:1599–604.
95. **Williams AE, Bowden AP.** Meeting the challenge for foot health in rheumatic diseases. *The Foot.* 2004;**14**:154–8.
96. **Brenton-Rule A, Hendry GJ, Barr G, Rome K.** An evaluation of seasonal variations in footwear worn by adults with inflammatory arthritis: a cross-sectional observational study using a web-based survey. *J Foot Ankle Res.* 2014;**7**:36.
97. **Thomas MJ, Moore A, Roddy E, Peat G.** 'Somebody to say "come on we can sort this"': a qualitative study of primary care consultation among older adults with symptomatic foot osteoarthritis. *Arthritis Care Res.* 2013;**65**:2051–5.
98. **Goodacre LJ, Candy FJ.** 'If I didn't have RA I wouldn't give them the house room': the relationship between RA, footwear and clothing choices. *Rheumatology.* 2011;**50**:513–17.
99. **Turner DE, Woodburn J.** Characterising the clinical and biomechanical features of severely deformed feet in rheumatoid arthritis. *Gait Posture.* 2008;**28**:574–80.
100. **Dahmen R, Buijsmann S, Siemonsma PC, Boers M, Lankhorst GJ, Roorda LD.** Use and effects of custom-made therapeutic footwear on lower-extremity related pain and activity limitations in patients with rheumatoid arthritis: a prospective observational cohort study. *J Rehabil Med.* 2014;**46**:561–7.
101. **Fransen M, Edmonds J.** Off the shelf orthopaedic footwear for people with rheumatoid arthritis. *Arthritis Care Res.* 1997;**10**:250–6.
102. **Cham MB, Ghasemi MS, Forogh B, Sanjari MA, Yeganeh MZ, Eshraghi A.** Effect of rocker shoes on pain, disability and activity limitation in patients with rheumatoid arthritis. *Prosthetics Orthotics Int.* 2014;**38**:310–15.
103. **Cho NS, Hwang JH, Chang HJ, Koh EM, Park HS.** Randomized controlled trial for clinical effects of varying types of insoles combined with specialized shoes in patients with rheumatoid arthritis of the foot. *Clin Rehabil.* 2009;**23**:512–21.
104. **Williams AE, Nester CJ, Ravey MI.** Rheumatoid arthritis patients' experiences of wearing therapeutic footwear—a qualitative investigation. *BMC Musculoskeletal Dis.* 2007;**8**:104.
105. **Menz HB, Auhl M, Tan JM, Levinger P, Roddy E, Munteanu SE.** Effectiveness of foot orthoses versus rocker-sole footwear for first metatarsophalangeal joint osteoarthritis: randomized trial. *Arthritis Care Res.* 2016;**68**:581–9.

106. **Woodburn J, Helliwell PS, Barker S.** Changes in 3D joint kinematics support the continuous use of orthoses in the management of painful rearfoot deformity in rheumatoid arthritis. *J Rheumatol.* 2003;**30**:2356–64.

107. **Woodburn J, Barker S, Helliwell PS.** A randomized controlled trial of foot orthoses in rheumatoid arthritis. *J Rheumatol.* 2002;**29**:1377–83.

108. **Chalmers AC, Busby C, Goyert J, Porter B, Schulzer M.** Metatarsalgia and rheumatoid arthritis: a randomized, single blind, sequential trial comparing 2 types of foot orthoses and supportive shoes. *J Rheumatol.* 2000;**27**:1643–7.

109. **Hodge MC, Bach TM, Carter GM.** Orthotic management of plantar pressure and pain in rheumatoid arthritis. *Clin Biomech (Bristol, Avon).* 1999;**14**:567–75.

110. **Conceicao CS, Neto MG, Mendes SMD, Sa KN, Baptista AF.** Systematic review and meta-analysis of effects of foot orthoses on pain and disability in rheumatoid arthritis patients. *Disability Rehabil.* 2015;**37**:1209–13.

111. **Hennessy K, Woodburn J, Steultjens MPM.** Custom foot orthoses for rheumatoid arthritis: a systematic review. *Arthritis Care Res (Hoboken).* 2012;**64**:311–20.

112. **Scottish Intercollegiate Guidelines Network.** *SIGN 123: Management of Early Rheumatoid Arthritis. A National Clinical Guideline.* Edinburgh: Royal College of Physicians; 2011.

113. **Forestier R, André-Vert J, Guillez P, et al.** Non-drug treatment (excluding surgery) in rheumatoid arthritis: clinical practice guidelines. *Joint Bone Spine.* 2009;**76**:691–8.

114. **Gossec L, Pavy S, Pham T, et al.** Nonpharmacological treatments in early rheumatoid arthritis: clinical practice guidelines based on published evidence and expert opinion. *Joint Bone Spine.* 2006;**73**:396–402.

115. **Luqmani R, Hennell S, Estrach C, et al.** British Society for Rheumatology and British Health Professionals in Rheumatology Guideline for the Management of Rheumatoid Arthritis (the first 2 years). *Rheumatology.* 2006;**45**:1167–69.

116. **Gibson KS, Woodburn J, Porter D, Telfer S.** Functionally optimized orthoses for early rheumatoid arthritis foot disease: a study of mechanisms and patient experience. *Arthritis Care Res.* 2014;**66**:1456–64.

117. **Halstead J, Chapman GJ, Gray JC, et al.** Foot orthoses in the treatment of symptomatic midfoot osteoarthritis using clinical and biomechanical outcomes: a randomised feasibility study. *Clin Rheumatol.* 2016;**35**:987–96.

118. **Rao S, Baumhauer J, Tome J, Nawoczenski D.** Orthoses alter in vivo segmental foot kinematics during walking in patients with midfoot arthritis. *Arch Phys Med Rehabil.* 2010;**91**:608–14.

119. **Ibuki A, Cornoiu A, Clarke A, Unglik R, Beischer A.** The effect of orthotic treatment on midfoot osteoarthritis assessed using specifically designed patient evaluation questionnaires. *Prosthet Orthot Int.* 2010;**34**:461–71.

120. **Otter SJ, Lucas K, Springett K, et al.** Foot pain in rheumatoid arthritis: prevalence, risk factors and management: an epidemiological study. *Clin Rheumatol.* 2010;**29**:255–71.

121. **Grondal L, Tengstrand B, Nordmark B, Wretenberg P, Stark A.** The foot: still the most important reason for walking incapacity in rheumatoid arthritis: distribution of symptomatic joints in 1,000 RA patients. *Acta Orthop.* 2008;**79**:257–61.

122. **van der Leeden M, Steultjens MP, Ursum J, et al.** Prevalence and course of forefoot impairments and walking disability in the first eight years of rheumatoid arthritis. *Arthritis Rheum.* 2008;**59**:1596–602.

123. **Smolen JS, Aletaha D.** Developments in the clinical understanding of rheumatoid arthritis. *Arthritis Res Ther.* 2009;**11**:204.

124. **Aletaha D, Huizinga TWJ.** The use of data from early arthritis clinics for clinical research. *Best Pract Res Clin Rheumatol.* 2009;**23**:117–23.

125. **Combe B.** Progression in early rheumatoid arthritis. *Best Pract Res Clin Rheumatol.* 2009;**23**:59–69.

126. **Otter SJ, Lucas K, Springett K, et al.** Comparison of foot pain and foot care among rheumatoid arthritis patients taking and not taking anti-TNFα therapy: an epidemiological study. *Rheumatol Int.* 2010;**31**:1515–19.

127. **Turner DE, Helliwell PS, Emery P, Woodburn J.** The impact of rheumatoid arthritis on foot function in the early stages of disease: a clinical case series. *BMC Musculoskelet Disord.* 2006;**7**:102.

128. **van der Leeden M, Fiedler K, Jonkman A, et al.** Factors predicting the outcome of customised foot orthoses in patients with rheumatoid arthritis: a prospective cohort study. *J Foot Ankle Res.* 2011;**4**:8.

129. **Hay SM, Moore DJ, Cooper JR, Getty CJM.** Diagnostic injections of the hindfoot joints in patients with rheumatoid arthritis prior to surgical fusion. *Foot.* 1999;**9**(1): 40–3.

130. **D'Agostino MA, Ayral X, Baron G, Ravaud P, Breban M, Dougados M.** Impact of ultrasound imaging on local corticosteroid injections of symptomatic ankle, hind-, and mid-foot in chronic inflammatory diseases. *Arthritis Rheum.* 2005;**53**(2):284–92.

131. **Cunnington J, Marshall N, Hide G, et al.** A randomized, double-blind, controlled study of ultrasound-guided corticosteroid injection into the joint of patients with inflammatory arthritis. *Arthritis Rheum.* 2010;**62**(7):1862–9.

132. **Chakravarty K, Pharoah PD, Scott DG.** A randomized controlled study of post-injection rest following intra-articular steroid therapy for knee synovitis. *Br J Rheumatol.* 1994;**33**(5):464–8.

133. **Dixon A St.J, Graber J.** *Local Injection Therapy in Rheumatic Diseases.* Basile: EULAR Publishers; 1981.

134. **Canoso JJ.** Aspiration and injection of joints and periarticular tissues. In: Klippel JH, Dieppe PA (eds). *Rheumatology*, 2nd edn. London: Mosby, 1998; pp. 2.12.1–2.12.12.

135. **Falsetti P, Frediani B, Fioravanti A, et al.** Sonographic study of calcaneal entheses in erosive osteoarthritis, nodal osteoarthritis, rheumatoid arthritis and psoriatic arthritis. *Scand J Rheumatol.* 2003;**32**(4):229–34.

136. **Arner A, Lindblom U, Meyerson BA, Molander C.** Prolonged relief of neuralgia after regional anesthetic clocks. A call for further experimental and systematic studies. *Pain.* 1990;**43**:287–97.

137. **Lemmey AB.** Rheumatoid cachexia: the undiagnosed, untreated key to restoring physical function in rheumatoid arthritis patients? *Rheumatology (Oxford).* 2016;**55**(7):1149–50.

138. **Rall LC, Roubenoff R.** Body composition, metabolism, and resistance exercise in patients with rheumatoid arthritis. *Arthritis Care Res.* 1996;**9**(2):151–6.

139. **de Jong Z, Munneke M, Zwinderman AH, et al.** Is a long-term high-intensity exercise program effective and safe in patients with rheumatoid arthritis? Results of a randomised controlled trial. *Arthritis Rheum.* 2003;**48**(9):2415–24.

140. **de Jong Z, Munneke M, Lems WF, et al.** Slowing of bone loss in patients with rheumatoid arthritis by long-term high-intensity exercise: results of a randomised controlled trial. *Arthritis Rheum.* 2004;**50**(4):1066–76.

141. **Lemmey AB, Marcora SM, Chester K, Wilson S, Casanova F, Maddison PJ.** Effects of high-intensity resistance training in patients with rheumatoid arthritis: a randomized controlled trial. *Arthritis Rheum.* 2009;**61**(12):1726–34.

142. **Hurley MV, Walsh N, Bhavnani V, Britten N, Stevenson F.** Health beliefs before and after participation on an exercised-based rehabilitation programme for chronic knee pain: doing is believing. *BMC Musculoskelet Disord.* 2010;**11**:31.

143. **Hurley MV, Walsh NE, Mitchell H, Nicholas J, Patel A.** Long-term outcomes and costs of an integrated rehabilitation program for chronic knee pain: a pragmatic, cluster randomized, controlled trial. *Arthritis Care Res (Hoboken).* 2012;**64**(2):238–47.

144. **Hurley MV, Carter A.** ESCAPE-into the community—a community-based rehabilitation programme for elderly people with chronic joint pain. *Perspect Public Health.* 2016;**136**(2):67–9.

145. **Bearne LM, Scott DL, Hurley MV.** Exercise can reverse quadriceps sensorimotor dysfunction that is associated with rheumatoid arthritis without exacerbating disease activity. *Rheumatology (Oxford).* 2002;**41**(2):157–66.

146. **Sharma L, Dunlop DD, Hayes KW.** Is a strong quadriceps muscle bad for a patient with knee osteoarthritis? *Ann Intern Med.* 2004;**140**(2):150.

Chapter 15

Surgery

Mike Backhouse and Nick Harris

Introduction

Although surgery is sometimes considered as a failure of conservative care, its ability to provide often dramatic improvements means it has an important role in the management of foot and ankle problems. Indeed, surgery is recommended in most guidelines for the management of rheumatic and musculoskeletal disease (RMD), yet many clinicians are unaware of surgical options in the foot and ankle or their outcomes, so are unable to consider them fully as part of a patient's management plan.

Rates of surgery vary greatly between and within different health services and are also influenced by a range of patient factors, including socioeconomic variables, race, and sex, which have been shown to influence a patient's willingness to undergo surgery (1–3). A patient's likelihood of having orthopaedic surgery increases with disease duration owing to the accumulation of joint damage and deformity over time, but it is important to acknowledge that improvements in the pharmacological management of inflammatory arthritis have played an important role in reducing the extent of joint damage we see today. As a result, rates of orthopaedic surgery in people with rheumatoid arthritis (RA) are decreasing internationally (4, 5) but, in the UK, approximately one-third of people with RA have orthopaedic surgery during the course of their disease, with the majority of this conducted on large joints such as the hip and knee (5). Providing accurate data on the rate of foot surgery is more difficult, as such information is rarely adequately captured in national cohorts or registers. However, data from the UK indicates that 4% of people with RA have surgery within the first 9 years of their disease, whereas figures as high as 58% have been reported at 20 years in a Swedish cohort (6, 7).

The evidence base for foot and ankle surgery is increasing, especially with the growing use of validated patient-reported outcome measures (PROMs), but large-scale prospective multi-centre studies remain rare, as indeed they do for many aspects of foot care. The majority of evidence for foot surgery in rheumatology relates to osteoarthritis (OA), and there is little in the inflammatory arthritides other than RA. However, in this chapter we will provide the reader with an overview of common surgical procedures and their outcomes that draws upon the available evidence and current practice.

Surgical considerations

Surgery can produce dramatic benefits, but it is also important to acknowledge that, as with all treatments, it comes with a risk of side-effects and complications, which vary depending on a multitude of factors. The patient's own preferences must be central to this decision process and the final decision to operate, as well as the specific procedure used, will be taken by the patient and the surgeon. Although referral paths and staff provision will vary considerably depending on local arrangements, foot surgeons should be considered a vital part of the multidisciplinary team (MDT). We strongly encourage clinicians who regularly treat foot and ankle problems to build links with their local foot surgeons, as improved communication and understanding will ultimately improve patient care.

Before considering when to refer a patient and how to optimize outcomes, it is important to consider what 'a good outcome' actually means. Although use of PROMs is increasing, these are developed on a group level, and truly patient-centred care requires clinicians to delve beyond these standardized measures and explore issues that are important to individual patients during a consultation. Patients interpret the outcome of foot and ankle surgery in the context of a complex array of factors in relation to their life context and underlying disease. Qualitative work in RA has shown that these factors include functional ability, participation in valued activities, appearance (of the foot itself and footwear), and the surgeon's appraisal of the procedure (8). Interestingly, despite being a major motivator for patients to seek surgery, pain appeared less important when interpreting outcome and was raised in conjunction with other factors during the interviews.

There is only limited guidance on indications for surgery and the available guidelines are not specific to the foot and ankle. The National Institute for Health and Care Excellence (NICE) states that surgery plays an important part in the management of OA that is unresponsive to core non-surgical treatments. It recommends that referral for surgical consideration should be sought before there is prolonged and established functional limitation with severe pain, but that symptoms should have a substantial impact on the person's quality of life and be refractory to non-surgical therapies (9). In RA, NICE recommends that a specialist surgical opinion should be offered for persistent pain caused by joint damage, worsening joint function, and progressive deformity in people who fail to respond to optimal conservative management (10). Patient-specific factors such as age, sex, obesity, and comorbidity should not be a barrier to referral for surgical consideration (9), although severe peripheral vascular disease and current infection are considered contraindications for elective surgery by most.

Over recent years, a number of studies have identified factors that can predict which individuals with RA are likely to undergo surgery during the course of their disease (11, 12). Most of this research has focused on large-joint surgery and factors identified here are also predictors of disease severity. There is much less research into predicting which patients will receive foot surgery and only one study has explored use of conservative and surgical care. This suggested that female patients with later-onset disease were more likely to receive conservative care, whereas female patients with earlier disease onset were more likely to have foot surgery (6).

Although predicting future surgery can potentially be used to stratify intensive conservative therapies with the hope of avoiding surgery, it does not help clinicians when considering whether to refer individual patients. Unfortunately, there is even less evidence to determine whether an individual patient will benefit from surgery, but people with RA tend to have worse outcomes for the same orthopaedic procedure than those with OA (13, 14). To date, one study has conducted exploratory prognostic modelling on a multi-centre cohort of people with RA undergoing foot surgery, although, as with all prognostic models, this now needs validating in external cohorts (15). Patient outcome was measured using the Foot Impact Scale and the key factors identified in the qualitative interviews described above (8, 15). The study identified three key constructs that predicted people with better outcomes: people with higher levels of preoperative pain improved better than those with less pain; those with worse deformity failed to improve as much as people with lower levels of deformity; and those with tighter disease control improved more than those with higher disease activity (15). This suggests that operating on people before they develop severe deformity may improve outcomes and that it is important to control disease activity in the perioperative period.

The demands of recovery and rehabilitation in the postoperative period are also an important consideration for people with RMD, particularly those who may be unable to use crutches owing to concurrent upper limb involvement. Some procedures require a person to avoid weightbearing through their foot for a prolonged period of time. In the case of ankle arthrodesis, for example, people are usually advised to avoid weightbearing on their operated limb completely for 6–8 weeks, and then wear an off-loading boot for another 6 weeks. Dealing with this requires appropriate planning, assessment for additional aids, and, potentially, additional support.

Perioperative management of disease activity

The most common complication of elective orthopaedic surgery in people with RA is surgical site infection, and this holds true in foot surgery (15, 16). In fact, foot and ankle surgery has itself been found to have a higher rate of post-operative infections than orthopaedic surgery on other joints in people with RA (16). As is often the case, much of the discussion in this section relates to RA as there is a lack of evidence in the other RMDs. However, many of the principles appear to hold true in other RMDs, although clinicians should always take into account the features of each specific condition and liaise with the wider MDT as understanding and treatment of these diseases continues to evolve.

Exactly why foot and ankle surgery should carry a higher risk of infection is yet to be explored empirically, but people with RA have an increased risk of infection generally. This is due to a combination of the disease itself and its impact beyond the musculoskeletal system, as well as the immunosuppressive medication used to treat the primary disease processes (17, 18). Fortunately, the majority of infections following foot and ankle surgery are superficial soft-tissue infections that respond well to therapy (15). Clinicians should remain vigilant, though, as infections can quickly spread to deeper tissues at incision sites, and a combination of immunosuppression and peripheral vascular disease can mask the classic signs of infection.

It is, of course, possible to reduce the level of immunosuppression ahead of elective surgery by adjusting a person's medication. However, a balance must be struck, as a reduction in immunosuppression can lead to a flare in disease activity with effects throughout the body and ultimately a worse outcome for the patient. There is still limited evidence to advise clinicians on perioperative disease control and practice varies for different drug classes.

It is common to increase the corticosteroid dose around the time of surgery in people with RA who already take these drugs to control disease activity (19). This is done to prevent adrenal insufficiency precipitated by the stress of surgery. The European League Against Rheumatism (EULAR) recommends that this should be anticipated in people receiving a more than 7.5 mg of prednisolone equivalent daily dose for more than 3 weeks (20).

Randomized controlled trial evidence demonstrates that there is no increase in infection risk or risk of delayed wound healing in patients who continue their methotrexate compared with those who suspended their methotrexate (21). In fact, there were more flares and wound complications in those who discontinued their medication and ultimately these patients had worse outcomes. There is little evidence for other synthetic disease-modifying antirheumatic drugs (DMARDs), but their use is generally considered safe and it is standard practice to continue their perioperative use.

Biologic DMARDs (biologics) are potent immunosuppressive agents and so there is greater concern about their potential to cause surgical site infections; guidelines are deliberately cautious. Tumour necrosis factor-alpha (TNF-α) inhibitors, for example, have been linked to higher rates of serious skin infections in people with RA who are not undergoing surgery (18). However, TNF-α also has an important role in normal wound healing (22) and the topical application of a TNF-α inhibitor in animal models has shown improved wound healing (19). In the absence of robust prospective studies, the available data appear to support the discontinuation of TNF-α inhibitors prior to surgery, although these retrospective studies are inherently confounded. Data for other biologics is even sparser, with the exception of rituximab, where the limited evidence suggests it has little impact on the likelihood of surgical site infection (19, 23). While the current evidence base does not permit the formulation of definitive guidelines, stopping biologics between two and five half-lives ahead of planned surgery is considered a prudent conservative approach (19).

Owing to interpatient variability, comorbidities, differing postoperative rehabilitation demands, and the ongoing development of new drugs, the rheumatology MDT (usually the rheumatologist or specialist nurse) should be consulted well in advance of the planned surgery. The wound should be fully healed and show no evidence of infection before a biologic is restarted.

Selected procedures and common indications

Ankle and rearfoot

Ankle arthroscopy

Ankle arthroscopy is a minimally invasive surgical technique used to deal with intraarticular and periarticular pathologies around the ankle (Figure 15.1). The use of smaller incisions minimizes soft-tissue complications and allows quicker recovery. Ankle arthroscopy can be used to treat a variety of conditions, including soft-tissue and bony impingement lesions (24) (Figure 15.2), as

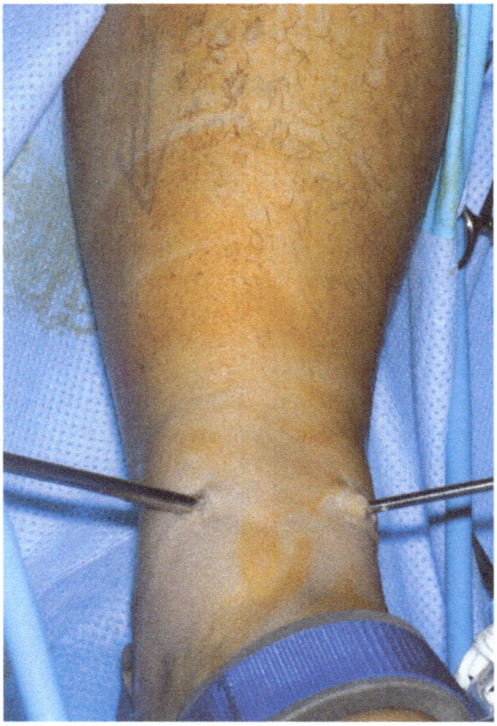

Figure 15.1 Intraoperative view of ankle arthroscopy using an anterior approach.

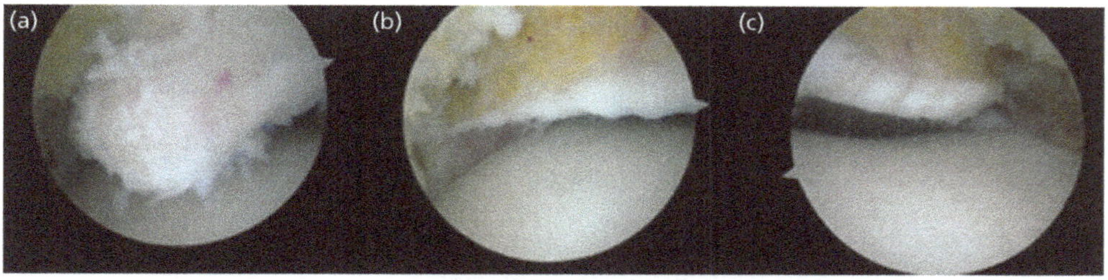

Figure 15.2 Intraoperative views of ankle arthroscopy. (a) Large osteophyte protruding from the tibia. (b, c) Images following resection of the osteophyte.

well as osteochondral lesions (25). Ankle arthroscopy can be performed either anteriorly (most commonly) or posteriorly depending on the location of the pathology. Usually, two small incisions are used, one for the camera and one for the arthroscopic instruments. A tensile load is often applied across the ankle joint to distract the joint as this increases the space available to conduct the procedure.

Ankle arthroscopy is usually performed as a day-case procedure. Postoperatively patients are immobilized in a walker boot until the wounds/portals are dry and then physiotherapy is commenced.

Tol et al. (24) reported the long-term outcomes of arthroscopic debridement procedures to treat anterior impingement in the ankle. At a mean follow-up of 6.5 years all patients with soft-tissue impingement alone reported good or excellent results. Of patients with grade 1 OA (osteophytes without joint space narrowing), 77% had good or excellent results, and 53% of patients with grade 2 OA (narrowing of the joint space with or without osteophytes) had good or excellent results.

Ferkel et al. (25) reported 72% good or excellent results following arthroscopic treatment of osteochondral lesions of the talus at a mean follow-up of 71 months. Treatment included excision of the osteochondral lesion, abrasion arthroplasty, or drilling.

Complications related to ankle arthroscopy include damage to the cutaneous nerves that cross the ankle, especially the superficial peroneal nerve, and tendon injury. Careful placement of the incisions reduces the risks.

Ankle arthrodesis

Ankle fusion remains the most reliable long-term treatment for symptomatic ankle arthritis not responding to conservative treatments. Over 40 different techniques have been described. Broadly they can be divided into open and arthroscopic. Open ankle fusion can be performed through anterior, lateral, or posterior incisions or a combination. Arthroscopic ankle arthrodesis is usually performed anteriorly, but posterior arthroscopic arthrodesis has been described as well.

Arthroscopic techniques aim to reduce soft-tissue complications and speed recovery but are restricted to well-aligned joints. Patients with severe deformity around the ankle still often require an open approach both to correct the deformity and achieve fusion. Fixation of the arthrodesis also varies but includes screws and plates (Figure 15.3). External fixation devices have also been described in revision and infected cases.

The average time to fusion is somewhere in the region of 12–14 weeks. Immediately postoperatively patients are kept non-weightbearing for 6–8 weeks, followed by another 6 weeks of protected weightbearing in a walker boot.

In most series union rates are high, at 80–90% (26–28). Complications include wound breakdown and infection, delayed union, non-union, and prominent metalwork. Longer-term

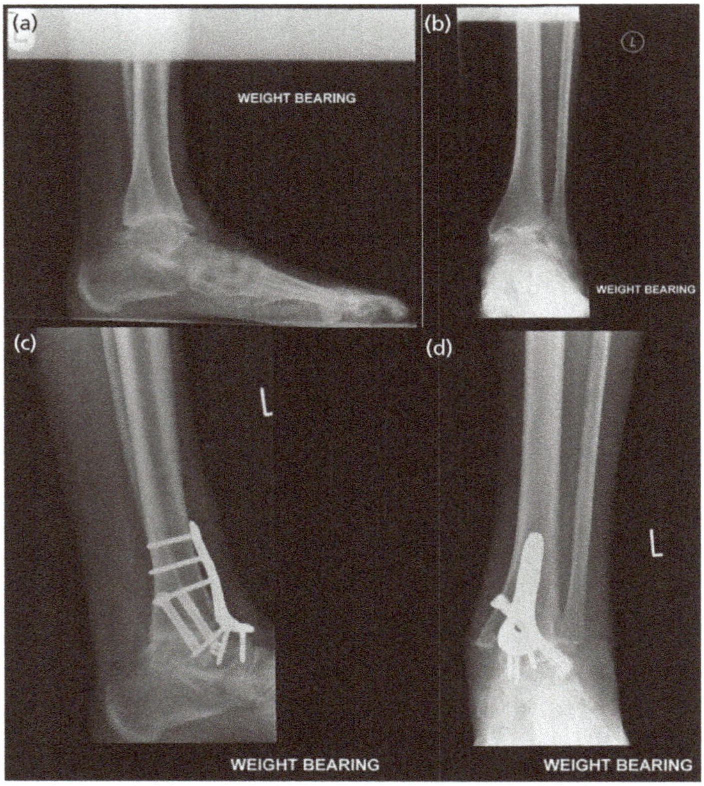

Figure 15.3 Ankle arthrodesis. (a, b) Preoperative radiographs showing severe ankle arthritis. (c, d) Postoperative images following arthrodesis with screws and plates.

complications include juxta-articular arthritis, especially of the talonavicular, subtalar, and calcaneocuboid joints (28). Complications are much higher in diabetic patients.

Ankle arthroplasty

Total ankle replacement is an alternative to ankle fusion in the management of end-stage symptomatic ankle arthritis. Approximately 1300 total ankle replacements are implanted in the UK each year, so these are not as widely used as hip or knee prostheses. Ten-year survival rates for ankle replacements vary between 69% and 94% (29–31). Preserving ankle movement has functional advantages over fusion, but total ankle replacement has a higher reoperation rate. Complications include edge loading and osteolysis or loosening of the implant (Figure 15.4). Newer designs are emerging all the time, embracing new technology and materials trying to improve survivorship and reduce complications. The Rebalance Total Ankle Replacement (Zimmer; Biomet) is one of the newest designs, using 'E' polyethylene, a vitamin E-infused polyethylene bearing with 7.5 times lower wear rates compared to conventional polyethylene; long-term clinical follow-up studies are in progress, but initial results appear promising (Figure 15.5). There is also renewed interest in fixed bearing implants, where the polyethylene bearing is attached to the tibial component, and cemented implants.

Total ankle replacement tends to be reserved for older, lower-demand patients and patients with inflammatory arthritis. For the best results, total ankle replacement requires a well-aligned

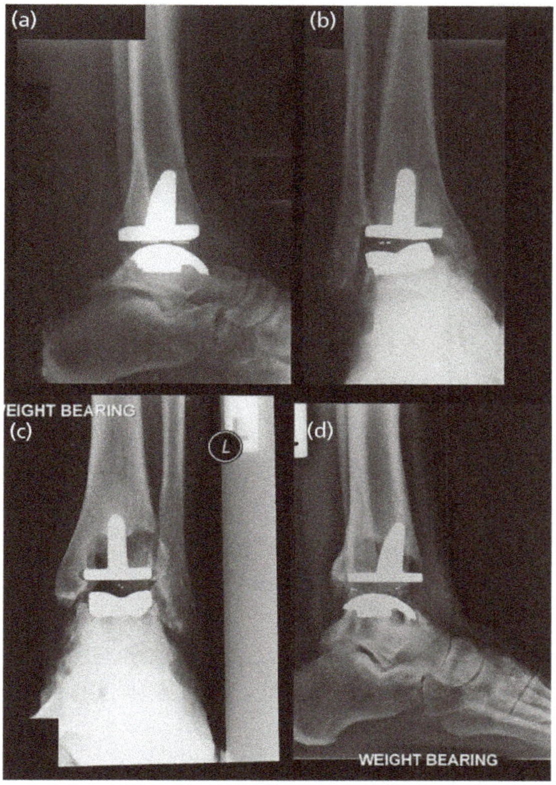

Figure 15.4 Complications in total ankle replacement. (a, b) Varus edge loading. (c, d) Large osteolysis around the tibial components, which is a cause of early failure.

joint and a preoperative range of movement of at least 20° to achieve best results. Postoperatively patients are allowed to start weightbearing as soon as the wounds have healed, which allows a quicker recovery compared to a fusion.

The most reliable treatment for a failed total ankle replacement is removal of the implant and conversion to a fusion. Owing to the lack of talar bone stock, an intramedullary nail is often used, fusing the subtalar joint as well (Figure 15.6). This results in some shortening, but fusion rates of 90% have been reported (32).

Subtalar, talonavicular, and calcaneocuboid arthrodesis

The subtalar, talonavicular, and calcaneocuboid joints can all be affected by arthritis or deformity, or both. Inflammatory arthritis such as RA often affects these joints. Calcaneal fractures can lead to post-traumatic arthritis of the subtalar and calcaneocuboid joints. Tibialis posterior tendon dysfunction can result in a valgus deformity of these joints and neurological conditions such as Charcot–Marie–Tooth can result in cavovarus deformities. If conservative measures fail (such as orthoses, physiotherapy, and image-guided injections), one, two, or all three joints can be fused. A fusion can be used to correct fixed deformity, treat arthritis, or both. A fusion of two of these joints is called a double fusion (Figure 15.7) and a fusion of all three joints is called a triple fusion. Following a fusion, patients are kept non-weightbearing for 6–8 weeks and are then allowed to weightbear partially in a walker boot for another 6 weeks.

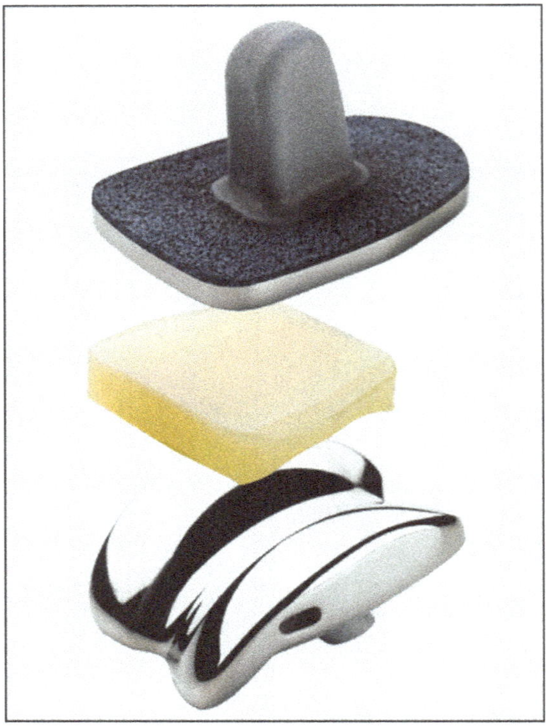

Figure 15.5 The Rebalance Total Ankle Replacement using 'E' poly as a bearing surface with the characteristic brown appearance.

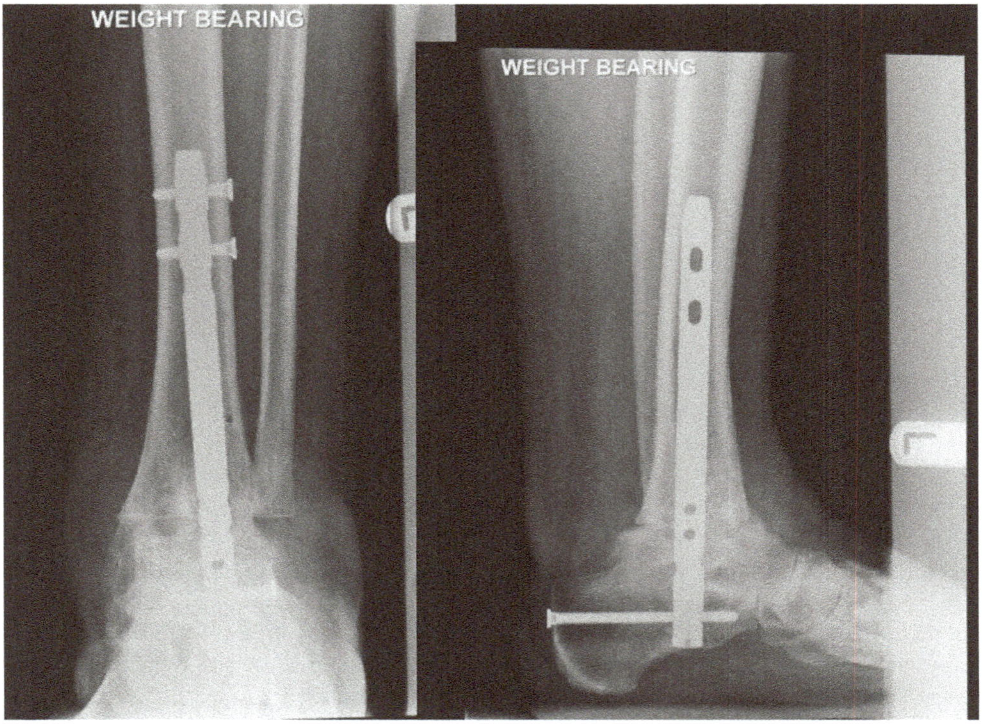

Figure 15.6 Conversion of a failed ankle replacement to a fusion with an intramedullary nail.

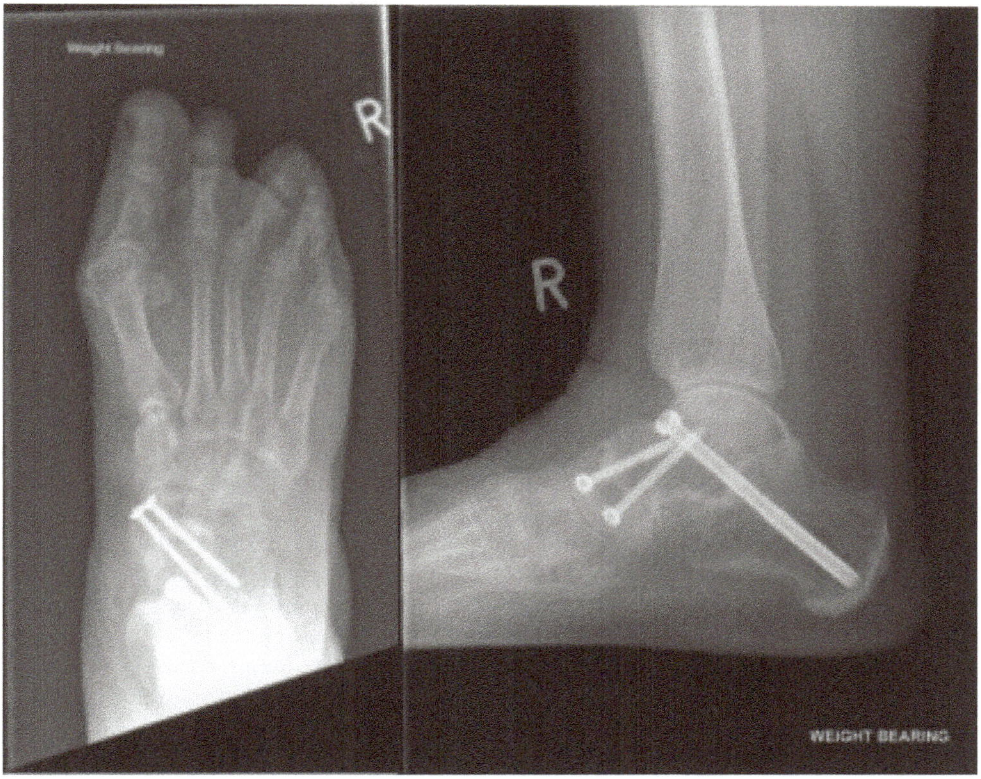

Figure 15.7 Double fusion of the talonavicular and subtalar joints.

Complications include wound healing problems, non-union, and juxta-articular arthritis of other midfoot joints (33–35).

Midfoot

Tarsometatarsal joint fusions

Tarsometatarsal (TMT) joint fusions are performed for painful arthritis or deformity, or both. The TMT joints are divided into three columns. The medial column consists of the first metatarsal and medial cuneiform. The second column consists of the second and third metatarsals and the intermediate and lateral cuneiforms. The third column consists of the fourth and fifth metatarsals and the cuboid. Good results have been reported following fusions of the first, second, and third TMT joints. Fusion of the fourth and fifth TMT joints is more controversial, and motion-sparing procedures have also been described, such as peroneus tertius interposition and the use of ceramic spheres as spacers. Fusion rates range from 83% to 97% with screws and/or plates (36, 37).

Forefoot

Procedures for hallux valgus

This is a common progressive deformity in which the first metatarsophalangeal (MTP) joint is progressively subluxed through a lateral deviation of the hallux and medial deviation of the first metatarsal (38). As the deformity progresses, lateral deviation of the hallux begins to interfere with the normal alignment of the lesser toes, causing hammer or claw deformities and accentuating changes in gait. Pressure from footwear can cause painful hyperkeratotic lesions (corns and calluses) on both the plantar and dorsal aspects of the foot, and may also lead to the development of an adventitious bursa on the medial prominence of the bunion (39).

Hallux valgus may be as much as nine times more common in women, and its prevalence is known to increase with age (38). Prevalence estimates vary but, typically, approximately one-third are thought to have some degree of hallux valgus. Despite being so common, hallux valgus should not be seen as a benign condition. It can be painful and has been shown to have a marked impact on patients' quality of life (40–42). The condition has also been shown to have a significant impact on balance (43) and gait patterns (43), as well as being an independent risk factor for falls in older people (44, 45).

Surgery is therefore very common, with hallux valgus corrections accounting for the majority of foot operations (46, 47). Although the vast majority of reported outcomes are very positive in terms of reducing pain and deformity, some reports suggest that around 30% of patients appear to be dissatisfied with the outcome (48). This has recently been linked to women's perceptions of the postoperative appearance of their foot and the range of footwear they are able to wear (48). More than 100 procedures to correct hallux valgus have been described in the literature, but they can be broadly categorized depending on their position on the first metatarsal.

Distal osteotomies such as the chevron osteotomy are often used to correct mild to moderate hallux valgus. In the chevron osteotomy, a V-shaped cut is made through the distal aspect of the first metatarsal neck. The distal fragment (metatarsal head) is then translated laterally to correct the deformity and held in place with a screw before the excess bone on the medial aspect of the metatarsal is resected. In case-series, good or excellent results have been reported in 80–90% of people who have had the procedure. However, recurrence or undercorrection have been reported in 10–14% of cases (49–51).

The scarf osteotomy is probably the most commonly performed procedure to correct hallux valgus. Case-series of this mid-shaft osteotomy report positive results with high levels of pain relief, patient satisfaction, and maintained correction reported up to 9 years postoperatively (52–54). Various optional modifications make this a highly adaptable technique capable of correcting deformity in all planes and adjusting the length of the first metatarsal (55, 56). After removing the medial eminence of the first metatarsal, a longitudinal Z-shaped cut is made through the distal two-thirds of the first metatarsal. The longitudinal cut is made along the length of the diaphysis, then the cut up through the dorsal aspect of the metatarsal is made at the distal end of the metatarsal. Finally, a cut is made through the plantar aspect at the proximal end of the metatarsal. Changing the orientation of these cuts provides the surgeon with the flexibility to correct other aspects of the deformity such as metatarsal length. The dorsal fragment is then translated medially to reduce the intermetatarsal angle and is usually held in place with two screws (Figure 15.8). The large surface area of the opposing osseous fragments is inherently stable and allows for a good environment for primary bone healing as well as an early return to weightbearing and normal activities (54).

Proximal procedures at the base of the first metatarsal are traditionally reserved for larger intermetatarsal angles. They have the ability to correct large deformities but are complex (57). The Lapidus procedure is perhaps the most established procedure and combines a laterally based closing wedge osteotomy at the base of the first metatarsal, lateral transposition of the metatarsal, and arthrodesis of the first metatarsocuneiform joint (58, 59). The bones are fixed in place with either screws or a locking plate. Published case-series suggest the procedure produces stable results, with non-union rates between 3% and 7% (57, 59) and an increase of less than 1° in both average intermetatarsal and hallux valgus angles up to 4 years postoperatively (59). Reported patient satisfaction levels are typically high, with only 7% expressing dissatisfaction with the procedure (58).

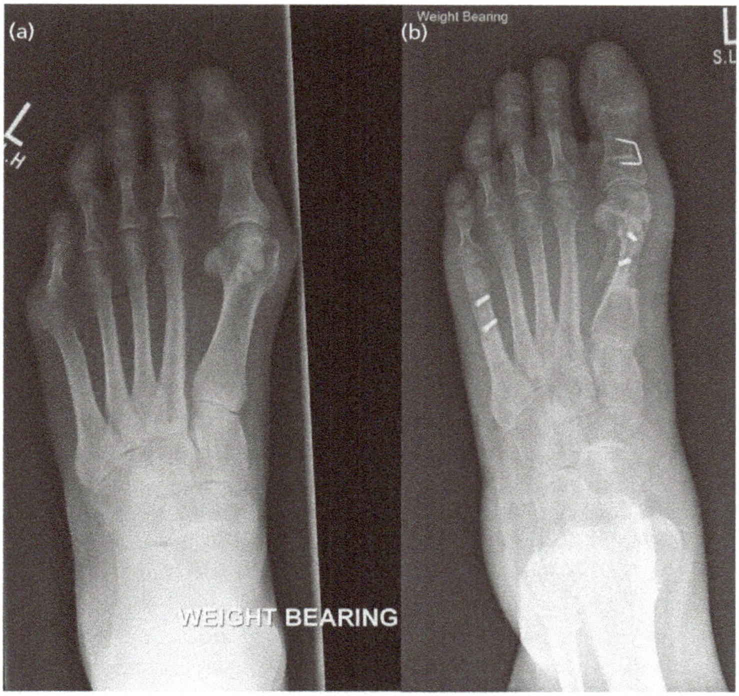

Figure 15.8 Hallux valgus correction. (a) Preoperative appearance. (b) Postoperative radiograph showing a scarf osteotomy performed on the first metatarsal. This is held in place by two screws and an Akin on the proximal phalanx of the hallux, which used a staple.

Severe hallux valgus deformities can also be reliably treated with a realignment and fusion of the first MTP joint.

In practice, it is common for the procedures listed above to be combined with a second osteotomy of the proximal phalanx of the hallux, such as an Akin osteotomy. This is a simple closing wedge osteotomy where a medially based wedge is cut through the proximal phalanx of the hallux and then removed. The two fragments are then held in place with a single screw or staple.

More recently there has been growing interest in minimally invasive forefoot surgery. This involves the use of specialized instruments through small incisions. Theoretically this reduces soft-tissue complications, but the surgery is technically demanding with a steep learning curve.

First metatarsophalangeal joint procedures

Involvement of the first MTP joint is common, particularly in OA, and there are many surgical procedures that have been suggested to alleviate symptoms. These procedures can be performed in isolation or combined with metatarsal osteotomies to correct deformities such as hallux valgus. Although surgeon preference varies, selection of the exact procedure largely depends on the extent of damage within the joint. Joint-preserving techniques such as cheilectomy are generally used in milder cases, whereas arthrodesis (joint fusion) is used when joint-preserving techniques fail or joint damage is more extensive.

Cheilectomy can be performed either endoscopically or, more commonly, as an open procedure (60), but is generally reserved for cases where loss of articular cartilage is limited (61). The procedure removes dorsal and medial osteophytes and up to one-third of the dorsal articular surface from either side of the MTP joint, which aims to reduce symptoms and improve range of motion (ROM). Although studies have shown good symptomatic relief in the short and medium term (62) and an increase in passive non-weightbearing ROM, similar improvements of ROM have not been demonstrated during gait (63, 64). It is not possible to predict how long symptom relief will last in individual patients, but it is unlikely that such a procedure would stop future joint degeneration. Importantly, cheilectomy maintains most of the joint surface, so future surgical options remain open if the joint deteriorates and symptoms persist. To our knowledge the cost-effectiveness of this procedure has not been explored robustly, which perhaps limits is use in some settings.

At the other end of the spectrum, first MTP joint arthrodesis is used in severe cases of joint damage or where other procedures have failed (61). It is frequently regarded as the gold standard procedure for first MTP joint arthritis owing to its long track record and predictable results. A variety of techniques has been described in the literature (65), but they all consist of removal of periarticular osteophytes and removal of the articular surfaces and subchondral bone from both the first metatarsal and proximal phalanx. The opposing bony surfaces are then positioned with the hallux in slight dorsiflexion and valgus so that, with the foot in a plantar grade position, the hallux pulp just engages the floor. It is then fixed in place, typically using a low-profile dorsal locking plate. Thus, the procedure removes the joint and any motion between the first metatarsal and proximal phalanx. Reported outcomes for first MTP joint arthrodesis are broadly positive: successful fusion occurs in approximately 98% of cases, with 90–95% of cases having excellent outcomes (61, 65).

Motion-preserving options include Keller's excisional arthroplasty and first MTP joint replacement. Keller's excisional arthroplasty is perhaps the best-known procedure but is now less frequently performed. It consists of resection of the proximal third of the proximal phalanx of the hallux and does not require long periods of immobilization. However, removal of a substantial portion of the proximal phalanx results in an inherently unstable joint, which is associated with higher rates of recidivistic deformity and also reduces subsequent options when salvaging failed procedures (66).

Several different replacement implants have been developed since first being described in the literature in 1877 (67). The most common designs are either a hinged double-stemmed silicone implant or a two-part implant made of metal or ceramic, but even these are now used sparingly and are often reserved for less active patients. Silicone implants were initially used following successful results in the metacarpophalangeal joints of the hands and early results showed promise, with high levels of patient satisfaction (68). Unfortunately, problems have since been noted with osteolysis, silicone wear, and foreign body reactions to the silicone itself (69). In addition, silicone implants often snapped and were unable to cope with the forces put through the joint during gait (70).

Subsequent development of more robust metal total joint replacements again showed early promise and the stronger implants were able to withstand the mechanical forces at the joint. However, they have been linked with poor osseous integration on the implant stems, early osteolysis, subsidence, and fracture of the metatarsal neck (71). Similar problems have been reported with ceramic implants, but with the added complication that failure can lead to shattering of the implant and production of many sharp shards of ceramic (72). After first MTP prosthesis failure, salvage is normally attempted through arthrodesis. These salvage arthrodeses are more difficult and have higher complication rates than primary arthrodesis. This is because of the relatively large volume of bone removed when inserting the primary implant, which is then compounded by removing additional bone that has been damaged when the implant fails (73). This therefore often requires a bone graft to enable effective arthrodesis and maintain the length of the first ray.

The high complication rates of most arthroplasty procedures have led to interest in the recent development of small implants described as synthetic cartilage implants. These are in fact made from poly (vinyl alcohol) hydrogels that manufacturers claim have similar mechanical properties to hyaline cartilage. The small circular implant (8 mm or 10 mm in diameter) is placed into the articular surface of the metatarsal head and protrudes 1–2 mm above the surface. Although still a relatively new product, a prospective randomized non-inferiority study of 202 patients with moderate to severe first MTP joint OA from 12 sites across Canada, USA, and the UK showed non-inferior pain and functional outcomes of the synthetic implant when compared to arthrodesis 2 years postoperatively (74). Proponents of the implant state that the minimal bone resection required when inserting the implant makes subsequent arthrodesis less complex, but, ultimately, more clinical studies with longer-term follow-up are still required.

Forefoot reconstruction

Whilst there are a great number of forefoot procedures described in the literature for people with RA, these can be seen as falling into two main categories: joint-preserving surgery and the more common, but destructive or joint-sacrificing, techniques (75).

Joint-sparing surgery aims to correct forefoot deformity through a combination of osteotomies of the metatarsals, which allow decompression of the MTP joint and correction of the deformity. The most commonly advocated approach uses a scarf osteotomy on the first metatarsal and Weil osteotomies on the lesser metatarsals (76). This approach appears to be gaining popularity, with supporters advocating that it can be used to compliment other procedures (77), and they expect it to become particularly useful as improved disease control reduces the extent of deformity (78). Although studies typically report levels of pain relief and patient satisfaction in the region of 70–80% (76, 77, 79), recurrence of deformity also appears to be common, affecting 15–38% of patients, with higher levels in studies with longer-term follow-up (76, 79). To date, though, there remains a lack of quality long-term studies in people with RA, with many authors combining cases with OA and RA in their analyses.

Reconstructive forefoot procedures that sacrifice the MTP joints were first reported in the literature in 1912 (80). The original procedure has evolved since then, with a number of modifications, but the basic principle remains unchanged, and it continues to be the mainstay of reconstructive forefoot surgery in RA (81). Called forefoot arthroplasty, pan met head resection, or forefoot reconstruction, the basic principles of the procedure are outlined in Figure 15.9. There are many variations described in the literature, and different surgeons will have their own preference of technique but perhaps most debate is around the main incision. A plantar incision allows direct access to the metatarsal heads and allows repositioning of the plantar fat pad. Concerns have been raised about the potential for painful scarring to be problematic following plantar incision, so some surgeons prefer a dorsal approach. This can be through a transverse incision or multiple longitudinal incisions about the metatarsal heads. Critics of this approach cite its limited access to the metatarsal heads, which is particularly problematic in severe deformity, and an inability to reposition the plantar fat pad. Both approaches continue to be used in practice.

Typically, studies of forefoot arthroplasty report that 70–90% of patients do well, or very well, and patient satisfaction has a similar range when reported (82–86). The number of patients reported as having poor outcomes or being dissatisfied is generally low (0–13%), but it is not always clear whether this is the patient or surgeon's opinion (82–84, 86). Few studies have attempted to take a more holistic approach when reporting surgical outcomes by reporting different aspects of outcome. In a cohort of patients with a mean follow-up of 11 years, 84% of patients had reduced pain, 71% had increased mobility, 64% could wear normal shoes with or without insoles, and 50% were satisfied with cosmesis (87, 88).

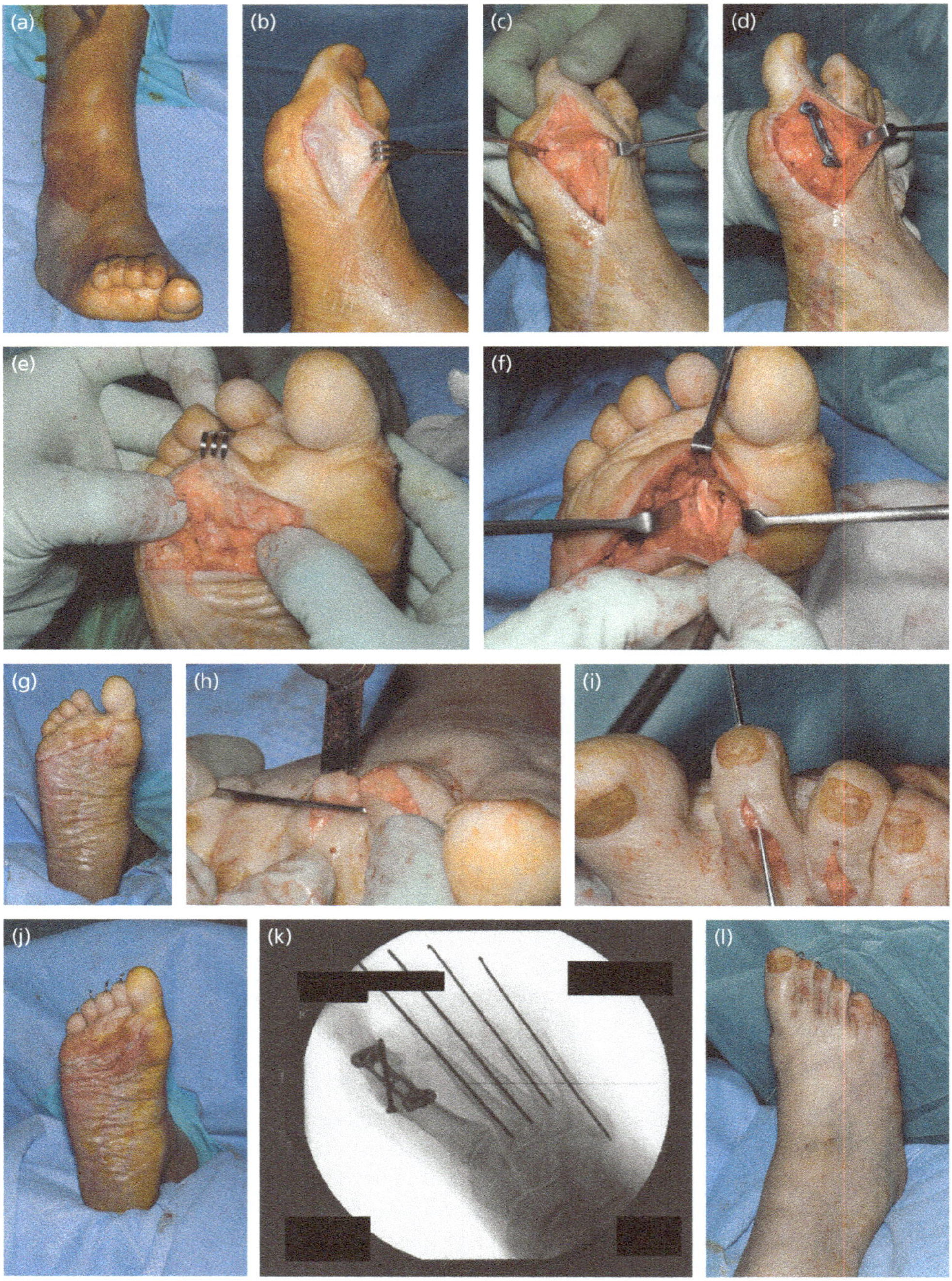

Figure 15.9 Forefoot arthroplasty. (a) Preoperative appearance showing forefoot deformity. (b, c) Medial incision of first metatarsophalangeal joint. (d) Dorsal locking plate and compression screw holding metatarsal and proximal phalange in place for fusion. (e) Plantar incision revealing eroded metatarsal heads. (f) Metatarsal heads removed. (g) Plantar view after closure of plantar incision. (h, i) Proximal interphalangeal joint arthrodesis showing removal of articular surfaces (h) and positioning of a temporary K-wire to hold toe in position and allow fusion (i). These are removed at a later outpatient appointment. (j, l) Postoperative appearance prior to leaving theatre. (k) Intraoperative radiograph showing all fixation in place at the end of the procedure.

Suboptimal patient outcomes have been linked with recidivistic deformities, callosities, and pain (89). Although rates of recurrent plantar hyperkeratosis and transfer metatarsalgia are rarely reported, objective measures of plantar pressure demonstrate significant reduction in plantar pressure under the metatarsal heads on a group level (84, 90). Transfer metatarsalgia has been linked to localized areas of high plantar pressure under the metatarsal stumps if they have been inadequately resected (84, 85). Clinicians should also be aware that 'bony regeneration at the metatarsal head' or 'metatarsal remodelling' has been reported in some patients and this leads to focal areas of increased pressure (91, 92). Although rare, this can present many years after surgery and can lead to ulceration in extreme cases if not addressed. Conservative measures include off-loading and appropriate footwear, but abnormal bone growth can also be successfully removed surgically if required.

Despite being over 100 years old, the forefoot arthroplasty remains the mainstay of reconstructing severe forefoot deformity in patients with RA (78, 93).

Within the past 20 years, an alternative to the forefoot arthroplasty described above has been reported in the literature (94). The Stainsby procedure acknowledges the hypothesized role of dorsal displacement of the plantar plate in lesser toe deformity and aims to restore its normal function by returning it under the metatarsal head (95, 96). Through angled dorsal incisions the proximal phalanx is divided through the neck and the proximal 25–33% is excised. The plantar plate is then identified, freed, and repositioned under the remaining fragment of the proximal phalanx. Once repositioned, the plantar plate subsequently relocates the plantar fat pad under the metatarsal heads by virtue of its attachment to the fat pad and plantar fascia. The toes are then stabilized through intramedullary K-wires, which are placed through the toes before being passed back into the metatarsal heads. The distal end of the severed extensor tendon is then transferred down to the flexor tendon and fixated with absorbable sutures to prevent recurrent dorsal displacement.

Although the Stainsby procedure acknowledges the pathological role of periarticular soft-tissue structures in forefoot deformity seen in RA and seems very logical, it has yet to be examined through robust scientific enquiry. Published results are largely positive, with patient satisfaction rates typically being in the region of 90% (97–99), although one study also reports revision rates of 20% at a mean of 32 months postoperatively (99). As such, the long-term outcome of this procedure is undetermined and concerns about recurrent deformity appear to limit its widespread use.

Soft tissue

Achilles tendon repair

Achilles tendon ruptures occur most commonly in men between the ages of 30 and 40 years and women between the ages of 60 and 80 years. Most ruptures are associated with sporting activities such as squash or tennis. Risk factors include corticosteroid use and fluoroquinolones (100). Patients usually describe being hit at the back of the leg or ankle with sudden pain. The calf squeeze test is the most sensitive clinical test for a ruptured Achilles tendon. With the patient in the prone position the calf is gently squeezed. On the affected side there will be no passive plantar flexion of the foot in a complete rupture. Where there is doubt, an ultrasound or magnetic resonance imaging scan are the investigations of choice.

There remains a wide range of opinion regarding the best management of Achilles tendon ruptures. In 1993, Cetti et al. published a prospective study comparing operative repair of a ruptured Achilles tendon with non-operative treatment in plaster (101). In the group treated operatively there was a 5% re-rupture rate and two deep infections. In the group treated conservatively there was a 15% re-rupture rate and one extreme overlengthening. Patients treated operatively also had a significantly higher rate of returning to sports at the same level, less calf atrophy, and better ankle movement compared to patients treated in plaster.

More recently, however, there has been a shift away from long periods of immobilization in plaster when treating ruptures conservatively owing to the use of a functional orthosis such as a VACOped or Aircast boot and early weightbearing in dedicated clinics. Re-rupture rates of only 1% have been reported (102).

With such low re-rupture rates using a functional orthosis there is now a shift to treat more and more ruptures non-operatively. The focus of current research is whether or not treatment with a functional orthosis results in a quicker and better functional recovery than surgery. The role of tendon gaps seen on ultrasound remains unclear. A gap of more than 1 cm may be associated with a poorer functional outcome in conservatively treated patients (103). Lastly, consideration should be given to venous thromboembolism prophylaxis during immobilization, especially in older patients.

Tibialis posterior tendon dysfunction

Failure of the tibialis posterior tendon and spring ligament are associated with an acquired flat foot deformity. Johnson and Strom (104) classified tibialis posterior tendon dysfunction into three types:

1. Inflammation of the tendon but no significant deformity.
2. Tibialis posterior tendinopathy or rupture with a flexible flatfoot deformity.
3. Subtalar arthritis and a fixed flat foot deformity.

This classification is helpful in planning treatment. Type 1 is usually treated conservatively with activity modification, non-steroidal anti-inflammatory drugs (NSAIDs), physiotherapy, and orthoses. Type 2 is usually treated operatively with a flexor digitorum longus tendon transfer or split tibialis anterior tendon transfer combined with repair of the spring ligament and medial displacement calcaneal osteotomy (Figure 15.10). Type 3 is usually treated with a double or triple fusion.

Myerson (105) introduced type 4 tibialis posterior tendon dysfunction, which involves ankle arthritis as well. This is usually treated with a pantalar fusion.

Pasapula et al. have recently postulated that there is a failure of the spring ligament before the tibialis posterior tendon based on some emerging cadaveric work and have termed this 'type 0' (106).

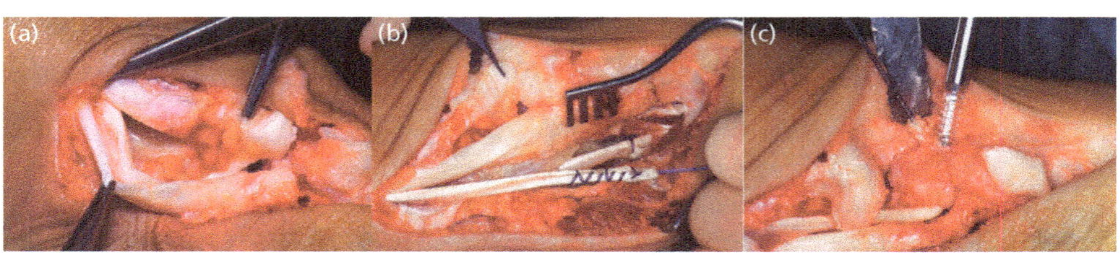

Figure 15.10 Flexor digitorum longus tendon transfer. (a) tendinopathic tibialis posterior tendon in a type 2 flatfoot deformity. (b) Harvesting the flexor digitorum longus tendon in preparation for transfer to the navicular. The distal end has been transferred to the flexor hallucis longus tendon. (c) Transfer of the flexor digitorum longus tendon into the navicular and fixation.

Haglund's deformity

A Haglund's deformity is a bony prominence arising from the posterior superior aspect of the calcaneus (Figure 15.11). The bony prominence can sometimes rub on the retrocalcaneal bursa and insertion of the Achilles tendon, leading to a bursitis and insertional Achilles tendinitis. Treatment is initially conservative, including activity modification, NSAIDs, physiotherapy, orthotics, and the avoidance of a tight heel counter in shoes. Sometimes an ultrasound-guided steroid injection into the retrocalcaneal bursa can be helpful. In recalcitrant cases the Haglund's deformity can be excised either open (107) or endoscopically (108) (Figure 15.11). Open techniques are more straightforward but are reported to have higher soft-tissue complications compared to endoscopic techniques.

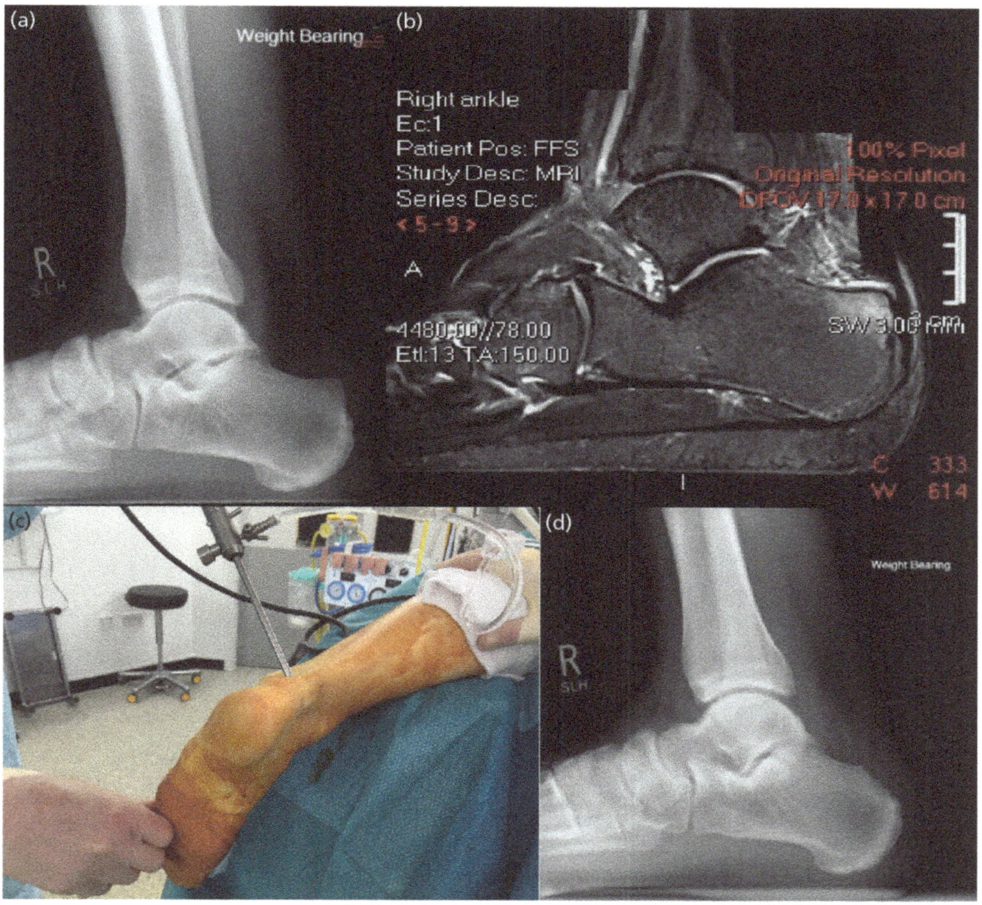

Figure 15.11 Haglund's deformity. (a) Radiograph. (b) Magnetic resonance image showing the bony prominence. (c) Endoscopic resection of a Haglund's deformity. (d) Postoperative X-ray showing resected deformity.

Toe amputation and partial toe amputation

Toe amputation and partial toe amputation may be performed for a broad range of indications, although most commonly it is likely to be for either deep-set infection and osteomyelitis or vascular compromise, particularly in people with diabetes. In RMDs there are still a number of indications for amputations, including deformity, trauma, ulceration, and, rarely, tumour. However, the procedure is most commonly performed when more extensive corrective surgery is contraindicated or not wanted by the patient, and tends to be conducted in older frail patients where quick recovery and minimal disruption is prioritized above long-term correction of deformity. Amputation can easily be performed under local anaesthetic which, again, reduces the burden on elderly patients and those with multiple comorbidities. For example, amputation of the second toe can be performed in severe hallux valgus with crossover of the second toe, as this is a shorter operation and allows quicker mobilization than a procedure to correct the deformity.

Toe amputations can either be performed by disarticulation at the MTP joint or a partial amputation through an osteotomy of part of the phalanges. A viable plantar flap is drawn over the amputation and closed without any tension (109). A single toe or multiple toes may be amputated depending upon the indication.

Conclusion

Foot and ankle surgery is a highly specialized field with a broad range of procedures available. Despite advances in the pharmacological therapy of inflammatory arthritis, surgery remains an important option in the management of foot and ankle problems across the spectrum of RMDs. As such, foot and ankle surgeons should be seen as important members of the MDT, and well-integrated services will benefit patient care.

References

1. **Loza E, et al.** Variability in the use of orthopedic surgery in patients with rheumatoid arthritis in Spain. *J Rheumatol.* 2007;**34**(7):1485–90.
2. **Barton JL.** The role of race in patient preferences for treatment in rheumatoid arthritis. *Arthritis Rheum.* 2009;**61**(4):411–12.
3. **Constantinescu F, et al.** Understanding why rheumatoid arthritis patient treatment preferences differ by race. *Arthritis Rheum.* 2009;**61**(4):413–18.
4. **Nystad TW, et al.** Reduction in orthopaedic surgery in patients with rheumatoid arthritis: a Norwegian register-based study. *Scand J Rheumatol.* 2016;**45**(1):1–7.
5. **Nikiphorou E, et al.** Hand and foot surgery rates in rheumatoid arthritis have declined from 1986 to 2011 but large-joint replacement rates remain unchanged: results from two UK inception cohorts. *Arthritis Rheum.* 2014;**66**(5):1081–9.
6. **Backhouse MR, et al.** Use of conservative and surgical foot care in an inception cohort of patients with rheumatoid arthritis. *Rheumatology.* 2011;**50**(9):1586–95.
7. **Kapetanovic MC, et al.** Orthopaedic surgery in patients with rheumatoid arthritis over 20 years: prevalence and predictive factors of large joint replacement. *Ann Rheum Dis.* 2008;**67**(10):1412–16.
8. **Backhouse MR, et al.** Interpreting outcome following foot surgery in people with rheumatoid arthritis. *J Foot Ankle Res.* 2016;**9**:20.
9. **National Institute for Health and Care Excellence.** *Osteoarthritis: Care and Management in Adults.* London: NICE; 2014.
10. **National Institute for Health and Care Excellence.** *Rheumatoid Arthritis: National Clinical Guideline for Management and Treatment in Adults.* London: NICE; 2009.

11. **James D, et al.** Orthopaedic intervention in early rheumatoid arthritis Occurrence and predictive factors in an inception cohort of 1064 patients followed for 5 years. *Rheumatology (Oxford).* 2004;**43**(3):369–76.
12. **Eberhardt K, et al.** Associations of HLA-DRB and -DQB genes with two and five year outcome in rheumatoid arthritis. *Ann Rheum Dis.* 1996;**55**(1):34–9.
13. **Goodman SM, et al.** Patients with rheumatoid arthritis are more likely to have pain and poor function after total hip replacements than patients with osteoarthritis. *J Rheumatol.* 2014;**41**(9):1774–80.
14. **Ravi B, et al.** Increased risk of complications following total joint arthroplasty in patients with rheumatoid arthritis. *Arthritis Rheum.* 2014;**66**(2):254–63.
15. **Backhouse MR.** *Factors Predicting the Outcome of Foot and Ankle Surgery in People with Rheumatoid Arthritis in School of Medicine.* Leeds: University of Leeds; 2011.
16. **den Broeder AA, et al.** Risk factors for surgical site infections and other complications in elective surgery in patients with rheumatoid arthritis with special attention for anti-tumor necrosis factor: a large retrospective study. *J Rheumatol.* 2007;**34**(4):689–95.
17. **Doran MF, et al.** Frequency of infection in patients with rheumatoid arthritis compared with controls: a population-based study. *Arthritis Rheum.* 2002;**46**(9):2287–93.
18. **Dixon WG, et al.** Rates of serious infection including site-specific and bacterial intracellular infection in rheumatoid arthritis patients receiving anti-tumor necrosis factor therapy: results from the British Society for Rheumatology Biologics Register. *Arthritis Rheum.* 2006;**54**(8):2368–76.
19. **Goodman SM.** Optimizing perioperative outcomes for older patients with rheumatoid arthritis undergoing arthroplasty: emphasis on medication management. *Drugs Aging.* 2015;**32**(5):361–9.
20. **Duru N, et al.** EULAR evidence-based and consensus-based recommendations on the management of medium to high-dose glucocorticoid therapy in rheumatic diseases. *Ann Rheum Dis.* 2013;**72**(12):1905–13.
21. **Grennan DM, et al.** Methotrexate and early postoperative complications in patients with rheumatoid arthritis undergoing elective orthopaedic surgery. *Ann Rheum Dis.* 2001;**60**(3):214–17.
22. **Chen CA, et al.** New MR imaging methods for metallic implants in the knee: artifact correction and clinical impact. *J Magn Reson Imaging.* 2011;**33**(5):1121–7.
23. **Godot S, et al.** Safety of surgery after rituximab therapy in 133 patients with rheumatoid arthritis: data from the autoimmunity and rituximab registry. *Arthritis Care Res (Hoboken).* 2013;**65**(11):1874–9.
24. **Tol JL, Verheyen CP, van Dijk CN.** Arthroscopic treatment of anterior impingement in the ankle. *J Bone Joint Surg Br.* 2001;**83**(1):9–13.
25. **Ferkel RD, et al.** Arthroscopic treatment of chronic osteochondral lesions of the talus: long-term results. *Am J Sports Med.* 2008;**36**(9):1750–62.
26. **Briggs PJ, Stainsby GD.** The Thomas method of ankle arthrodesis: 2 to 20 year follow-up. *The Foot.* 1997;**7**:14–18.
27. **Felix NA, Kitaoka HB.** Ankle arthrodesis in patients with rheumatoid arthritis. *Clin Orthop Relat Res.* 1998;**349**:58–64.
28. **Coester LM, et al.** Long-term results following ankle arthrodesis for post-traumatic arthritis. *J Bone Joint Surg Am.* 2001;**83-A**(2):219–28.
29. **Haddad SL, et al.** Intermediate and long-term outcomes of total ankle arthroplasty and ankle arthrodesis. A systematic review of the literature. *J Bone Joint Surg Am.* 2007;**89**(9):1899–905.
30. **Henricson A, Nilsson JA, Carlsson A.** 10-year survival of total ankle arthroplasties: a report on 780 cases from the Swedish Ankle Register. *Acta Orthop.* 2011;**82**(6):655–9.
31. **Jastifer JR, Coughlin MJ.** Long-term follow-up of mobile bearing total ankle arthroplasty in the United States. *Foot Ankle Int.* 2015;**36**(2):143–50.
32. **Ali AA, O'Connor P, Harris N.** Revision total ankle replacement to a hind-foot fusion with a nail: the experience from Leeds. *Bone Joint J.* 2015;**97-B**(Suppl. 14):19.
33. **DeVries JG, Scharer B.** Hindfoot deformity corrected with double versus triple arthrodesis: radiographic comparison. *J Foot Ankle Surg.* 2015;**54**(3):424–7.

34. **Pell RFt, Myerson MS, Schon LC.** Clinical outcome after primary triple arthrodesis. *J Bone Joint Surg Am.* 2000;**82**(1):47–57.
35. **Knupp M, et al.** Triple arthrodesis in rheumatoid arthrtis. *Foot Ankle Int.* 2008;**29**(3):293–7.
36. **Komenda GA, Myerson MS, Biddinger KR.** Results of arthrodesis of the tarsometatarsal joints after traumatic injury. *J Bone Joint Surg Am.* 1996;**78**(11):1665–76.
37. **Kulkarni A, Soomro T, Sidique M.** Tarsometatarsal joint fusion results in 100 people using a low profile dorsal locking plates. *Bone Joint J.* 2012;**94(B)**(Suppl. XXII):31.
38. **Mann RA, Coughlin MJ.** Hallux valgus—etiology anatomy treatment and surgical considerations. *Clin Orthop Rel Res.* 1981;**157**:31–41.
39. **Spink MJ, Menz HB, Lord SR.** Distribution and correlates of plantar hyperkeratotic lesions in older people. *J Foot Ankle Res.* 2009;**2**(1):8.
40. **Menz HB, et al.** Impact of hallux valgus severity on general and foot-specific health-related quality of life. *Arthritis Care Res (Hoboken).* 2011;**63**(3):396–404.
41. **Lazarides S, et al.** Association amongst angular deformities in hallux valgus and impact of the deformity in health-related quality of life. *Foot Ankle Surg.* 2005;**11**(4):193–6.
42. **Thordarson D, et al.** Age-adjusted baseline data for women with hallux valgus undergoing corrective surgery. *J Bone Joint Surg Am.* 2005;**87**(1):66–75.
43. **Menz H, Lord S.** Gait instability in older people with hallux valgus. *Foot & Ankle International/ American Orthopaedic Foot and Ankle Society (and) Swiss Foot and Ankle Society.* 2005;**26**(6):483–9.
44. **Menz HB, Morris ME, Lord SR.** Foot and ankle risk factors for falls in older people: a prospective study. *J Gerontol A Biol Sci Med Sci.* 2006;**61**(8):866–70.
45. **Mickle KJ, et al.** ISB Clinical Biomechanics Award 2009: toe weakness and deformity increase the risk of falls in older people. *Clin Biomech (Bristol Avon).* 2009;**24**(10):787–91.
46. **Menz HB, Gilheany MF, Landorf KB.** Foot and ankle surgery in Australia: a descriptive analysis of the Medicare Benefits Schedule database 1997–2006. *J Foot Ankle Res.* 2008;**1**(1):10.
47. **Saro C, et al.** Surgical treatment of hallux valgus and forefoot deformities in Sweden: a population-based study. *Foot Ankle Int.* 2008;**29**(3):298–304.
48. **Dawson J, et al.** Factors associated with satisfaction with bunion surgery in women: a prospective study. *Foot.* 2007;**17**(3):119–25.
49. **Torkki M, et al.** Surgery vs orthosis vs watchful waiting for hallux valgus: a randomized controlled trial. *JAMA.* 2001;**285**(19):2474–80.
50. **Ferrari J, Higgins JP, Prior TD.** Interventions for treating hallux valgus (abductovalgus) and bunions. *Cochrane Database Syst Rev.* **2004**(1):CD000964.
51. **van Groningen B, et al.** Outcomes in chevron osteotomy for hallux valgus in a large cohort. *Foot.* 2016;**29**:18–24.
52. **Blair S, Ong M, Gregori A.** The scarf osteotomy for hallux valgus: a clinical and radiological review. *Foot.* 2001;**11**:140–3.
53. **Crevoisier X, et al.** The scarf osteotomy for the treatment of hallux valgus deformity: a review of 84 cases. *Foot Ankle Int.* 2001;**22**(12):970–6.
54. **Kilmartin TE, O'Kane C.** Combined rotation scarf and Akin osteotomies for hallux valgus: a patient focussed 9 year follow up of 50 patients. *J Foot Ankle Res.* 2010;**3**:2.
55. **O'Kane C, Kilmartin TE.** The rotation Scarf osteotomy for the correction of severe hallux valgus. *Foot.* 2002;**12**(4):203–12.
56. **McCarthy AD, et al.** Three-dimensional analysis of different first metatarsal osteotomies in a hallux valgus model. *Foot Ankle Int.* 2008;**29**(6):606–12.
57. **Metzdorf A, Strehle JK.** Early complications of the modified lapidus procedure for hallux valgus treatment in adults. *Foot.* 2001;**11**:38–44.
58. **Rink-Brüne O.** Lapidus arthrodesis for management of hallux valgus—a retrospective review of 106 cases. *J Foot Ankle Surg.* 2004;**43**(5):290–5.

59. **Coetzee JC, Wickum D.** The Lapidus procedure: a prospective cohort outcome study. *Foot Ankle Int.* 2004;**25**(8):526–31.
60. **Iqbal MJ, Chana GS.** Arthroscopic cheilectomy for hallux rigidus. *Arthroscopy.* 1998;**14**(3):307–10.
61. **Coughlin MJ, Shurnas PS.** Hallux rigidus. *J Bone Joint Surg Am.* 2004;86-A Suppl. 1(Pt 2):119–30.
62. **Beertema W, et al.** A retrospective analysis of surgical treatment in patients with symptomatic hallux rigidus: long-term follow-up. *J Foot Ankle Surg.* 2006;**45**(4):244–51.
63. **Canseco K, et al.** Quantitative motion analysis in patients with hallux rigidus before and after cheilectomy. *J Orthop Res.* 2009;**27**(1):128–34.
64. **Kuni B, et al.** Foot kinematics in walking on a level surface and on stairs in patients with hallux rigidus before and after cheilectomy. *J Foot Ankle Res.* 2014;**7**(1):13.
65. **Coughlin MJ, Abdo RV.** Arthrodesis of the first metatarsophalangeal joint with Vitallium plate fixation. *Foot Ankle Int.* 1994;**15**(1):18–28.
66. **Perler AD, et al.** End-stage osteoarthritis of the great toe/hallux rigidus: a review of the alternatives to arthrodesis: implant versus osteotomies and arthroplasty techniques. *Clin Podiatr Med Surg.* 2013;**30**(3):351–95.
67. **Hueter C.** *Klinik der Gelenkkrankheiten mit Einschluß der Orthopädie,* Vol. **2**. Leipzig: Vogel; 1877.
68. **Swanson AB, Lumsden RM, Swanson GD.** Silicone implant arthroplasty of the great toe. A review of single stem and flexible hinge implants. *Clin Orthop Relat Res.* 1979;**142**:30–43.
69. **Patel DC, Frascone ST, DeLuca A.** Synovitis secondary to silicone elastomeric joint implant. *J Foot Ankle Surg.* 1994;**33**(6):628–32.
70. **Freed JB.** The increasing recognition of medullary lysis cortical osteophytic proliferation and fragmentation of implanted silicone polymer implants. *J Foot Ankle Surg.* 1993;**32**(2):171–9.
71. **Fuhrmann RA, Wagner A, Anders JO.** First metatarsophalangeal joint replacement: the method of choice for end-stage hallux rigidus? *Foot Ankle Clin.* 2003;**8**(4):711–21, vi.
72. **Nixon MF, Taylor GJS.** Early failure of the Moje implant when used to treat hallux rigidus: the need for regular surveillance. *The Foot* 2008;**18**(1):1–6
73. **Gross CE, et al.** Revision MTP arthrodesis for failed MTP arthroplasty. *Foot Ankle Spec.* 2013;**6**(6):471–8.
74. **Baumhauer JF, et al.** Prospective randomized multi-centered clinical trial assessing safety and efficacy of a synthetic cartilage implant versus first metatarsophalangeal arthrodesis in advanced hallux rigidus. *Foot Ankle Int.* 2016;**37**(5):457–69.
75. **Myerson MS.** Foreword. *Foot Ankle Clin N Am.* 2007;**3**(12):ix–x.
76. **Barouk LS.** Joint-preserving surgery in rheumatoid forefoot: preliminary study with more-than-two-year follow-up. *Foot Ankle Clin N Am.* 2007;**12**(3):435–54.
77. **Berg RP, et al.** Scarf and Weil osteotomies for correction of rheumatoid forefoot deformities: a review of 20 cases. *Foot and Ankle Surgery*, 2007;**13**(1):35–40.
78. **Jeng C, Campbell J.** Current concepts review: the rheumatoid forefoot. *Foot Ankle Int.* 2008;**29**(9):959–68.
79. **Hanyu T, et al.** Arthroplasty for rheumatoid forefoot deformities by a shortening oblique osteotomy. *Clin Orthop Rel Res.* 1997;**338**:131–8.
80. **Hoffman MD.** An operation for severe grades of contracted or clawed toes. *Am J Orthop Surg.* 1912;**9**:441–9.
81. **Myerson MS.** Foreward. *Foot Ankle Clin N Am.* 2007;**12**(3):ix–x.
82. **Brattström H, Brattström M.** Resection of the metatarsophalangeal joints in rheumatoid arthritis. *Acta Orthop Scand.* 1970;**41**:213–24.
83. **van der Heijden KW, et al.** Kates forefoot arthroplasty in rheumatoid arthritis. A 5-year follow up study. *J Rheumatol.* 1992;**19**(10):1545–50.
84. **Harris N, et al.** A prospective 10–16 year clinical and pedobarographic evaluation of forefoot arthroplasty. *Foot.* 1997;**7**(3):166–9.

85. **Stockley I, et al.** A prospective study of forefoot arthroplasty. *Clin Orthop Rel Res.* 1989;**248**:213–18.
86. **Coughlin MJ.** Rheumatoid forefoot reconstruction. A long-term follow-up study. *J Bone Joint Surg Am.* 2000;**82**(3):322–41.
87. **Betts RP, et al.** Foot pressure studies in the assessment of forefoot arthroplasty in the rheumatoid foot. *Foot Ankle.* 1988;**8**(6):315–26.
88. **Harris N, et al.** A prospective 10–16 year clinical and pedobarographic evaluation of forefoot arthroplasty. *Foot.* 1997;**7**(3):166–9.
89. **Vahvanen V, Piirainen H, Kettunen P.** Resection arthroplasty of the metatarsophalangeal joints in rheumatoid arthritis. A follow-up study of 100 patients. *Scand J Rheumatol.* 1980;**9**(4):257–65.
90. **Stockley I, et al.** The importance of the valgus hindfoot in forefoot surgery in rheumatoid arthritis. *J Bone Joint Surg–Br.* 1990;**72**(4):705–8.
91. **Petrov O, et al.** Recurrent plantar ulceration following pan metatarsal head resection. *J Foot Ankle Surg.* 1996;**35**(6):573–7.
92. **Diez E, et al.** Metatarsal remodelling following surgery on the rheumatic forefoot. A long-term study. *Foot.* 2002;**12**:83–7.
93. **Matricali GA, et al.** The presence of forefoot problems and the role of surgery in patients with rheumatoid arthritis. *Ann Rheum Dis.* 2006;**65**(9):1254–5.
94. **Stainsby GD, Briggs PJ.** Modified Keller's type procedure for the lateral four toes. *J Bone Joint Surg–Br.* 1990;**72**:530.
95. **Stainsby GD.** Pathological anatomy and dynamic effect of the displaced plantar plate and the importance of the integrity of the plantar plate-deep transverse metatarsal ligament tie-bar. *Ann R Coll Surg Eng.* 1997;**79**(1):58–68.
96. **Briggs PJ.** Controversies and perils: reconstruction of the rheumatoid forefoot. *Tech Orthop.* 2003;**18**(3):303–10.
97. **Briggs PJ, Stainsby GD.** Metatarsal head preservation in forefoot arthroplasty and the correction of severe claw toe deformity. *Foot Ankle Surg.* 2001;7:93–101.
98. **Mangaleshkar SR, Rajesh MB, Tandon RK.** Surgical correction of severe claw toe deformity: a review of the Stainsby procedure. *Foot.* 2001;**11**:126–31.
99. **Hassan K, et al.** Forefoot reconstruction: effectiveness of Stainsby operation in treating disclocated lesser toes. *Foot.* 2007;**17**:136–42.
100. **Vyas H, Krishnaswamy G.** Images in clinical medicine. Quinolone-associated rupture of the Achilles' tendon. *N Engl J Med.* 2007;**357**(20):2067.
101. **Cetti R, et al.** Operative versus nonoperative treatment of Achilles tendon rupture. A prospective randomized study and review of the literature. *Am J Sports Med.* 1993;**21**(6):791–9.
102. **Hutchison AM, et al.** The treatment of a rupture of the Achilles tendon using a dedicated management programme. *Bone Joint J.* 2015;**97-B**(4):510–15.
103. **Lawrence JE, et al.** Functional outcomes of conservatively managed acute ruptures of the Achilles tendon. *Bone Joint J.* 2017;**99-B**(1):87–93.
104. **Johnson KA, Strom DE.** Tibialis posterior tendon dysfunction. *Clin Orthop Relat Res.* 1989;**239**:196–206.
105. **Myerson MS.** Adult acquired flat foot deformity. *J Bone Joint Surg.* 1996;**78A**:780–92.
106. **Pasapula C, Shariff S, Fischer NC.** *The Resistance to Failure of Spring Ligament Reconstruction.* San Diego: Orthopaedic Research Society; 2017: pp PS1–067.
107. **Anderson JA, et al.** Surgery for retrocalcaneal bursitis: a tendon-splitting versus a lateral approach. *Clin Orthop Relat Res.* 2008;**466**(7):1678–82.
108. **Jerosch J, et al.** (Endoscopic calcaneoplasty (ECP) in Haglund's syndrome Indication surgical technique surgical findings and results.) *Z Orthop Unfall.* 2012;**150**(3):250–6.
109. **Richardson DR.** Amputations of the foot. In: ST Canale and J Beaty (eds). *Campbell's Operative Orthopaedics.* Philadelphia: Mosby; 2012 pp 613–35.

Chapter 16

Organizing care

Jane McAdam and Maggie Helliwell

Introduction

Whilst the organization of any health system is often in a state of flux, the principles of organizing services remain constant. This chapter will lay out those principles in the current health system within the English National Health Service (NHS), which is publicly funded. The authors acknowledge that international health systems will vary but planning of those services contain standard principles. At its best the organization of any health service is the key driver of quality, efficiency, and the optimum outcomes for patients. In simple terms commissioning any disease service within the NHS is the process of planning, agreeing, and monitoring services. However, this simple statement hides a complex world, which is dependent on an understanding of epidemiology of populations both nationally and locally, an understanding of complex datasets within those populations, health needs assessments of those populations, a clear understanding of best evidence within clinical conditions, an awareness of patient pathways (i.e., the right care for the right patient in the right place at the right time), a knowledge of service specification, contracting, negotiating, and procurement before one even reaches the continuous quality assessment that improves outcomes.

Burden of rheumatology and musculoskeletal disorders

Health priorities vary across countries and are complicated by political imperatives and mandatory requirements. Despite their prevalence, morbidity, and complexity, as chronic health conditions rheumatology, musculoskeletal (MSK), and podiatry services often do not appear in the top 20 locality services perceived as requiring either attention or planned change—they could be perceived as Cinderella services. This is despite the fact that they contribute to more years lived with disability in the UK than heart conditions, cancer, and diabetes. Around 10 million people have some form of arthritis. Over 1 million have an inflammatory arthritis, of which over two-thirds have rheumatoid arthritis (RA), and 50,000 people have a form of lupus. Upon diagnosis, approximately 16% of people with RA have foot involvement, and in 15% of cases the forefoot is the first part of the body to become symptomatic. By 10 years, 90% of patients with RA have some form of disease-related foot and ankle involvement. In the main these inflammatory conditions are diseases of youth and working age; people in the prime of their lives. The working days lost in 2006–7 because of rheumatic disease were estimated to be worth £5.7 million; this did not include the cost contributed by informal carers. A relatively recent report from the 2015/16 national audit of inflammatory arthritis (www.rheumatology.org.uk) showed that the UK is an outlier in Europe in terms of management of these conditions with delays in referral and treatment. This is particularly emphasized by people only entering care in the severe stages of disease. Delays occur along all parts of the patient pathway and completely reflect the position of these diseases (with podiatry particularly ignored) amongst local health priorities.

Planning data

Planning services requires good-quality data and information. In most rheumatological conditions, although hospital data (Hospital Episode Statistics [HES] data) is collected there is no standardized coding for these conditions within SnoMed (systematized nomenclature of medical clinical terms). The ICD10 (International Statistical Classification of Diseases and related health problems, 10th edn) codes used in the UK for the commissioning of MSK services focus on orthopaedic services, with many rheumatological costs falling outside this budget. Hospital outpatient codes only cover 75% of rheumatological and MSK medical conditions and it is alleged that only 5% are actually collected (www.rheumatology.org.uk/resources/commissioning-support). Hospital data do not reflect the complexity of information required or the majority of care for these patients. Ambulatory care data and primary care data, even if collected, are not coordinated with hospital data and are not standardized. Podiatry data are also not standardized across hospital, primary care, community, and individual private practitioner data. Individual consultant rheumatologists have often built up rich datasets connected to their routine care and ongoing research, but these have rarely been integrated into hospital datasets.

There are now substantial electronic patient records (ePRs) within primary care, but these are not routinely replicated in daily routine hospital care although some primary care computer systems (SystmOne being an example) integrate hospital outpatient and rheumatological specialist nurse consultation appointments into the primary care record. Apart from the pockets of rheumatological data within the primary care Quality and Outcomes Framework (QOF) there is no national standardization of required coded data within these primary care records for any rheumatological diseases and the QOF data contain no reference to podiatry, assistive equipment, orthotics, or physiotherapy.

Some primary care systems integrate podiatry consultations within the patient record, but this is not standardized and may not contain any reference to the patient's underlying reason for the specific podiatry appointment. The College of Podiatry (https://www.evidence.nhs.uk/search?q=podiatry, Accessed 02/12/18) carried out a 1-day snapshot survey in 2015 amongst their members. This uncovered a plurality of settings, both NHS and private. Among the appointments, 8% were for patients with RA and 18% were for patients with osteoarthritis and included direct treatment and orthotic advice. Fifty-three per cent of the patients were under long-term follow-up but the survey did not delineate how many of those patients had long-term rheumatological conditions. This emphasized the dearth of real-time information on which to plan services and demonstrated very little information on outcomes for those patients either within hospital or at podiatry appointments within primary and community care of all types. This may improve if personal care budgets are utilized throughout the whole patient pathway, as the coding will have to match the service provided in all settings for contractual and financial monitoring.

Audit data

National audits can also be a basis for understanding service gaps and, therefore, key priorities for future planning, improvement, and workforce needs across the whole multidisciplinary team (MDT). The British Society of Rheumatology (BSR), in association with the Health Quality Improvement Partnership (HQIP), produced two key national audits in 2015 and 2016 based on the implementation of the Rheumatoid Arthritis NHS Quality Standards across 124 hospital trusts in England and Wales (www.rheumatology.org.uk/resources/audits/defaultaspx). Both reports make for sobering reading and are an excellent proxy for service needs, particularly in podiatry. The first report's key findings were that Standard 1—referral by a general practitioner (GP) within 3 days of first presentation—was only adhered to in 17% of cases. For Standard 2, where patients are supposed to be seen within 3 weeks of referral, only 38% of trusts achieved the target, and only 53% of patients were on disease-modifying drugs 6 weeks from their first outpatient appointment. Within these figures there was considerable variation at local level, and some patients waited more than 1 year for their first treatment.

The second audit (2016) was completed by 88% of all providers in England and Wales, and covered compliance with all the quality standards rather than just two. There was very little improvement in relation to the two standards audited in 2014/15. A key finding was that only 51% of providers had access to specialist podiatry, and some providers did not offer any education or self-management for patients. Again, there was enormous variation in standards both locally and nationally.

Currently the same organization is running a similar audit in relation to early inflammatory arthritis, which aims to complete its first report in 2019 (https://www.rheumatology.org.uk/Knowledge/Excellence/Audits/Reports).

Patient-led resources

Patient organizations also have a voice in health needs assessment and support for podiatry. Amongst them are Psoriasis and Psoriatic Arthritis Alliance (PAPAA; www.papaa.org), Arthritis Research UK (www.arthritisresearchuk.org), and the National Rheumatoid Arthritis Society (www.nras.org.uk). NRAS provides support for Commissioning for Quality on Rheumatoid Arthritis (CQRA). They have developed key commissioning metrics based on best quality evidence. They have also captured and improved the patient experience in respect of validated patient-reported experience measures (PREMs). Their website also supplies the tools for these metrics. The BSR have formed a Musculoskeletal Solution Alliance with Arthritis Care and have also produced a range of commissioning tools (www.rheumatology.org.uk/resources/commisioning-support).

Organizing for quality

Guidelines can be used to demonstrate possible good clinical and value outcomes when developing MSK and podiatry services. The current gold standard is provided by NICE (National Institute for Health and Care Excellence; www.nice.org.uk) and their quality standards are used in contract monitoring. NICE has also provided information through their pathways for other conditions for which they have not provided specific disease clinical guidelines. These include

- Specific individual drug management of systemic lupus erythematosus (SLE).
- Specific individual drug management of vasculitis.
- Specific individual drug management of ankylosing spondylitis.

The current NICE guidance related to MSK disorders of all types is:

- NG100 Rheumatoid arthritis.
- CG177 Osteoarthritis.
- CG161 Falls.
- CG146 Osteoporotic fragility fractures.

- NG65 Spondyloarthritis.
- CG153 Psoriasis contains references to psoriatic arthritis.

NICE has associated quality standards. They are derived from high-quality guidance such as that from NICE or other sources accredited by NICE, which includes the BSR. For example, there is a NICE-accredited BSR guideline in development on the management of foot health in inflammatory arthritis. Each standard consists of a prioritized set of specific, concise, and measurable statements. They are designed to support the measurement of improvement.

The current available NICE quality standards (available from www.nice.org.uk) are:

- QS 33 RA in over 16s.
- QS 87 Osteoarthritis.
- QS 40 Psoriasis.
- QS 149 Osteoporosis.
- QS 170 Spondyloarthritis.

Other organizations, both national and international, produce excellent guidance for care of rheumatological and, specifically, foot and ankle problems. These include:

- The College of Podiatry (cop.org.uk).
- Arthritis and Musculoskeletal Alliance (ARMA)—e.g., standards of care for people with MSK foot health problems (http://arma.uk.net/resources/standards-of-care/).
- BSR (www.rheumatology.org.uk).
- European League Against Rheumatism (EULAR; www.eular.org).
- American College of Rheumatology (ACR; www.rheumatology.org).
- Podiatry Rheumatic Care Association (PRCA; www.prcassoc.org.uk/standards-project).

Information can also be obtained through the NHS evidence portal (evidence.nhs.uk).

The other key driver of commissioned quality comes through Commissioning for Quality and Innovation (CQUINS; www.england.nhs.uk/nhs-standard-contract/cquin). These are applied to monitor the performance of provider organizations, e.g., hospitals. These consist of two types: those for the specialized services and those for local services. The CQUINS for local services are subdivided into nationally prescribed local targets and those priorities that are locally agreed. These therefore vary between localities and may not include any specific reference to rheumatology or foot and ankle services.

Currently the specialized rheumatology CQUINS for 2017–18 include three indicators. The first, GE2, is systematic measurement of self-management of patients using a recognized patient activation measure. This is to be used to improve outcomes by rating self-management and by stratification of support. This indicator should include reference to foot and ankle services. The second indicator, IM3, is related to multi-system autoimmune rheumatic disease MDT clinics. There should be systematic review of cases to ensure policy compliance, with data flowing to registries. Those for localized services are agreed between local commissioners and local providers. The derived data for this indicator should include access to foot and ankle management. This indicator is also to support the development of coordinated MDT clinics. The third indicator, GE5, relates to shared decision-making resources specific to specific conditions, which could include MSK disease. The national local CQUINS for 2017–18 do not include any indicators related to any long-term condition.

The QOF is a contractual means of paying primary care in England through achievement of quality targets within various domains. In the past targets have concentrated on RA. The maintenance of a practice register, annual face-to-face review, assessment of cardiovascular risk in those patients with RA, assessment of fracture risk using a recognized tool. Currently the planned targets for 2018–19 (www.nhsemployers.org) are the maintenance of a register and an annual face-to-face review. Unfortunately, the coding does not include individual subsets within this care and the level of service and degree of compliance with good foot and ankle care is not known.

In 2005 the NHS produced the National Service Frameworks for Long Term Conditions (www.gov.uk/government/publications/). It was intended to be the template for a framework for commissioning and planning quality services across all long-term conditions and its principles still hold strong for all rheumatological and MSK conditions. It defined 12 quality standards, which followed any possible patient journey and, within those standards, defined contractual quality markers and indicators that still reflect and expand those separate quality standards more recently developed by NICE.

Access to patient-centred care

One of the key tenets of NHS England's current strategy is the concept of patients being at the centre of their healthcare and the fundamental partner in all decisions made about their care: 'No care for me without me'. All care should also be achieved through shared decision-making between the health professional and the patient.

People access care for foot and ankle problems via a multiplicity of routes. There is now a plethora of healthcare information via online NHS statutory services, social media, patient organizations, and charities. Despite this and despite most healthcare services being free at the point of delivery there appear to be barriers to accessing healthcare. These barriers are both organizational—a combination of inefficient systems and a lack or absence of local resources—and personal. The personal barriers are a combination of lack of knowledge, both by health professionals and patients pre- and post-diagnosis, which leads to the acceptance that 'nothing can be done'. Not everyone is aware of the transformation of health outcomes and possible therapeutic treatment options in podiatry in the past 30 years within rheumatological conditions and still perceive inflammatory conditions to be more disabling than they now are. This lack of knowledge is compounded by low levels of health literacy (1, 2). Services may appear to provide clear information via leaflets and websites; however, this recent study of health information materials reveal them to be generally too complex. Forty-three per cent of people between 15 and 65 were unable to understand and use everyday healthcare information effectively. This figure rose to 61% when the information required numeracy skills. This finding may also be compounded when English is not a patient's first language. It is vital that service users and members of the public are engaged in co-developing patient information to a level that can be understood by all.

To aid the need for increasing awareness, The College of Podiatry has produced a series of videos that are aimed at improving understanding of podiatric care amongst other healthcare practitioners and the public (https://cop.org.uk/foot-health/what-is-podiatry/). The BSR national audit for RA agreed that elevating awareness within the general public would be of benefit. There are numerous national campaigns in other disease areas (e.g., 'Be clear on Cancer'), which encourage patients to seek advice if they have certain key symptoms—this has been extended to rheumatological conditions via the inflammatory arthritis awareness campaign, also known as the S Factor Campaign. This work was developed by the Rheumatology Futures project and was endorsed by Arthritis Research UK, the Royal College of General Practioners (RCGP) and the Primary Care Rheumatology Society. This campaign was transmitted through posters to be displayed in GP surgeries, libraries, pharmacies, and other suitable public places. Resources permitting, this could be amplified by focused regional campaigns in areas—mapped to emphasize that seeking podiatric care for foot and ankle disorders could focus on the benefits of improved health outcomes such as pain reduction, mobility improvement, a return to work, and improved ability to take part in social activities.

Organizational barriers also exist. The existing silos of hospital versus community versus private care within podiatry and rheumatology need to be broken down into one service with the patient and their advocates orchestrating their care. NHS England is hoping that this will be achieved through sustainable transformation partnerships (STPs) using the 'vehicle' of integrated care systems (ICSs). New planning guidance from the NHS was issued in 2018 (https://www.england.nhs.uk/integrated care/integrated-care-system) and covered the development of ICSs. There are 44 STPs, which now include 18 pilot ICSs. These organizations aim to eliminate previous silos between commissioners, primary and secondary healthcare providers, community care, local authority, social care, voluntary organizations, patients, and carers, and cover large geographical areas across the country. Within the footprint of the STPs are further new smaller 'placed-based' groupings: these include accountable care organizations, the vanguards and collaborations of acute hospitals, and 'place'-based coalitions of organizations. From April 2017 STPs became the single application and approval mechanism for accessing NHS transformation funding, with the best plans set to receive funds the soonest, so local success in collaborative planning and meaningful consultation is essential.

Other organizational barriers include the lack of data standardization in relation to NHS podiatry services and the absence of standard national evidence-based criteria for access. This applies to both initial and ongoing access. Many community services still restrict access on the basis of age and narrowly defined medical conditions, which often do not extend beyond RA. This is balanced by other services that focus on appropriate medical and podiatric needs but, again, often only treat those 'at risk' or at 'high risk' with no standardized definitions. This lack of resources extends beyond community services into specialized services where a majority of hospitals have no access to specialized podiatry within their rheumatological teams.

One solution to ease these barriers could be self-referral in primary and community care. This, however, depends on well-defined evidence-based and standardized triage at initial assessment. This would filter out those patients who can manage with self-care and those who might require simple solutions from healthcare assistants, from those who require a more specialized ongoing foot protection service, which would recognize the need for ongoing care, crisis management, and the ability to dip in and out for appropriate episodes of more acute care. This footcare service would also contain links into community- and hospital-based orthotics and equipment services, which would obviate the need for unnecessary GP appointments merely to gain referral permission. The College of Podiatry Guide to the Benefits of podiatry to patient care (https://www.evidence.nhs.uk/search?q=podiatry, Accessed 02/12/18) demonstrates the benefits of a skills-based service needed for such triage.

All of this is predicated on a sustainable workforce. The College of Podiatry Report (2014) 'Towards a sustainable Podiatry Workforce for the UK towards 2030' https://evidence.nhs.uk graphically demonstrates the current and potential need and current and future provision required to build this type of service.

Person-centred systems

Currently, most countries have a national illness service rather than a national health service. Transformation from a hospital-centred and illness-based system towards a patient-centred and health-based system will require a gradual but seismic cultural change. However, it should benefit most patients with long-term rheumatological and foot and ankle conditions, as the majority of their care takes place outside hospital and they require solutions that are community, work, housing, and 'life' based. Bringing together all these budgets to self-management at the individual level has been shown to be a success both at a population level and amongst individual people narratives (3). Several key opinion leaders published a new 'NHS Manifesto' in the Lancet in December 2016 (4), which outlined this evidence.

A key lever for the facilitation of self-referral, particularly for those patients with an inflammatory arthritis, is that of personal health budgets. Within current national commissioning plans there are various government targets. The most relevant of these for all rheumatological patients and those with MSK problems is that of personal health budgets (www.england.nhs.uk/healthbudgets). Adults who are eligible for NHS continuing healthcare and children in receipt of continuing care have had the right to have a personal health budget since 2014. Since April 2015, commissioners of care have been mandated to look at expanding their local personal health budget offer to others who could benefit, and NHS England and the Department of Health Social Care are currently (2018) consulting on extending the legal rights to have a personal health budget. The mandate from the government to NHS England in 2016/17 set out a clear expectation that, by 2020, 50–100,000 people will have a personal health budget or a personal budget that combines NHS funding with social care. To achieve this, commissioners should engage widely with their local communities and patients, including with their local Healthwatch, and include those plans in their local joint health and wellbeing strategy and their STP.

Patients can use this budget to plan their own health and social care needs. This budget can be managed by themselves or a third party and can be used for therapies, including podiatry and physiotherapy, personal care, and equipment such as orthotics and wheelchairs. Patients will need to be informed of the optimum patient pathways in their area, but they are not confined to these and can use their budget to buy other care from the private or the voluntary sector—this might be particularly relevant in relation to podiatry and equipment. Patients will have access to various resources, including 'Peoplehub' (www.peoplehub.org.uk), a resource for people with long-term conditions, and patients, carers, and families have been welcomed to and encouraged to apply for the Peer Leadership Academy for 2016/17 (https://www.england.nhs.uk/personal-health-budgets/, Accessed 02/12/18), which will 'allow them to be more involved in shaping the national programme'. This type of initiative can only encourage confidence in self-care, which leads to better health outcomes.

This personal health budget is confined to the specifics of a patient's long-term condition. It is not intended to cover emergency care or the normal care from a patient's GP.

The patient at the centre of the multidisciplinary team

In 2011 the BSR, in conjunction with the Royal College of Physicians and using NICE guidance, produced an excellent 'Patient centred service wheel' (Figure 16.1) with orthotics and podiatry services as essential components. In addition, the College of Podiatry produced a model for a step-wise integration of services in podiatry (Figure 16.2).

A true patient-centred MDT should cross current care boundaries and contain clinical professionals who work with the patient in multiple settings and through multiple means. Access to each layer of this team should be through evidence-based referral understandable to the patient and their carers. Traditional face-to-face encounters may not always be cost-effective and, increasingly, clinics, practitioners, community practices, and patients avail themselves of telephone contact and telemedicine in its various forms.

There are many advantages to a team skills-based approach. The right care in the right place by the right practitioner at the right time for each patient is the essence. Each member can focus

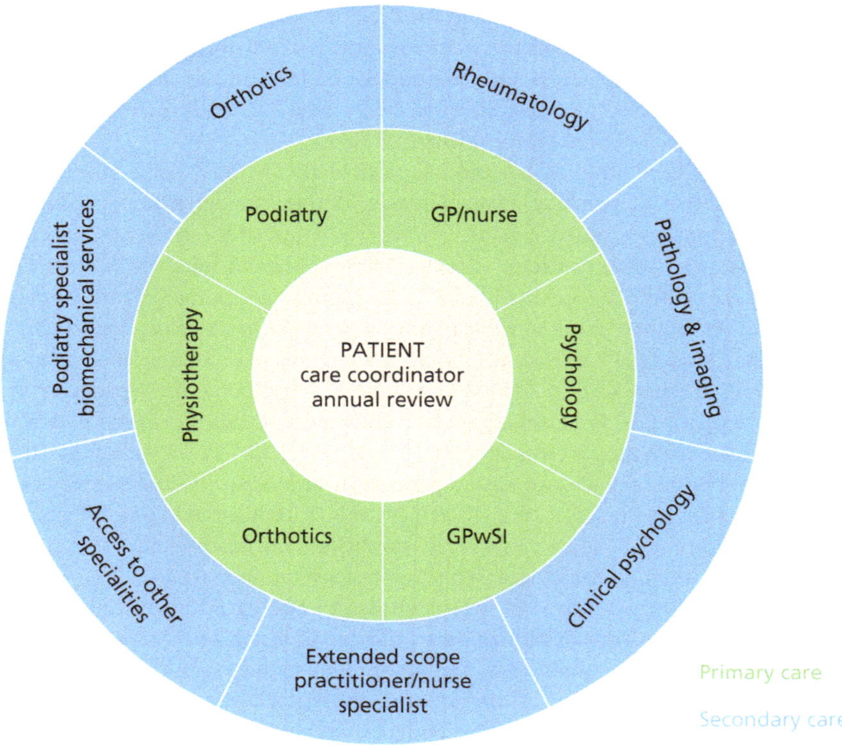

Figure 16.1 Patient-centred service wheel.
GPwSI = GP with a Special Interest

on providing the right competencies for the patient and will gain professional peer support and education during the process. The patient will benefit from that right care and the education and support that a team can offer. Treatment planning for all patients will place them at the centre of their care. With appropriate inter- and extra-team referral criteria and the opportunity for case discussion, the patient can be seen and given optimum management, not only by his or her rheumatology team but by other services that they might require to improve their health holistically.

Those patients requiring regular preventive foot care and review can be managed by a foot protection team. This term captures the role of the team more clearly than describing the care provided as 'in the community'. Defining the type of care rather than the setting is essential. The foot protection team is a subset of the MDT and specialist podiatry, providing the majority of care for foot disorders and is key in preventing crises. The team can support the implementation of service and care standards and is in a prime position to identify people with primary inflammatory conditions and disease flares. With the right referral pathways and criteria these patients can be referred urgently to more specialized care, thus complying with NICE quality standards. The team is also able to contribute to the public health agenda by encouraging patients with rheumatological conditions to engage in weight reduction and appropriate physical activity.

When this integrated model includes a specialist podiatrist it complies with the NICE quality standards and elevates the importance of this specialty within the care of those patients with

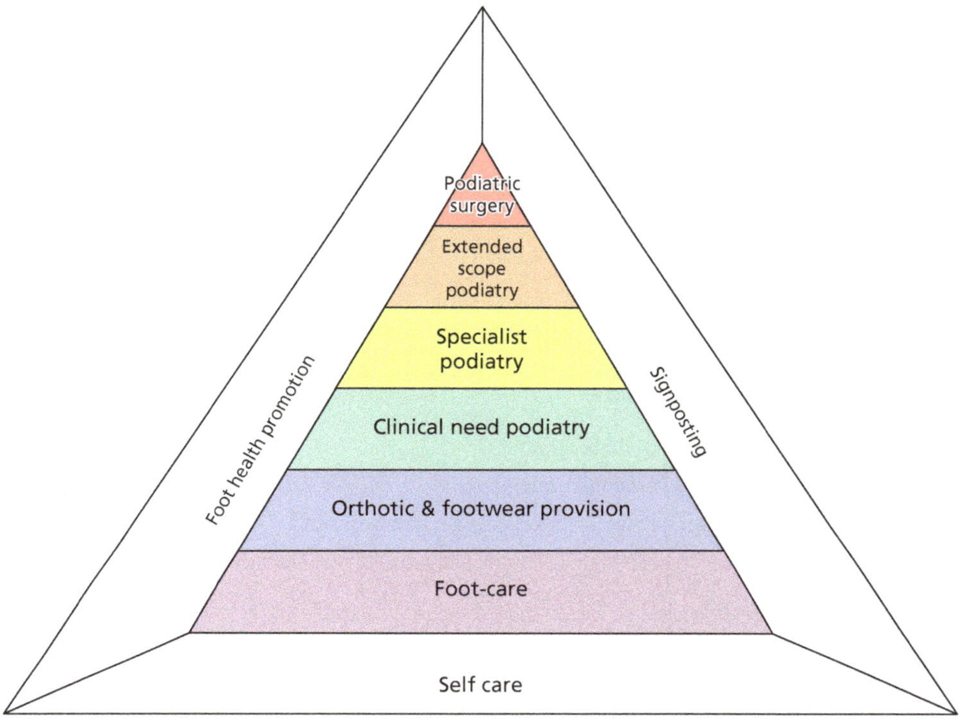

Figure 16.2 The foot health spectrum of care.

Adapted from Boden, Christopher (2007) Older people and 'person-centred' podiatry: a critical evaluation of two models of care. PhD thesis, University of Gloucestershire.

rheumatic diseases. This role combines education, advice, and comprehensive management in a timely fashion at the right points in the patient pathway. Appropriately commissioned to provide resources in primary, community, and hospital care, with self-management and patient-held records at the centre of the model, care for patients can only be improved. The specialized members of the whole MDT can also contribute clinical leadership and resource and support. The whole team, which includes the foot care team and the patients, should contribute to local referral and care pathways. The team should aim for continual improvement in care. This should be achieved by reviewing pathways, examining and implementing evidence-based care, and delivering education and training to the whole team. Local teams should also be enhanced by engagement with voluntary and charitable organizations as well as their professional bodies. Patient organizations can be essential allies in championing the need for service and will provide crucial local evidence of experience and need.

What to include in an outline business case

Box 16.1 comprises the ideal approach. It is recognized that the local data baseline might not currently provide the required information. The first steps may need to include planning on how to obtain this data.

Box 16.1 What to include in an outline business case

1. Establish need for the service
   - Use local epidemiological data on foot problems in general
   - Use epidemiological data on high-risk rheumatology groups
   - Provide local existing data on use of services in primary, community, secondary, and private healthcare
2. Identify existing resources
   - Rheumatology, musculoskeletal orthopaedic clinics in primary and secondary care
   - Podiatry services
3. Identify existing costs
   - Is there an identifiable podiatry budget?
   - Is there an identifiable orthotic budget?
   - What are the podiatry costs for the existing client groups?
   - What are the indirect costs? Inefficient travelling time/cost for professionals and patients?
4. Identify lead purchaser and providers in your locality
   - These are the organizations with whom you will have to negotiate
5. Identify any possible quality and cost benefits
   - e.g., savings from self-management for routine podiatry care put into high-risk care
   - More patient-focused experience
   - Raised staff morale and retention of high-quality staff
   - Concentration of skills in the right place and, potentially, cross-fertilization with other specialities, e.g., diabetes
   - A service in line with National Institute for Health and Care Excellence and National Service Frameworks quality standards

Conclusions

Teamwork across patients and health professionals in the locality multidisciplinary service is essential to achieve the required quality outcomes. Changes can and should be made to current UK services for those patients with foot and ankle disorders. The current silos in planning, organizing, and providing patient foot and ankle services should be eliminated and healthcare professionals in all sites should communicate with each other and their commissioners to provide an efficient and effective service within their locality.

Further research/audit suggestions

- Continuation of the national audit into implementation of NICE quality standards.
- Re-audit of podiatry contacts across a representative private, community, and hospital locality using more focused categories of contact.

- Consideration of standardized coding across all podiatry contacts.
- Consideration of standardized triage for access to podiatry across the NHS.
- Pilot study into the use and uptake of person-centred budgets within rheumatology and podiatry.

References

1. **Rowlands G, Protheroe J, Price H, Gann B, Rafi I.** *Health Literacy Report from an RCGP-led Health Literacy Workshop*. London: Royal College of General Practitioners; 2014.
2. **Rowlands G, Protheroe J, Winkley J, Richardson M, Seed P, Rudd R.** A mismatch between population health literacy and the complexity of health information: an observational study. *Br J Gen Pract*. 2015;**65**:e379–86.
3. **Forder J, Jones K, Glendinning C, et al.** *Evaluation of the Personal Health Budget Pilot Programme*. London: Department of Health; 2012.
4. **Crisp N, Stuckler D, Horton R, et al.** Manifesto for a healthy and health creating society. *Lancet*. 2016;**388**(10062):PE24–E27.

Index

Note: figures, tables, and boxes are indicated by *f, t,* and *b* following the page number. For example, 221*f* indicates a figure on page 221.